Selected Bibliography of Pediatric Orthopaedics With Commentary

Edited by
James H. Beaty, MD
Professor of Orthopaedics
Director of Residency Program
University of Tennessee
Campbell Clinic
Memphis, Tennessee

Charles T. Price, MD
Surgeon in Chief
Nemours Children's Clinic, Orlando
Director of Pediatric Orthopaedics
Orlando Regional Health Care System
Orlando, Florida

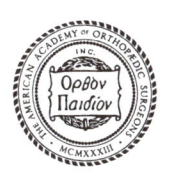

American Academy of Orthopaedic Surgeons
6300 North River Road
Rosemont, Illinois 60018

American Academy of Orthopaedic Surgeons

Committee on Pediatric Orthopaedics 1996

James H. Beaty, MD, Chairman
John G. Birch, MD
E. Dennis Lyne, MD
William L. Oppenheim, MD
Charles T. Price, MD
George T. Rab, MD
Angela B. Smith, MD
Carl L. Stanitski, MD
Elizabeth A. Szalay, MD
George H. Thompson, MD

Board of Directors 1996

Kenneth E. DeHaven, MD
John J. Callaghan, MD
Richard D. Coutts, MD
James D. Heckman, MD
James H. Herndon, MD
Serena S. Hu, MD
Douglas W. Jackson, MD
Richard F. Kyle, MD
George L. Lucas, MD
David R. Mauerhan, MD
Bernard F. Morrey, MD
Edward A. Rankin, MD
Scott B. Scutchfield, MD
James W. Strickland, MD
D. Eugene Thompson, MD
Roger A. Winquist, MD
William W. Tipton, Jr., MD,
 (*ex officio*)

Copyright © 1996 by the American Academy of Orthopaedic Surgeons

Publications Staff

Director of Publications:
 Marilyn L. Fox, PhD
Senior Editor:
 Bruce A. Davis
Associate Senior Editor:
 Joan Abern
Associate Senior Editor:
 Lisa Moore
Production Manager:
 Loraine Edwalds
Production Coordinator:
 Sophie Tosta
Production Assistant:
 Jana Ronayne
Layout and Text Design:
 Geraldine Dubberke
Cover Design:
 Pamela Erickson

The material presented in Selected Bibliography of Pediatric Orthopaedics with Commentary has been made available by the American Academy of Orthopaedic Surgeons for educational purposes only. This material is not intended to present the only, or necessarily best, methods or procedures for the medical situations discussed, but rather is intended to represent an approach, view, statement, or opinion of the author(s) or producer(s), which may be helpful to others who face similar situations.

Furthermore, any statements about commercial products are solely the opinion(s) of the author(s) and do not represent an Academy endorsement or evaluation of these products. These statements may not be used in advertising or for any commercial purpose.

All rights reserved. No part of this publication may be reproduced, stored in a retrieval system, or transmitted, in any form, or by any means, electronic, mechanical, photocopying, recording, or otherwise, without prior written permission from the publisher.

Contributors

Benjamin A. Alman, MD
Assistant Professor
Pediatric Orthopaedic Surgeon
The Hospital for Sick Children
University of Toronto Faculty of
  Medicine
Toronto, Ontario, Canada

Robert M. Bernstein, MD
Orthopaedic Surgeon
Shriners Hospital for Crippled
  Children
Los Angeles Unit
Los Angeles, California

John G. Birch, MD
Assistant Chief of Staff
Texas Scottish Rite Hospital
  for Children
Dallas, Texas

John A. Churchill, MD
Pediatric Orthopedist
Virginia Center for Orthopedics
Norfolk, Virginia

R. Jay Cummings, MD
Chairman, Department of
  Orthopaedics
Nemours Children's Clinic
Jacksonville, Florida

Peter A. DeLuca, MD
Associate Professor of
  Orthopaedic Surgery
University of Connecticut
Connecticut Orthopaedic
  Specialists
New Haven, Connecticut

Michael J. Goldberg, MD
Professor and Chairman,
  Orthopaedics
Tufts-New England
  Medical Center
Boston, Massachusetts

Walter B. Greene, MD
Chairman, Department of
  Orthopaedic Surgery
University of Missouri/Columbia
Columbia, Missouri

Stephen D. Heinrich, MD
Associate Professor
Division of Pediatric
  Orthopaedic Surgery
Department of Orthopaedic
  Surgery
Louisiana State University
  Medical Center
New Orleans, Louisiana

John A. Herring, MD
Chief of Staff
Texas Scottish Rite Hospital
  for Children
Dallas, Texas

Laurie O. Hughes, MD
Assistant Professor of
  Orthopedic Surgery
The University of Arkansas for
  Medical Sciences
Little Rock, Arkansas

John T. Killian, MD
Chief of Pediatric Orthopedics
Children's Hospital
Birmingham, Alabama

John M. Mazur, MD
Nemours Children's Clinic
Jacksonville, Florida

Richard E. McCarthy, MD
Arkansas Spine Center
Little Rock, Arkansas

William L. Oppenheim, MD
Professor and Chief
Pediatric Orthopedics
UCLA School of Medicine
Los Angeles, California

George T. Rab, MD
Chief, Pediatric Orthopaedics
University of California, Davis
Sacramento, California

Angela D. Smith, MD
Assistant Professor of
 Orthopaedics and Pediatrics
Case Western Reserve
 University
Cleveland, Ohio

Carl L. Stanitski, MD
Professor
Wayne State University
Detroit, Michigan

Deborah F. Stanitski, MD
Associate Professor
Wayne State University
Detroit, Michigan

Elizabeth A. Szalay, MD
Pediatric Orthopedic Surgeon
Beaumont Bone and Joint Clinic
Beaumont, Texas

George H. Thompson, MD
Professor, Orthopaedic Surgery
 and Pediatrics
Case Western Reserve
 University
Cleveland, Ohio

William C. Warner, Jr, MD
Associate Professor, Orthopaedic
 Surgery
University of Tennessee
Campbell Clinic, Inc.
Germantown, Tennessee

Peter Waters, MD
Clinical Director
Hand and Upper Extremity
 Clinics
Childrens Hospital
Boston, Massachusetts

Stuart L. Weinstein, MD
Ponseti Professor of
 Orthopaedic Surgery
University of Iowa Hospitals
 and Clinics
Iowa City, Iowa

Table of Contents

Preface	xv
1. History of Orthopaedics	1
2. Growth and Development of the Musculoskeletal System	5
Intrauterine, Infant, and Childhood Bone Growth and Development	5
Muscle Growth	8
Psychomotor Skills Development: Achieving Motor Milestones	8
Normal Milestones	9
Development of Gait	10
Development of Complex Psychomotor Skills	10
Factors Related to Normal Growth and Development	11
3. Genetics and Syndromes	13
Larsen Syndrome	14
Freeman-Sheldon Whistling Face Syndrome	15
Pterygium Syndromes	15
Congenital Contractural Arachnodactyly	16
Neurofibromatosis	17
Proteus Syndrome	20
Down Syndrome	21
de Lange Syndrome	23
Progeria (Hutchinson-Gilford Syndrome)	23
Familial Dysautonomia	24
Noonan Syndrome	24
Prader-Willi Syndrome	24
Fetal Alcohol (and Other Abused Substances)	25
Fetal Acquired Immunodeficiency Syndrome	26
Rett Syndrome	27
TAR (Thrombocytopenia With Absent Radii) Syndrome	27
VATER (Vertebral, Anal, Tracheoesophageal, Renal, and Radial Limb Anomalies) Association	28
Femoral Hypoplasia-Unusual Facies	28
Connective Tissue Disorders	29
Biochemistry	29

v

Marfan Syndrome	29
Homocystinuria	30
Osteogenesis Imperfecta	31
Other Syndromes	33

4. Cervical Spine — 35
Basilar Impression	35
Occipitoatlantal Complex	37
Atlantoaxial Instability	39
Os Odontoideum	43
Klippel-Feil Syndrome	44
Torticollis	45
Miscellaneous	49

5. Vertebral Column — 51
Adolescent Idiopathic Scoliosis	51
Prevalence and Natural History	51
School Screening	53
Etiology	54
Nonsurgical Treatment	55
Surgical Treatment	56
Juvenile Idiopathic Scoliosis	61
Infantile Idiopathic Scoliosis	61
Congenital Scoliosis and Kyphosis	61
General	61
Natural History	62
Etiology	63
Treatment	63
Scheuermann's Disease and Postural Roundback	65
Miscellaneous Spine Deformities	67
Cerebral Palsy and Neuromuscular Scoliosis	67
Postlaminectomy Spinal Deformity	69
Skeletal Dysplasia	69
Herniated Nucleus Pulposus	69
Spondylolysis and Spondylolisthesis	70

	Spinal Cord Monitoring	73
	Miscellaneous	74
	Sacral Agenesis	74
6.	**Upper-Extremity Deformities**	**75**
	Shoulder	75
	Congenital Pseudarthrosis of the Clavicle	75
	Cleidocranial Dysplasia	75
	Sprengel's Deformity	76
	Obstetric Brachial Plexopathy	77
	Elbow and Forearm	78
	Radioulnar Synostosis	78
	Congenital Radial Head Dislocation	79
	Congenital Pseudarthrosis of the Forearm	79
	Wrist	80
	Radial Club Hand	80
	Ulnar Club Hand	80
	Madelung's Deformity	81
	Hand	81
	Polydactyly	81
	Syndactyly	81
	Camptodactyly	82
	Cleft Hand	82
	Constriction Band Syndrome	82
	Thumb	82
	Syndromes	84
	Apert's Syndrome	84
	Arthrogryposis	85
7.	**The Hip**	**87**
	Developmental Dysplasia of the Hip	87
	Vascular Supply	87
	Screening, Evaluation, and Detection	88
	Nonsurgical Treatment	91
	Closed Reduction and Traction	92
	Open Reduction	95

Pelvic and Femoral Osteotomy	96
Osteonecrosis	98
Long-term Results	99
Slipped Capital Femoral Epiphysis	100
Detection and Pathoanatomy	100
Treatment	101
Acute Slips	104
Long-term Results	104
Legg-Calvé-Perthes Disease	106
Etiology	106
Evaluation	107
Treatment	108
Remodeling and Long-term Prognosis	111
Transient Synovitis of the Hip	113
Arthrodesis of the Hip	113
8. The Knee	**115**
Knee Dislocation	115
Patella	116
Menisci	119
General	119
Osteochondritis Dissecans	122
Ligament Injuries	123
Plica	126
Osgood-Schlatter Disease	126
9. The Foot and Ankle	**129**
Normal Feet	129
Clubfoot	129
Pathologic Anatomy	129
Genetics	131
Nonsurgical Treatment	131
Surgical Treatment: Soft-Tissue Release	132
Surgical Treatment: Tendon Transfers	134
Surgical Treatment: Bony Operations	135
Miscellaneous	136

Metatarsus Adductus	136
Flatfoot	138
Congenital Vertical Talus	139
Tarsal Coalition	140
Adolescent Bunions	142
Congenital Short Achilles Tendon	144
Osteochondroses of the Foot	145
Peroneal Tendon Instability	147
Toe Deformity	148
Miscellaneous Foot Deformities	149

10. Limb-Length Discrepancy and Angular Deformity — 151

Limb-Length Discrepancy	151
General	151
Evaluation	152
Shortening/Epiphysiodesis	154
Lengthening	155
Angular Deformity	157
General	157
Evaluation	159
Treatment	160
Partial Physeal Arrest	163
Epiphysiolysis	164

11. Congenital Limb Deficiency and the Child Amputee — 165

General	165
Classification	166
Congenital Constriction Band Syndrome	166
Proximal Femoral Focal Deficiency	167
Surgical Management	169
General	169
Upper-Extremity Surgery	170
Lower-Extremity Surgery/Tibial and Fibular Hemimelia	171
Prosthetic Management	175

12. Fractures of the Spine and Spinal Cord Injuries — 179

ix

13. Trauma: Upper Extremity — 185
 Sternoclavicular Joint — 185
  Anterior Dislocations — 185
  Posterior Dislocations — 185
 Fractures of the Clavicle — 186
 Fractures of the Proximal Humerus — 187
 Shoulder Dislocations — 187
 Elbow: General — 188
 Supracondylar Humeral Fractures — 189
  Nonsurgical Treatment — 190
  Closed Reduction and Percutaneous Pinning — 190
  Open Reduction — 192
  Complications (Neurovascular) — 193
  Complications (Deformity) — 194
 Fractures of the Lateral Humeral Condyle — 195
 Fractures of the Medial Humeral Condyle — 197
 Fractures of the Medial Humeral Epicondyle — 197
 T-condylar Fractures of the Distal Humerus — 198
 Distal Humeral Epiphyseal Separation — 199
 Elbow Dislocation — 200
 Monteggia Fracture-Dislocation — 201
 Fractures of the Radial Neck — 202
 Fractures of the Olecranon — 203
 Nursemaid Elbow — 203
 Fractures of the Forearm — 203
 Galeazzi Fracture-Dislocation — 207
 Wrist Injuries — 208
 Fractures of the Hand — 209
 Miscellaneous — 210
  Injuries to the Physis — 211
  Child-Abuse Syndrome — 211
  Overuse Syndromes — 212

14. Fractures of the Pelvis and Lower Extremities — 215
 Hip Dislocations — 216
 Fractures of the Femoral Neck and Peritrochanteric Region — 217

Femoral Shaft Fractures	218
Patellar Fractures	223
Fractures of the Distal Femoral Epiphysis	224
Fractures of the Intercondylar Eminence of the Tibia	224
Fractures Involving the Proximal Tibial Physis and Tuberosity	226
Fractures of the Proximal Tibial Metaphyses	227
Fractures of the Tibial Shaft	227
Fractures of the Distal Tibial Metaphysis and Physis	229
Fractures of the Foot	230
Polytrauma/Multiple Fractures	232

15. Bone and Joint Infections — 233

Etiology	233
Evaluation	234
Miscellaneous	235
Treatment	238
Outcome Studies	239

16. Neuromuscular Diseases — 241

General	241
Duchenne Muscular Dystrophy	242
Other Muscular Dystrophies	245
Spinal Muscular Atrophy	246
Charcot-Marie-Tooth Disease	247
Friedreich's Ataxia	249
Arthrogryposis Multiplex Congenita	250
Miscellaneous	253

17. Cerebral Palsy — 255

General	255
Upper Extremity	256
Selective Posterior Dorsal Rhizotomy	258
Foot Deformities	259
Varus Foot	259
Valgus Foot	261
Hip	263

Ankle Equinus Deformity	266
Knee Dysfunction	267
Gait Analysis	269
Miscellaneous	270

18. Myelomeningocele — **271**

General Overview	271
Fractures	275
Ambulation-Rehabilitation	276
Spine	278
Hip	283
Knee and Lower Limb	285
Ankle and Foot	286

19. Inflammatory Conditions — **289**

Juvenile Rheumatoid Arthritis	289
Etiology	289
Growth Abnormalities and Nutrition	290
Radiology	290
Medical Management	291
Physical Therapy	292
Other Systems	292
Impairment Evaluation	292
Orthopaedic Aspects	292
Pregnancy	295
Spondyloarthropathy	295
Juvenile Psoriatic Arthritis	296
Lyme Disease	296

20. Disorders of the Hematopoietic System — **299**

Sickle Cell Disease	299
Thalassemia	303
Diamond-Blackfan (Congenital Hypoplastic) Anemia	304
Fanconi Anemia	304
Chronic Granulomatous Disease	305
Shwachman-Diamond Syndrome	305
Acquired Immunodeficiency Syndrome (AIDS)	306

Gaucher Disease	307
Langerhans Cell Histiocytosis (Eosinophilic Granuloma of Bone)	309
Thrombocytopenia With Absent Radius (TAR) Syndrome	311
Hemophilia	311
Leukemia	314

21. Tumors **317**
    Evaluation and Diagnosis 317
        General 317
        Biopsy 319
        Imaging 319
        Staging 320
        Allografts 320
    Benign Tumors 321
        Aneurysmal Bone Cyst 321
        Chondroblastoma 321
        Chondromyxoid Fibroma 322
        Enchondroma 322
        Eosinophilic Granuloma 322
        Fibrous Cortical Defect/Nonossifying Fibroma 323
        Giant Cell Tumor 323
        Osteoblastoma 323
        Osteochondroma 324
        Osteoid Osteoma 325
        Unicameral Bone Cyst 326
    Malignant Tumors 327
        Adamantinoma 327
        Ewing's Sarcoma 328
        Chondrosarcoma 328
        Osteosarcoma 329
        Soft-Tissue Sarcomas 331
        Malignant Fibrous Histiocytoma 332
        Rehabilitation 332

Preface

This fourth edition of the *Selected Bibliography of Pediatric Orthopaedics* continues the tradition begun with the first edition in 1970. We have again attempted to provide a broad overview of the pediatric orthopaedic literature, focusing in this edition on publications of 1991 through early 1996. Some older, classic articles also have been retained.

A work of this magnitude would not, of course, have been possible without the diligence of the many contributors who searched the literature, made decisions about exclusions and inclusions, and prepared the commentaries. We would like to thank them for their cooperation and expertise.

A special thanks to Campbell Foundation personnel, Kay Daugherty, Linda Jones, and Joan Crowson, who provided editorial, clerical, and research assistance; and to Pamela Banister for her assistance in manuscript preparation.

The American Academy of Orthopaedic Surgeons Department of Publications, directed by Marilyn Fox, PhD, deserves much credit for the finished product. We are most grateful for the infinite patience and excellent work of Joan Abern, Associate Senior Editor, and for the contributions of others in the Department of Publications, including Bruce Davis, Senior Editor and Geraldine Dubberke, who did all of the manuscript inputting and page layout.

JAMES H. BEATY, MD
CHARLES T. PRICE, MD

Section 1

History of Orthopaedics

Elizabeth A. Szalay, MD

Bick EM: *Source Book of Orthopaedics.* New York, NY, Hafner, 1968.

This is an extensive reference for history of orthopaedic practice and literature.

Rang M: *Anthology of Orthopaedics.* Edinburgh, Scotland, Churchill Livingstone, 1966.

This book provides biographic information about early orthopaedists.

Shands AR Jr: *The Early Orthopedic Surgeons of America.* St. Louis, MO, CV Mosby, 1970.

This book provides biographic information.

Wenger DR, Rang M: *The Art and Practice of Children's Orthopaedics.* New York, NY, Raven Press, 1993.

In addition to practical advice on the treatment of common pediatric orthopaedic disorders, this book contains vignettes of pioneers in the field and brief histories of selected procedures and devices.

Since 1963, with few exceptions, each volume of *Clinical Orthopaedics and Related Research* has been introduced with a classic article related to the subject of its symposium. Originally published from the late 17th century onward, some appear for the first time in English. Some have been collated into a volume entitled *Classics of Orthopaedics.* Selected articles pertaining to pediatric orthopaedics follow, listed in alphabetical order according to their authors.

Calvé J: On a particular form of pseudo-coxalgia associated with a characteristic deformity of the upper end of the femur. *Clin Orthop* 1980;150:4–7.

This is a 1910 French paper. The new technique of roentgenography contributed to the definition of a juvenile hip disease that was distinctly different from the then-common tuberculosis of the hip.

Codivilla A: On the means of lengthening, in the lower limbs, the muscles and tissues which are shortened through deformity. *Clin Orthop* 1994; 301:4–9.

This 1904 Italian paper published in AJOS contains a discussion of the "difficulties encountered in lengthening a shortened limb," a description of techniques then used, and an introduction of the concept of staged distraction delivered via a skeletal pin.

Ekman OJ: Congenital osteomalacia. *Clin Orthop* 1981;159:3–5.

This 1788 Swedish paper provides perhaps the first clinical description of osteogenesis imperfecta, with "proof of the softness of the bones being . . . inherited from parents to offspring."

Ewing J: Diffuse endothelioma of bone. *Clin Orthop* 1984;185:2–5.

This 1921 American paper is Ewing's description and clinical cases of the "round cell sarcoma" that has come to bear his name.

Foucher JTE: Separations of the epiphyses. *Clin Orthop* 1984;188:3–9.

This 1867 French dissertation on the anatomy and mechanism of injury of physeal fractures is based on clinical observation and cadaveric experimentation.

Lange F: Support for the spondylitic spine by means of buried steel bars, attached to the vertebrae. *Clin Orthop* 1986;203:3–6.

The author of this 1910 German paper published in AJOS speaks of "Replacing parts of the living organs . . . (for) mechanical purposes . . . by inorganic materials." This is a discussion of properties of different metals and reactions to implantation with a description of implantation of a steel rod secured with silk suture.

le Damany PGM: Technique of tibial tropometry. *Clin Orthop* 1994; 302:4–10.

The author of this 1903 French paper describes clinical and cadaveric measurements of tibial torsion in humans and other animals, theorizing causation from structural consequences of bipedalism and in utero "packing."

Legg AT: An obscure affectation of the hip joint, in Bick EM (ed): *Classics of Orthopaedics*. Philadelphia, PA, JB Lippincott, 1976, pp 385–388.

This American paper, read in 1909 and published 1910, provides the first description of the childhood affliction that now shares the author's name. It contains speculations on etiology, which contrast the disease with other known entities.

Little WJ: Deformities of the human frame. *Clin Orthop* 1978;131:3–9

This 1843 British paper provides a clinical description of cerebral palsy, to become known as "Little's disease," with speculations regarding etiology and recommendations for surgical and nonsurgical treatment.

Paget J: Ununited fractures in children. *Clin Orthop* 1982;166:2–4.

This 1891 British article indicates that pseudarthrosis of the tibia is outlined from clinical observation. Most treatment modalities attempted resulted in ultimate amputation.

Pavlik A: The functional method of treatment using a harness with stirrups as the primary method of conservative therapy for infants with congenital dislocation of the hip. *Clin Orthop* 1992;281:4–10.

This paper was first published in 1957 in Czechoslovakia. It is a translation of the rationale and description of the nonsurgical treatment of hip dislocation to avoid osteonecrosis.

Perthes GC: Concerning arthritis deformans juvenilis. *Clin Orthop* 1981;158:5–9.

In this 1910 German paper, the author describes a nontubercular hip disease from a clinical, radiologic, prognostic, and pathologic viewpoint.

Scheuermann HW: Kyphosis dorsalis juvenilis. *Clin Orthop* 1977; 128:5–7.

This 1921 Danish paper provides the initial description of the juvenile kyphosis to subsequently bear his name; little has changed in our data base since then.

Still GF: On a form of chronic joint disease in children. *Clin Orthop* 1990;259:4–10.

This 1896 British paper provides a definition of juvenile rheumatoid arthritis (later known as "Still's disease") that differentiates the pathology seen in children from the distinctly different disease seen in adults.

von Volkmann R: Ischaemic muscle paralyses and contractures, in Bick EM (ed): *Classics of Orthopaedics*. Philadelphia, PA, JB Lippincott, 1976, pp 168–169.

This 1881 German paper describes "paralysis and contraction of the limb" directly attributed to "prolonged blocking of arterial blood (and) . . . simultaneous massive venous stasis."

Section 2

Growth and Development of the Musculoskeletal System

Angela D. Smith, MD

Intrauterine, Infant, and Childhood Bone Growth and Development

Blimkie CJR, Chilibeck PD, Davison KS: Bone mineralization: Endocrine, nutrition, and physical activity influences during the lifespan, in Bar-Or O, Lamb D, Clarkson P (eds): *Perspectives in Exercise Science and Sports Medicine: Exercise and the Female—A Life Span Approach.* Carmel, IN, Cooper Publishing Group, 1996.

This excellent and exhaustive review of the current knowledge on bone mass accretion through childhood and adolescence includes the controversies concerning the possible positive effects of calcium supplements and weightbearing or impact-loading physical activity and the possible negative effects of excessive exercise that may be related to endocrine changes.

Eckhoff DG: Effect of limb malrotation on malalignment and osteoarthritis. *Orthop Clin North Am* 1994;25:405–414.

This article reviews evidence that rotational malalignment is a potential source of arthrosis.

Fabry G, MacEwen GD, Shands AR Jr: Torsion of the femur: A follow-up study in normal and abnormal conditions. *J Bone Joint Surg* 1973;55A: 1726–1738.

The authors studied 1,148 patients, determining their femoral anteversion by the Dunlap-Shands biplanar radiography method in addition to performing clinical examinations of the hips. Instructions to stop sitting with the hips internally rotated; use of Denis Browne splints, twister cables, and/or lateral sole wedges; or any combination of these did not lead to improvement compared to the untreated group.

Golding JS: The mechanical factors which influence bone growth. *Eur J Clin Nutr* 1994;48(suppl 1):S178–S185.

This is an historical development of concepts related to Wolff's law, with interesting, although mostly anecdotal, examples of situations that illustrate mechanical adaptations during bone growth.

Langenskiöld A: Partial closure of the epiphyseal plate: Principles of treatment. *Clin Orthop* 1993;279:4–6.

This reprint of the classic article discusses the treatment of partial physeal closure.

Nilsson A, Ohlsson C, Isaksson OG, et al: Hormonal regulation of longitudinal bone growth. *Eur J Clin Nutr* 1994;48(suppl 1):S150–S158.

The authors discuss the relationships of the hormones that regulate postnatal somatic growth (growth hormone, thyroid hormones, and the sex steroids) and the other mediators of bone growth (cytokines, etc).

Ogden JA: The uniqueness of growing bones, in Rockwood CA Jr, Wilkins KE, Beaty JH (eds): *Fractures in Children,* ed 4. Philadelphia, PA, Lippincott-Raven, 1996, vol 3.

This chapter on bone growth distills much that is in the literature. A "must-read" for orthopaedic residents.

Price JS, Oyajobi BO, Russell RG: The cell biology of bone growth. *Eur J Clin Nutr* 1994;48(suppl 1):S131–S149.

This is an excellent, well organized, current review of mediators of bone growth, including the cytokines and insulin-like growth factors.

Salenius P, Vankka E: The development of the tibiofemoral angle in children. *J Bone Joint Surg* 1975;57A:259–261.

The study includes 1,279 patients, 111 of whom were followed longitudinally for 2 or more radiographs 6 months apart. At birth, marked varus angulation was the rule, with the tibiofemoral angle straightening around 18 months of age, then progressing into valgus. Maximum valgus was apparent near 3 years of age.

Silverman FN (ed): The bones, in *Caffey's Pediatric X-Ray Diagnosis: An Integrated Imaging Approach*, ed 8. Chicago, IL, Year Book Medical Publishers, 1985, pp 389–915.

Silverman discusses normal ossification and remodeling of developing bone and provides the age-at-appearance percentiles for the major postnatal ossification centers. He describes the study populations used to generate the Greulich and Pyle and Tanner-Whitehouse methods for determining maturity, with their strengths and limitations. Included are tables of the lengths of the long bones of the limbs by age and gender. To assist in prenatal diagnosis of dwarfing conditions, the mean prenatal femoral lengths (as determined by ultrasound examination) related to gestational age are provided.

Slemenda CW, Miller JZ, Hui SL, et al: Role of physical activity in the development of skeletal mass in children. *J Bone Miner Res* 1991;6: 1227–1233.

This prospective study of 118 children provides important evidence linking physical activity and bone mass. However, the amount and types (impact-loading versus weightbearing or resistance exercise) of physical activity required for the positive effect remain controversial and are discussed in the chapter by Blimkie, et al.

Staheli LT: Rotational problems in children, in Schafer M (ed): *Instructional Course Lectures Volume 43*. Rosemont, IL, American Academy of Orthopaedic Surgeons, 1993, pp 199–209.

This is an excellent review of natural history, treatment options, and long-term concerns of torsional problems.

Staheli LT, Corbett M, Wyss C, et al: Lower-extremity rotational problems in children: Normal values to guide management. *J Bone Joint Surg* 1985;67A:39–47.

This classic study of clinical changes in the rotational profile of 500 subjects presents data on individuals from infancy through the eighth decade. Graphs include changes by age in foot progression angle, tibial version, and femoral version, and provide mean ± 2 standard deviations for each parameter at each age.

Tetsworth K, Paley D: Malalignment and degenerative arthropathy. *Orthop Clin North Am* 1994;25:367–377.

This is an excellent review of normal mechanical alignment and joint alignment and a review of the literature regarding malalignment and development of arthrosis.

Muscle Growth

Heslinga JW, te Kronnie G, Huijing PA: Growth and immobilization effects on sarcomeres: A comparison between gastrocnemius and soleus muscles of the adult rat. *Eur J Appl Physiol* 1995;70:49–57.

Using a rat soleus model, the authors found that the number of sarcomeres in series within fibers increased after growth and decreased after immobilization. For fibers of the gastrocnemius, these changes were not observed. The authors proposed that muscle architecture is an important factor in these results. They suggest that increases in bone length during growth affect the length of soleus fibers more than those of gastrocnemius fibers because gastrocnemius is more pennate than soleus. During immobilization, atrophy of gastrocnemius fibers was sufficient for the muscle length adaptation to meet the muscle length change induced by immobilization, but in the soleus muscle, atrophy had to be accompanied by decreases in the number of sarcomeres in series to achieve adequate muscle length adaptation.

Sun JS, Hou SM, Liu TK, et al: Analysis of neogenesis in rabbit skeletal muscles after chronic traction. *Histol Histopathol* 1994;9:699–703.

The authors concluded that traction neogenesis of the skeletal muscle during limb lengthening occurs mainly near the myotendinous junction.

Psychomotor Skills Development: Achieving Motor Milestones

Allen MC, Alexander GR: Gross motor milestones in preterm infants: Correction for degree of prematurity. *J Pediatr* 1990;116:955–959.

Children with birth weights of 490 to 1,770 g and gestational age 23 to 32 weeks were compared with a population of normal infants born at term. Infants with marked hypotonia, cerebral palsy, and so forth, were excluded. The authors concluded that very preterm infants can be expected to demonstrate sequential gross motor development at a rate expected for degree of prematurity.

Hack M, Taylor HG, Klein N, et al: School-age outcomes in children with birth weights under 750 g. *N Engl J Med* 1994;331:753–759.

Children with birth weights under 750 g were inferior in cognitive ability, psychomotor skills, and academic achievement to children with birth weights of 750 to 1,499 g and those born at term. The rates of cerebral palsy were 9%, 6%, and 0%, respectively. Major cerebral ultrasonographic abnormalities were associated with cerebral palsy (odds ratio, 15.2; 95% confidence interval, 3.0 to 77.4).

Harris SR: Early diagnosis of spastic diplegia, spastic hemiplegia, and quadriplegia. *Am J Dis Child* 1989;143:1356–1360.

A retrospective study of 399 infants with birth weights of 1,500 g or less or respiratory distress syndrome or "any other" high-risk factor, who were followed longitudinally in a high-risk infant follow-up clinic, examined early neurodevelopmental behaviors of children with spastic or athetoid disorders. The Movement Assessment of Infants was more than three times as sensitive as the Bayley Motor Scale in detecting motor abnormalities in 4-month-old infants with diplegia and more than twice as sensitive in detecting early abnormalities of hemiplegia. However, at 4 months of age, the Movement Assessment of Infants was only 63% specific. At 1 year of age, the Bayley Motor Scale was extremely sensitive in picking up motor deficits in children with all three types of cerebral palsy.

Normal Milestones

Tirosh E, Jaffe M, Marmur R, et al: Prognosis of motor development and joint hypermobility. *Arch Dis Child* 1991;66:931–933.

Fifty-nine infants were studied at age 18 months and again at 54 to 60 months with assessment of joint hypermobility and motor development. By approximately 5 years of age, 84% of the children with hypermobility but normal motor development had resolved their hypermobility. Only 40% of the hypermobile children who were found to have developmental delay at 18 months had resolved their hypermobility by the 5-year-old follow-up. The authors concluded that infants with joint hypermobility and motor delay are a subgroup associated with a less favorable motor outcome and careful follow-up is indicated. They note the relationship between hypermobility and delayed motor development, but state no hypothesis about which is cause and which is effect.

Development of Gait

Sutherland, DH, Olshen R, Cooper L, et al: The development of mature gait. *J Bone Joint Surg* 1980;62A:336–353.

This is the classic article on the development of human gait from toddler to mature gait. A mature gait pattern is well established by 3 years of age.

Tachdjian MO (ed): *Pediatric Orthopedics,* ed 2. Philadelphia, PA, WB Saunders, 1990, pp 4–27.

Good description of the phases of the gait cycle and the determinants of gait, with excellent illustrations of both. Also includes illustration of the times of activity of each lower extremity muscle during each phase of gait. Pathologic gait patterns in childhood are discussed.

Development of Complex Psychomotor Skills

Butterfield SA, Loovis EM: Influence of age, sex, balance, and sport participation on development of throwing by children in grades K-8. *Percept Mot Skills* 1993;76:459–464.

The development of throwing skill in 381 boys and 338 girls (ages 4 to 14) was studied. Mature throwing development was influenced by sport participation and sex. Boys performed better at all grades; this difference apparently was related to increased participation in sports.

Butterfield SA Loovis EM: Influence of age, sex, balance, and sport participation on development of kicking by children in grades K-8. *Percept Mot Skills* 1994;79:691–697.

The development of kicking skill by 379 boys and 337 girls (ages 4 to 14) was studied. Development of mature form was significantly related to sex (grade 6: boys outperformed girls), static and dynamic balance (grade 7), and age (grade 6).

Factors Related to Normal Growth and Development

Malina RM: Physical activity and training: Effects on stature and the adolescent growth spurt. *Med Sci Sports Exerc* 1994;26:759–766.

The author presents data that suggest that regular physical activity and sport participation do not affect an individual's final stature, timing of peak height velocity, or rate of longitudinal growth.

Malina RM, Ryan RC, Bonci CM: Age at menarche in athletes and their mothers and sisters. *Ann Hum Biol* 1994;21:417–422.

Age at menarche was obtained from 109 university athletes, their mothers, and 77 sisters of the athletes. The findings suggest that later menarche commonly observed in athletes is to a large extent familial rather than a result of their athletic training.

Section 3

Genetics and Syndromes

Benjamin A. Alman, MD

Michael J. Goldberg, MD

Goldberg MJ: *The Dysmorphic Child: An Orthopaedic Perspective.* New York, NY, Raven Press, 1987.

This book presents the musculoskeletal and significant nonorthopaedic aspects of the most frequently encountered syndromes. The author emphasizes the differential diagnosis of children with similar extremity and spine deformities.

Jones KL (ed): *Smith's Recognizable Patterns of Human Malformation*, ed 4. Philadelphia, PA, WB Saunders, 1988.

Previous editions of Smith's textbook established it as the standard of a beautifully illustrated and concise textbook of dysmorphology. This edition by Jones continues the tradition.

Jones KL, Robinson LK: An approach to the child with structural defects. *J Pediatr Orthop* 1983;3:238–244.

This article presents a systematic approach to the child with congenital anomalies. This approach allows a specific overall diagnosis to be made.

McKusick VA, Francomano CA, Antonarakis SE (eds): *Mendelian Inheritance in Man: Catalogs of Autosomal Dominant, Autosomal Recessive, and X-Lined Phenotypes*, ed 10. Baltimore, MD, Johns Hopkins University Press, 1992.

This is an encyclopedic listing of genetically transmitted disorders. It also includes essential basic clinical information, detailed biochemistry, and an up-to-date bibliography.

Pilarski RT, Pauli RM, Engber WD: Hand-reduction malformations: Genetic and syndromic analysis. *J Pediatr Orthop* 1985;5:274–280.

Of 61 patients sequentially evaluated for congenital amputations of portions of the hand, 25% were the result of single gene disorders, and 33% had multiple malformation syndromes.

Van Regemorter N, Dodion J, Druart C, et al: Congenital malformations in 10,000 consecutive births in a university hospital: Need for genetic counseling and prenatal diagnosis. *J Pediatr* 1984;104:386–390.

An extensive analysis details the high birth incidence of genetic and sporadic malformations, many of which are orthopaedic.

Larsen Syndrome

Bonaventure J, Lasselin C, Mellier J, et al: Linkage studies of four fibrillar collagen genes in three pedigrees with Larsen-like syndrome. *J Med Genet* 1992;29:465–470.

Results of this linkage study show that Larsen syndrome is unlikely to be due to a defect in collagen 1A1, 1A2, or 3A1.

Bowen JR, Ortega AK, Ray S, et al: Spinal deformities in Larsen's syndrome. *Clin Orthop* 1985;197:159–163.

A characteristic pattern of spinal deformity, including scoliosis and spondylolysis, was found in eight patients with Larsen syndrome. The cervical spine was the most severely involved area, with dysraphism and vertebral hypoplasia.

Laville MB, Lakermance P, Limouzy F: Larsen's syndrome: A review of the literature and analysis of thirty-eight cases. *J Pediatr Orthop* 1994; 14:63–73.

For patients with Larsen syndrome, the authors recommend early conservative treatment of clubfeet, with surgical treatment postponed until knee deformities have been corrected by plaster cast or early operation. They recommend surgical treatment of unilateral hip dislocation at 2 years of age, no treatment of bilateral hip dislocations, and lifetime monitoring of spinal status.

Stevenson GW, Hall SC, Palmieri J: Anesthetic considerations for patients with Larsen's syndrome. *Anesthesiology* 1991;75:142–144.

This series illustrates potential difficulties in achieving airway control in patients with Larsen sydrome. Problems can arise due to difficulty with airway visualization and with potential cervical subluxation. These issues are important in surgical planning in patients with Larsen syndrome.

Freeman-Sheldon Whistling Face Syndrome

Jones R, Dolcourt JL: Muscle rigidity following halothane anesthesia in two patients with Freeman-Sheldon syndrome. *Anesthesiology* 1992;77: 599–600.

Two children had malignant hyperthermia-like reactions to halothane anesthesia. Performance of a caffeine-halothane muscle contraction test, or avoidance of halothane and/or succinylcholine, is advised.

Malkawi H, Tarawneh M: The whistling face syndrome, or craniocapotarsal dysplasia: Report of two cases in a father and son and review of the literature. *J Pediatr Orthop* 1983;3:364–369.

The authors review this arthrogryposis-like syndrome involving hands and feet and note that the characteristic deformities do not improve spontaneously, but require surgery.

Pterygium Syndromes

Addison A, Webb PJ: Flexion contractures of the knee associated with popliteal webbing. *J Pediatr Orthop* 1983;3:376–379.

The authors present the results and technique of surgical correction of the flexion deformity in five children with pterygium syndromes. They distinguish between multiple pterygium syndrome and popliteal pterygium syndrome and emphasize the associated anatomic abnormalities.

Hall JG, Reed SD, Rosenbaum KN, et al: Limb pterygium syndromes: A review and report of eleven patients. *Am J Med Genet* 1982;12:377–409.

This is an introduction to the pterygium syndromes–multiple, popliteal, and lethal–with a discussion of genetics and associated findings.

Oppenheim WL, Larson KR, McNabb MB, et al: Popliteal pterygium syndrome: An orthopaedic perspective. *J Pediatr Orthop* 1990;10:58–64.

The authors reviewed four patients and the literature. The neurovascular bundle was located in the posterior subcutaneous margin of the web. Extension osteotomy with shortening of the femur is advocated as an early surgical procedure.

Congenital Contractural Arachnodactyly

Bawle E, Quigg MH: Ectopia lentis and aortic root dilatation in congenital contractural arachnodactyly. *Am J Med Genet* 1992;42:19–21.

This case report, which includes a review of the literature, points out that there is heterogeneity in patients with congenital contractural arachnodactyly. Some individuals have aortic abnormalities and ectopia lentis; thus, the authors advocate cardiac and ophthalmologic evaluation of these patients.

Langenskiöld A: Congenital contractural arachnodactyly: Report of a case and of an operation for knee contracture. *J Bone Joint Surg* 1985;67B:44–46.

The author describes this syndrome, which can mimic Marfan syndrome, and gives a technique for managing the knee deformity.

Tsipouras P, Del Mastro R, Sarfarazi M, et al: Genetic linkage of the Marfan syndrome, ectopia lentis, and congenital contractural arachnodactyly to the fibrillin genes on chromosomes 15 and 5: The International Marfan Syndrome Collaborative Study. *N Engl J Med* 1992;326:905–909.

Congenital contractural arachnodactyly, ectopic lentis, and Marfan syndrome are all due to defects in the fibrillin gene (two genes on chromosome 5 and 15). This linkage study shows that congenital contractural arachnodactyly was linked to a defect in the fibrillin gene located on chromosome 5, whereas the other two disorders are due to a defect in the fibrillin gene on chromosome 15. Fibrillin gene mutations produce different phenotypic disease depending on the location of the abnormality. Genetic analysis can be used in the differential diagnosis of these conditions.

Neurofibromatosis

Akbarnia BA, Gabriel KR, Beckman E, et al: Prevalence of scoliosis in neurofibromatosis. *Spine* 1992;17(suppl 8):S244–S248.

Twenty-three of 220 patients in a multispecialty neurofibromatosis clinic had structural scoliosis.

Calvert PT, Edgar MA, Webb PJ: Scoliosis in neurofibromatosis: The natural history with and without operation. *J Bone Joint Surg* 1989;71B:246–251.

This is a review of 47 patients with neurofibromatosis and dystrophic spinal deformities. Short angular thoracic curves are the commonest pattern. Deterioration is usual but the rate is unpredictable. Early surgical stabilization by combined anterior and posterior fusion is indicated for kyphotic deformities or dystrophic apical vertebral changes. Selected patients may require posterior fusion and instrumentation alone.

Craig JB, Govender S: Neurofibromatosis of the cervical spine: A report of eight cases. *J Bone Joint Surg* 1992;74B:575–578.

Patients presented in the second decade of life with a neurologic deficit, a mass in the neck, or increasing deformity. Posterior fusion alone failed. Anterior or combined anterior and posterior fusion had better results.

Crawford AH: Pitfalls of spinal deformities associated with neurofibromatosis in children. *Clin Orthop* 1989;245:29–42.

This excellent review article covers all aspects of spinal deformity in neurofibromatosis based on 74 patients (64%) of a series of 116 patients. It has an excellent bibliography.

Crawford AH Jr, Bagamery N: Osseous manifestations of neurofibromatosis in childhood. *J Pediatr Orthop* 1986;6:72–88.

This is a detailed review of the skeletal manifestations of neurofibromatosis in 116 children diagnosed before age 12 years and followed up for an average of 5 years.

Egelhoff JC, Bates DJ, Ross JS, et al: Spinal MR findings in neurofibromatosis types 1 and 2. *Am J Neuroradiol* 1992;13:1071–1077.

Twelve of 19 patients had spinal lesions demonstrated by magnetic resonance imaging (MRI) despite being asymptomatic. These data give further support to MR imaging of the entire spine before surgical intervention.

Funasaki H, Winter RB, Lonstein JB, et al: Pathophysiology of spinal deformities in neurofibromatosis: An analysis of seventy-one patients who had curves associated with dystrophic changes. *J Bone Joint Surg* 1994;76A:692–700.

In a study of 71 patients, risk factors for progression of the curve were identified: early age at onset, a high Cobb angle at first examination, an abnormal kyphosis, vertebral scalloping, severe rotation at the apex of the curve, location of the apex of the curve in the middle to caudal thoracic area, penciling of one or more ribs on the concave side or on both sides of the curve, and penciling of four ribs or more.

Gutmann DH, Collins FS: The neurofibromatosis type I gene and its protein product, neurofibromin. *Neuron* 1993;10:335–343.

This is an excellent review of the basic science that led to the identification of the neurofibromatosis gene (NF1) and its protein product (neurofibromin). The role of the NF1 in pathologic and normal biology is explored.

Hsu LCS, Lee PC, Leong JCY: Dystrophic spinal deformities in neurofibromatosis: Treatment by anterior and posterior fusion. *J Bone Joint Surg* 1984;66B:495–499.

This is a 7-year follow-up of 13 patients who underwent anterior-posterior combined fusion. Results were unsatisfactory in patients with sharply angled kyphoscoliosis and good in those with smooth or minimal kyphosis.

Mandell GA, Harcke HT, Scott CI, et al: Protusio acetabuli in neurofibromatosis: Nondysplastic and dysplastic forms. *Neurosurgery* 1992;30:552–556.

Twenty-one percent of patients with neurofibromatosis were found to have protrusio acetabuli. Patients with progressive protrusio usually had contiguous soft-tissue neurofibroma and lumbar dural ectasia. The patients with nonprogressive protrusio did not have lumbar dural ectasia.

Mathoulin C, Gilbert A, Azze RG: Congenital pseudarthrosis of the forearm: Treatment of six cases with vascularized fibular graft and a review of the literature. *Microsurgery* 1993;14:252–259.

Five of the reported cases were in individuals with neurofibromatosis. Vascularized grafts combined with forearm shortening resulted in healing in all. However, longer-term follow-up of these patients is needed.

Ostrowski DM, Eilert RE, Waldstein G: Congenital pseudoarthrosis of the ulna: A report of two cases and a review of the literature. *J Pediatr Orthop* 1985;5:463–467.

The authors describe pseudarthroses of the ulna in two teenagers with neurofibromatosis and discuss treatment options.

Sirois JL III, Drennan JC: Dystrophic spinal deformity in neurofibromatosis. *J Pediatr Orthop* 1990;10:522–526.

Twenty-three of 32 patients (72%) wth spinal deformity had dystrophic curve patterns; 38% of those undergoing isolated posterior fusion had pseudarthroses. The authors recommend combined anterior-posterior fusion for kyphoscoliotic curves.

Strong ML, Wong-Chung J: Prophylactic bypass grafting of the prepseudarthrotic tibia in neurofibromatosis. *J Pediatr Orthop* 1991;11:757–764.

Three of nine patients required additional surgical intervention. All of these patients were treated with braces, and it is unclear if the surgical procedure altered the results of brace treatment.

Wilde PH, Upadhyay SS, Leong JC: Deterioration of operative correction in dystrophic spinal neurofibromatosis. *Spine* 1994;19:1264–1270.

Patients with dystrophic spinal neurofibromatosis treated surgically were followed up for a mean of 9.7 years after surgery. The authors report that the deformity progresses despite the achievement of spinal arthrodesis in those with hyperkyphosis and short curves. The study shows that vertebral subluxation, disk wedging, and peripheral skeletal dystrophy are additional prognostic features that predict the progression of deformity after arthrodesis of the spine.

Winter RB, Lonstein JE, Anderson M: Neurofibromatosis hyperkyphosis: A review of 33 patients with kyphosis of 80 degrees or greater. *J Spinal Disord* 1988;1:39–49.

The authors review the natural history of the untreated deformity and the results of treatment, and they outline a plan of management for these patients.

Winter RB, Moe JH, Bradford DS, et al: Spine deformity in neurofibromatosis: A review of one hundred and two patients. *J Bone Joint Surg* 1979;61A:677–694.

The authors discuss problems of spinal deformity (scoliosis and kyphosis) in patients with neurofibromatosis.

Proteus Syndrome

Cohen MM Jr: Further diagnostic thoughts about the Elephant Man. *Am J Med Genet* 1988;29:777–782.

The author presents evidence that skeletal findings are more consistent with a diagnosis of proteus syndrome and hip trauma than with neurofibromatosis.

Stricker S: Musculoskeletal manifestations of Proteus syndrome: Report of two cases with literature review. *J Pediatr Orthop* 1992;12:667–674.

This is a case report of two patients plus a comprehensive review of the literature.

Vaughn RY, Selinger AD, Howell CG, et al: Proteus syndrome: Diagnosis and surgical management. *J Pediatr Surg* 1993;28:5–10.

Extensive soft-tissue resections and reconstructions were performed. Lymphatic leakage was common after the surgical procedures. Most patients required multiple surgeries.

Down Syndrome

Aprin H, Zink WP, Hall JE: Management of dislocation of the hip in Down syndrome. *J Pediatr Orthop* 1985;5:428–431.

The authors reviewed surgical treatment for dislocation of the hip in six patients with Down syndrome (ten hips). Those with dislocation and a normal acetabulum fared better than those with a dysplastic acetabulum.

Burke SW, French HG, Roberts JM, et al: Chronic atlanto-axial instability in Down syndrome. *J Bone Joint Surg* 1985;67A:1356–1360.

Thirty-two patients with Down syndrome had serial radiographs between 1970 and 1983. The average atlanto-dens interval increased and new instability developed in seven.

Dugdale TW, Renshaw TS: Instability of the patellofemoral joint in Down syndrome. *J Bone Joint Surg* 1986;68A:405–413.

The authors evaluated 210 institutionalized persons and 151 persons in the community with Down syndrome. Fewer than 10% had dislocated/dislocatable patellae and only three were unable to walk because of patellofemoral instability.

French HG, Burke SW, Roberts JM, et al: Upper cervical ossicles in Down syndrome. *J Pediatr Orthop* 1987;7:69–71.

Serial radiographs and radiographic anatomy in six young adults with Down syndrome suggest that the ossicles at C2 represent an avulsion of the dens rather than a developmental ossiculum terminale.

Goldberg MJ: Spine instability and the Special Olympics. *Clin Sports Med* 1993;12:507–515.

This is a review of the literature on spinal instability in patients with Down syndrome and recommendations for management based on the literature.

Selected Bibliography of Pediatric Orthopaedics

Jagjivan B, Spencer OA, Hosking G: Radiographical screening for atlanto-axial instability in Down's syndrome. *Clin Radiol* 1988;39:661–663.

Of 220 patients of all ages with Down syndrome, 156 (7%) had abnormal atlanto-dens intervals. Of these, 11 (70%) were younger than 25 years of age.

Mendez AA, Keret D, MacEwen GD: Treatment of patellofemoral instability in Down's syndrome. *Clin Orthop* 1988;234:148–158.

Sixteen patients with Down syndrome and patellofemoral dislocations were reviewed. If initial ambulatory ability was either fair or good, nonsurgical management maintained or improved ambulatory status. If initial ambulatory ability was poor, then surgery was needed, and ambulation improved in 85% of the surgically-treated patients.

Olive PM, Whitecloud TS III, Bennett JT: Lower cervical spondylosis and myelopathy in adults with Down's syndrome. *Spine* 1988;13:781–784.

In 105 patients with Down syndrome and normal upper cervical spines, there was a significant prevalence of lower cervical degenerative changes, and two patients had clinical myelopathy.

Pueschel SM, Moon AC, Scola FH: Computerized tomography in persons with Down syndrome and atlantoaxial instability. *Spine* 1992;17:735–737.

Computed tomography (CT) showed subtle abnormalities of the upper cervical spine that were not detected on plain radiographs. Measurement of the space available for the cord was smaller with CT than with plain radiographs.

Pueschel SM, Scola FH: Atlantoaxial instability in individuals with Down syndrome: Epidemiologic, radiographic, and clinical studies. *Pediatrics* 1987;80:555–560.

Of 404 people with Down syndrome, 59 (14.6%) had C1–C2 instability. Of these, 53 were asymptomatic and six required fusion for myelopathy. An additional 95 patients followed up longitudinally showed neither clinical nor radiographic changes.

Pueschel SM, Scola FH, Pezzullo JC: A longitudinal study of atlanto-dens relationships in asymptomatic individuals with Down syndrome. *Pediatrics* 1992;89:1194–1198.

Only minor changes in the atlanto-dens interval occurred over time in 144 asymptomatic patients who were followed up with serial radiographs.

Segal LS, Drummond DS, Zanotti RM, et al: Complications of posterior arthodesis of the cervical spine in patients who have Down syndrome. *J Bone Joint Surg* 1991;73A:1547–1554.

Every patient in this series had a major complication with posterior cervical arthrodesis. Six of the ten patients had graft resorption. The authors recommend nonsurgical management for asymptomatic individuals.

White KS, Ball WS, Prenger EC, et al: Evaluation of the craniocervical junction in Down syndrome: Correlation of measurements obtained with radiography and MR imaging. *Radiology* 1993;186:377–382.

A comparison of flexion and extension radiographs with flexion and extension MRI in children with Down syndrome showed that the neural canal width, as opposed to the atlanto-dens interval, correlated best with MRI findings.

de Lange Syndrome

Joubin J, Pettrone CF, Pettrone FA: Cornelia de Lange's syndrome: A review article (with emphasis on orthopedic significance). *Clin Orthop* 1982;171:180–185.

Six cases illustrate typical facial and skeletal features of this syndrome.

Progeria (Hutchinson-Gilford Syndrome)

Gamble JG: Hip disease in Hutchinson-Gilford progeria syndrome. *J Pediatr Orthop* 1984;4:585–589.

The author describes progressive symptomatic hip subluxation/dislocation in two preadolescents with progeria.

Moen C: Orthopaedic aspects of progeria. *J Bone Joint Surg* 1982;64A: 542–546.

The author reviews two current cases and 60 in the literature, with emphasis on the progressive hip dysplasia, osteolysis, and osteonecrosis seen in this syndrome.

Familial Dysautonomia

Ganz SB, Levine DB, Axelrod FB, et al: Physical therapy management of familial dysautonomia. *Phys Ther* 1983;63:1121–1124.

The authors outline techniques to manage spinal deformity and postural contractures often seen in this syndrome.

Mitnick JS, Axelrod FB, Genieser NB, et al: Aseptic necrosis in familial dysautonomia. *Radiology* 1982;142:89–91.

The osteonecrosis of the femoral head, talus, and distal femur that occurs in as many as 8% of patients with this syndrome is described.

Robin GC: Scoliosis in familial dysautonomia. *Bull Hosp Jt Dis Orthop Inst* 1984;44:16–26.

This is a review of surgical and nonsurgical management of the scoliosis and kyphosis that occur in 90% of patients with this syndrome.

Noonan Syndrome

Allanson JE: Noonan syndrome. *J Med Genet* 1987;24:9–13.

An extensive bibliography accompanies this overview of the Noonan syndrome. References to cases of malignant hyperthermia are of particular value.

Prader-Willi Syndrome

Cassidy SB: Prader-Willi syndrome. *Curr Probl Pediatr* 1984;14:1–55.

This monograph covers all aspects of this syndrome from historical notes to cytogenetics of chromosome 15, as well as management of the orthopaedic and nonorthopaedic manifestations.

Nicholls RD: Genomic imprinting and uniparental disomy in Angelman and Prader-Willi syndromes: A review. *Am J Med Genet* 1993;46:16–25.

Both Angelman syndrome and Prader-Willi syndrome are caused by the same chromosome abnormality (a defect on chromosome 15q11-q13). If the gene is of paternal origin, Prader-Willi syndrome develops, while Angelman syndrome develops if the gene is of maternal origin.

Rees D, Jones MW, Owen R, et al: Scoliosis surgery in Prader-Willi syndrome. *J Bone Joint Surg* 1989;71B:685–688.

The authors discuss problems encountered in scoliosis surgery in children with Prader-Willi syndrome.

Soriano RM, Weisz I, Houghton GR: Scoliosis in the Prader-Willi syndrome. *Spine* 1988;13:209–211.

Scoliosis occurs in 62% to 86% of patients with Prader-Willi syndrome. The authors report on management of five patients.

Tsuji M, Kurihara A, Uratsuji M, et al: Cervical myelopathy with Prader-Willi syndrome in a 13-year-old boy: A case report. *Spine* 1991;16:1342–1344.

A child with cervical instability and spinal cord compression is described. The cervical spine should be evaluated in symptomatic individuals with Prader-Willi syndrome.

Fetal Alcohol (and Other Abused Substances)

Ernhart CB, Sokol RJ, Martier S, et al: Alcohol teratogenicity in the human: A detailed assessment of specificity, critical period, and threshold. *Am J Obstet Gynecol* 1987;156:33–39.

A detailed prospective study of 359 neonates revealed that the critical period for alcohol teratogenicity is around the time of conception, and that certain anomalies, but not all, occur in a dose-response manner.

Graham JM Jr, Hanson JW, Darby BL, et al: Independent dysmorphology evaluations at birth and 4 years of age for children exposed to varying amounts of alcohol in utero. *Pediatrics* 1988;81:772–778.

The greater the levels of alcohol exposure during early pregnancy, the more likely the child will have recognizable, persistent fetal alcohol effects.

Jaffer Z, Nelson M, Beighton P: Bone fusion in the foetal alcohol syndrome. *J Bone Joint Surg* 1981;63B:569–571.

Carpal fusions and radioulnar synotosis were found in three of 15 patients with fetal alcohol syndrome.

Snodgrass SR: Cocaine babies: A result of multiple teratogenic influences. *J Child Neurol* 1994;9:227–233.

This review article documents the many reported malformations associated with maternal cocaine use. However, the author suggests that many of these malformations may be due to other confounding variables, such as poor maternal nutrition and maternal alcohol use.

Spiegel PG, Pekman WM, Rich BH, et al: The orthopedic aspects of the fetal alcohol syndrome. *Clin Orthop* 1979;139:58–63.

Cervical spine fusions, radioulnar synotosis, and contractures are the common orthopaedic complications of this syndrome.

Zimmerman EF: Substance abuse in pregnancy: Teratogenesis. *Pediatr Ann* 1991;20:541–547.

This is a review of proven and unproven teratogenic effects of legal and illegal substances of abuse.

Fetal Acquired Immunodeficiency Syndrome

Marion RW, Wiznia AA, Hutcheon RG, et al: Fetal AIDS syndrome score: Correlation between severity of dysmorphism and age at diagnosis of immunodeficiency. *Am J Dis Child* 1987;141:429–431.

Characteristic dysmorphic facial features of children born with human immunodeficiency virus (HIV) infection are evaluated in 37 children. These were found to be helpful in establishing the diagnosis prior to clinical acquired immunodeficiency syndrome (AIDS).

Rett Syndrome

Guidera KJ, Borrelli J Jr, Raney E, et al: Orthopaedic manifestations of Rett syndrome. *J Pediatr Orthop* 1991;11:204–208.

Orthopaedic manifestations of Rett syndrome in nine patients included scoliosis, lower extremity contracture, and coxa valga.

Naidu S, Murphy M, Moser HW, et al: Rett syndrome: Natural history in 70 cases. *Am J Med Genet* 1986;1(suppl):61–72.

This is a review of all aspects of this syndrome in 70 females ages 2-1/2 to 34 years, with emphasis on the time of appearance and severity of each characteristic. This is one of 40 articles in this supplement volume devoted to Rett syndrome.

TAR (Thrombocytopenia With Absent Radii) Syndrome

Alter BP: Arm anomalies and bone marrow failure may go hand in hand. *J Hand Surg* 1992;17A:566–571.

In this review of blood dyscrasias associated with congenital upper extremity anomalies, Fanconi, Diamond-Blackfan, and thromboctytopenia with absent radii are reviewed.

Brochstein JA, Shank B, Kernan NA, et al: Marrow transplantation for thrombocytopenia-absent radii syndrome. *J Pediatr* 1992;121:587–589.

Bone marrow transplant can be used to correct thrombocytopenia. A patient was able to undergo orthopaedic reconstructive procedures at 8 years of age after having received a marrow transplant at 2 years of age. However, thrombocytopenia tends to improve with age in these individuals, with many children achieving platelet counts of > 100,000 by age 5 years.

Schoenecker PL, Cohn AK, Sedgwick WG, et al: Dysplasia of the knee associated with the syndrome of thrombocytopenia and absent radius. *J Bone Joint Surg* 1984;66A:421–427.

Eighteen of 21 patients with thrombocytopenia with absent radii had developmental anomalies of the lower extremity and significant deformity of the knee. The difficulties of treatment are detailed.

VATER (Vertebral, Anal, Tracheoesophageal, Renal, and Radial Limb Anomalies) Association

Beals RK, Rolfe B: VATER association: A unifying concept of multiple anomalies. *J Bone Joint Surg* 1989;71A:948–950.

This review article ties together the multiple anomalies in terms of fetal development.

Chestnut R, James HE, Jones KL: The VATER association and spinal dysraphia. *Pediatr Neurosurg* 1992;18:144–148.

Six patients with VATER association with a lipoma or tethering of the spinal cord are reviewed. Tethered cord should be considered as a cause of subtle neurologic findings in individuals with VATER.

Femoral Hypoplasia-Unusual Facies

Baraitser M, Reardon W, Oley C, et al: Femoral hypoplasia unusual facies syndrome with preaxial polydactyly. *Clin Dysmorphol* 1994;3:40–45.

The authors present a case report and a review of the literature. Polydactyly can occur in this syndrome, and its existence should not preclude making this diagnosis.

Burn J, Winter RM, Baraitser M, et al: The femoral hypoplasia-unusual facies syndrome. *J Med Genet* 1984;21:331–340.

Features of this syndrome are delineated, including the dysgenesis of the proximal femur, the elbow, and the lumbar spine.

Johnson JP, Carey JC, Gooch WM III, et al: Femoral hypoplasia-unusual facies syndrome in infants of diabetic mothers. *J Pediatr* 1983;102:866–872.

The etiologic relationship of this syndrome to maternal diabetes is discussed.

Connective Tissue Disorders

Biochemistry

Cole WG: Etiology and pathogenesis of heritable connective tissue diseases. *J Pediatr Orthop* 1993;13:392–403.

This is a review of the molecular genetic mechanisms for several heritable connective tissue disorders. The genetic defects are correlated with the clinical findings in these disorders.

Treble NJ, Jensen FO, Bankier A, et al: Development of the hip in multiple epiphyseal dysplasia: Natural history and susceptibility to premature osteoarthritis. *J Bone Joint Surg* 1990;72B:1061–1064.

In 42 patients, premature osteoarthritis was frequent and almost inevitable before the age of 30 years in those with incongruent hips. The prognosis could be predicted in childhood: in sporadic cases from the type of immature hip (of two types identified), and in familial cases by the outcome of affected relatives.

Marfan Syndrome

Joseph KN, Kane HA, Milner RS, et al: Orthopaedic aspects of the Marfan phenotype. *Clin Orthop* 1992;277:251–261.

This is a review of 36 patients with phenotypic features of Marfan, who were grouped into three categories based on how many clinical signs of Marfan they exhibited. There was a 100% incidence of scoliosis in the group with the largest number of clinical signs. Other manifestations of the syndrome and their treatment are reviewed.

Pyeritz RE, Fishman EK, Bernhardt BA, et al: Dural ectasia is a common feature of the Marfan syndrome. *Am J Hum Genet* 1988;43:726–732.

Widening of the lumbar spinal canal was present in two thirds of patients with Marfan syndrome, some of whom had associated pedicle erosion, meningocele, and neurologic signs.

Smith MD: Large sacral dural defect in Marfan syndrome: A case report. *J Bone Joint Surg* 1993;75A:1067–1070.

Dural ectasia can occur in the sacral region, as well as in the more common lumbar and thoracic locations.

Sponseller PD, Hobbs W, Riley LH III, et al: The thoracolumbar spine in Marfan syndrome. *J Bone Joint Surg* 1995;77A:867–876.

Of 82 skeletally immature patients with Marfan syndrome, 52 (63%) had scoliosis; the thoracic portion of the curve was convex to the right in all but two patients. In a separate group of 56 patients with scoliosis, those with curves of more than 30° had mild progression and those with curves of more than 50° had marked progression. Thirty adult patients had pain in the region of the curve.

Homocystinuria

Boers GH, Polder TW, Cruysberg JR, et al: Homocystinuria versus Marfan's syndrome: The therapeutic relevance of the differential diagnosis. *Neth J Med* 1984;27:206–212.

This article contains a lucid discussion of the biochemistry and the rationale for treatment, and has excellent patient photographs. It is worth having the library search for it.

Mudd SH, Skovby F, Levy HL, et al: The natural history of homocystinuria due to cystathionine beta-synthase deficiency. *Am J Hum Genet* 1985;37:1–31.

This study of 629 patients with homocystinuria details the onset and natural history of the most common complications (osteoporosis, thromboembolism, optic lens dislocation). Comparison is made between B-6 (pyridoxine) responsive and nonresponsive individuals.

Skovby F: Homocystinuria: Clinical, biochemical and genetic aspects of cystathionine beta-synthase and its deficiency in man. *Acta Pediatr Scand* 1985;321(suppl):1–21.

This is an excellent review of the entire subject, including clinical features, but mainly details about the biochemistry and the rationale for therapy.

Osteogenesis Imperfecta

Alman B, Frasca P: Fracture failure mechanisms in patients with osteogenesis imperfecta. *J Orthop Res* 1987;5:139–143.

Biomechanical data revealed osteogenesis imperfecta bone to be more plastic ("taffy") with decreased work to failure.

Binder H, Conway A, Hason S, et al: Comprehensive rehabilitation of the child with osteogenesis imperfecta. *Am J Med Genet* 1993;45:265–269.

A comprehensive rehabilitation program resulted in increased involvement in school and social situations in children with osteogenesis imperfecta.

Cetta G, Ramirez F, Tsipouras P (eds): Third international conference on osteogenesis imperfecta. *Ann N Y Acad Sci* 1988;543:1–185.

This volume, devoted to osteogenesis imperfecta, has 21 articles by leaders in the field. They cover such wide ranging topics as: nosology and genetics (Sillence DO, pp 1-15); clinical heterogenicity (Maroteaux P, pp 16-29); collagen biochemistry (Hollister DW, pp 62-72); the molecular basis of clinical disease (Byers PH, pp 117-128); prenatal diagnosis (Sykes B, pp 136-141); and orthopaedic and medical treatment (Cole WG, pp 157-166; Finidori G, pp 167-169; and Brunelli PC, pp 170-179).

Cole DE: Psychosocial aspects of osteogenesis imperfecta: An update. *Am J Med Genet* 1993;45:207–211.

This is a review of potential factors facing individuals with osteogenesis imperfecta that may adversely affect their adjustment to social and work enviornments.

Dent JA, Paterson CR: Fractures in early childhood: Osteogenesis imperfecta or child abuse? *J Pediatr Orthop* 1991;11:184–186.

Radiographs of 194 fractures in children younger than 5 years of age with osteogenesis imperfecta (OI) were compared to radiographs of 84 fractures sustained by 69 normal children of the same age. The results do not support the view that a particular fracture pattern renders the diagnosis of OI unlikely.

Gamble JG, Rinsky LA, Strudwick J, et al: Non-union of fractures in children who have osteogenesis imperfecta. *J Bone Joint Surg* 1988;70A: 439–443.

Of 52 patients with osteogenesis imperfecta, 10 had 12 nonunions, all of which resulted in functional disability.

Hanscome DA, Winter RB, Lutter L, et al: Osteogenesis imperfecta: Radiographic classification, natural history, and treatment of spinal deformities. *J Bone Joint Surg* 1992;74A:598–616.

Based on the radiographic changes in 64 patients, six types of osteogenesis imperfecta (OI) were identified. These types were associated with differing natural histories, development of spinal deformities, and response to treatment.

Marini JC: Osteogenesis imperfecta: Comprehensive management. *Adv Pediatr* 1988;35:391–426.

In addition to a lucid discussion of classification, collagen biochemistry, and orthopaedic management, there are also details of caring for the associated neurologic, ocular, hearing, dental, growth, and cardiovascular problems.

Nicholas RW, James P: Telescoping intramedullary stabilization of the lower extremities for severe osteogenesis imperfecta. *J Pediatr Orthop* 1990;10:219–223.

Sixteen patients had 56 Bailey-Dubow nails placed in 48 long bones, including 18 revisions. Despite a high rate of complication, extendable nails provided correction of the angular deformities, decreased fracturing, and allowed most previously nonambulatory children to walk.

Other Syndromes

Ainsworth SR, Aulicino PL: A survey of patients with Ehlers-Danlos syndrome. *Clin Orthop* 1993;286:250–256.

A survey of 151 patients with Ehlers-Danlos syndrome showed a high percentage of types I, II, III, and IV (of 9 types). Bracing and fusion are the most commonly used orthopaedic treatments; surgical complications were common.

Andrisano A, Soncini G, Calderoni PP, et al: Critical review of infantile fibrous dysplasia: Surgical treatment. *J Pediatr Orthop* 1991;11:478–481.

A review of 65 patients demonstrated that "circumscribed" types of the disease usually do not require surgical treatment, while "extended" types, as well as Albright's syndrome, require early surgical treatment aimed at preventing development of skeletal deformities, which are difficult to correct later.

Brinker MR, Palutsis RS, Sarwark JF: The orthopaedic manifestations of prune-belly (Eagle-Barrett) syndrome. *J Bone Joint Surg* 1995;77A: 251–257.

Although prune-belly syndrome is uncommon, the diagnosis necessitates a thorough orthopaedic evaluation because of the high prevalence of associated musculoskeletal abnormalities. Of 40 children with the syndrome, 25 (63%) had musculoskeletal abnormalities, including congenital dislocation of the hip that was resistant to conventional treatment, pectus excavatum, and idiopathic-like scoliosis.

Field RE, Buchanan JA, Copplemans MG, et al: Bone-marrow transplantation in Hurler's syndrome: Effect on skeletal development. *J Bone Joint Surg* 1994;76B:975–981.

In 11 children with Hurler syndrome treated with bone-marrow transplantation, all had abnormal bone modeling, local failures of ossification, and an avascular disorder of the femoral head. Increasing valgus deformity of the knees and progressive generalized myopathy caused loss of mobility as the children entered adolescence. Bone-marrow transplantation as a treatment for Hurler syndrome is limited by the poor penetration of the musculoskeletal tissues by the enzyme derived from the leucocytes.

Green NE, Lowrey ER, Thomas R: Orthopaedic aspects of prune-belly syndrome. *J Pediatr Orthop* 1993;13:496–501.

Deformities observed in children with this syndrome included developmental dislocation of the hip (DDH), clubfeet, metatarsus adductus, vertical talus, and congenital muscular torticollis. The authors recommend aggressive treatment of these deformities because children with prune-belly syndrome can be expected to have a relatively normal life if their renal function is good. Surgery, however, should be delayed until children are old enough to be able to clear pulmonary secretions easily.

Guidera KJ, Satterwhite Y, Ogdan JA, et al: Nail patella syndrome: A review of 44 orthopaedic patients. *J Pediatr Orthop* 1991;11:737–742.

Nail patella syndrome is a rare dysplasia with characteristics of fingernail abnormalities, hypoplastic patellas, radial head dislocations, and iliac horns. All 44 patients were ambulatory, 20 had knee operations, and 24 had operations to correct foot and ankle deformities. Knee extensor realignments and foot posteromedial releases had overall good results.

McGroy BJ, Amadio PC, Dobyns JH, et al: Anomalies of the fingers and toes associated with Klippel-Treaunay syndrome. *J Bone Joint Surg* 1991;73A:1537-1546.

Of 108 patients with this syndrome, 126 anomalies were found in 29 patients, each of whom had 1 to 13 malformations of the fingers or toes or both, most commonly macrodactyly. The ratio of female to male patients was approximately 2 to 1.

Section 4

Cervical Spine

George H. Thompson, MD

Hensinger RN: Congenital anomalies of the cervical spine. *Clin Orthop* 1991;264:16–38.

The author presents a review of congenital malformations affecting the pediatric cervical spine. He emphasizes that those affecting the upper cervical spine have a greater propensity toward development of early instability and neurologic problems, whereas those of the lower cervical spine tend to produce degenerative osteoarthritis in adult life.

Menezes AH, Ryken TC: Craniovertebral junction abnormalities, in Weinstein SL (ed): *The Pediatric Spine: Principles and Practice.* New York, NY, Raven Press, 1994, pp 307–321.

This is an excellent review of the embryology, development, blood supply, and biomechanics of the occiput and upper cervical spine. It includes clinical presentation, radiographic features, and treatment of occipital malformations, basilar invagination (impression), assimilation of the atlas, and anomalies of the odontoid process.

Basilar Impression

Caetano de Barros M, Farias W, Ataide L, et al: Basilar impression and Arnold-Chiari malformation: A study of 66 cases. *J Neurol Neurosurg Psychiatry* 1968;31:596–605.

The authors compare the symptoms, radiographic findings, and results of treatment in children, adolescents, and adults with basilar impression with (33) and without (33) associated Arnold-Chiari malformation. Basilar impression without the Arnold-Chiari malformation tends to produce pyramidal tract involvement with proprioception disturbances. The combined form tends to present with cerebellar, vestibular, and cranial nerve involvement.

Harkey HL, Crockard HA, Stevens JM, et al: The operative management of basilar impression in osteogenesis imperfecta. *Neurosurgery* 1990; 27:782–786.

Four patients with osteogenesis imperfecta and neurologically significant basilar impression are discussed with respect to the disease process, neurologic involvement, radiologic findings, and modes of surgical therapy. The authors currently recommend extensive removal of the anterior bony compression by a transoral approach followed by a posterior rigid fixation that transfers the weight of the head to the thoracic spine.

Kohno K, Sakaki S, Nakamura H, et al: Foramen magnum decompression for syringomelia associated with basilar impression and Chiari I malformation: Report of three cases. *Neurol Med Chir Tokyo* 1991;31:715–719.

Results of anterior or posterior decompression of the foramen magnum in three patients were evaluated using pre- and postoperative magnetic resonance imaging. Postoperatively, all three had sustained shrinkage of the syrinx and rounding of the flattened cerebellar tonsils, and two showed upward movement of the herniated tonsils. Symptoms in all patients were improved during 2- to 4-year follow-up.

McRae DL: The significance of abnormalities of the cervical spine. *Am J Roentgenol* 1960;84:3–25.

This lecture, given to the American Roentgen Ray Society in 1959, covers everything from congenital anomalies to cervical disk disease and osteoarthritis. Although most of the patients presented are adults, many of the abnormalities developed or presented in childhood. The article describes neurologic symptoms and signs in patients with radiographic abnormalities of the cervical spine. The conclusion is to correlate clinical and radiographic findings to determine which patients require treatment.

Sillence DO: Craniocervical abnormalities in osteogenesis imperfecta: Genetic and molecular correlation. *Pediatr Radiol* 1994;24:427–430.

Basilar impression assessed by either plain lateral skull radiograph or computed tomography sagittal reconstruction of the craniocervical junction occurs in 25% of patients with osteogenesis imperfecta. It appears to occur most frequently in patients with mild to moderate liability to fractures, normal sclerae, and dentinogenesis imperfecta. Neurologic signs indicating compression of posterior fossa structures occur predominantly in these patients.

Wong VC, Fung CF: Basilar impression in a child with hypochondroplasia. *Pediatr Neurol* 1991;7:62–64.

Magnetic resonance imaging showed basilar impression with compression at the craniovertebral junction and mild degree of hydrocephalus in a 4-year-old boy with hypochondroplasia who had a delay in gross motor development. Posterior fossa decompression resulted in improvement in neurologic function and relief of hydrocephalus.

Occipitoatlantal Complex

Dormans JP, Drummond DS, Sutton LN, et al: Occipitocervical arthrodesis in children: A new technique and analysis of results. *J Bone Joint Surg* 1995;77A:1234–1240.

Fusion was successful in 15 of 16 patients. Wiring, autogenous bone graft, and halo immobilization were used. The authors concluded that early halo removal was possible with this method of stable fixation.

Georgopoulos G, Pizzutillo PD, Lee MS: Occipito-atlantal instability in children: A report of five cases and review of the literature. *J Bone Joint Surg* 1987;69A:429–436.

The authors describe five patients with occipitoatlantal instability, a rare disorder due to either trauma or congenital abnormalities. The clinical symptoms and radiographic findings are diffuse. An excellent discussion of the anatomy of the occiput and upper cervical spine is included. Surgical stabilization (occiput–C1 or occiput–C2 posterior arthrodesis) is recommended for both traumatic and congenital occipitoatlantal instability.

Koop SE, Winter RB, Lonstein JE: The surgical treatment of instability of the upper part of the cervical spine in children and adolescents. *J Bone Joint Surg* 1984;66A:403–411.

The authors describe a technique for occiput-upper cervical posterior arthrodesis that involves a cautious exposure, an osteogenic periosteal flap from the occiput, delicate decortication by an air-drill, placement of autogenous cancellous iliac grafts, and external immobilization by a halo cast. This minimizes the risk of neural damage and is a reliable way to obtain a solid arthrodesis. It eliminates the need for wiring and is especially useful when anomalous vertebrae are present. The authors report a solid arthrodesis in 12 of 13 children and adolescents and no reoperations using this technique.

Letts M, Kaylor D, Gouw G: A biomechanical analysis of halo fixation in children. *J Bone Joint Surg* 1988;70B:277–279.

The authors discuss the variability in the mechanics of halo pin fixation in young children, including forces applied during insertion, penetration of the inner table of the skull, friction at the pin-halo interface, and the variability of skull thickness as measured by computed tomography (CT). Skull thickness ranged from 1.1 to 4.3 mm in children younger than 6 years of age. CT scanning of the skull prior to halo application is recommended to ascertain the safest pin sites.

Letts M, Slutsky D: Occipitocervical arthrodesis in children. *J Bone Joint Surg* 1990;72A:1166–1170.

The authors describe a technique for posterior occipitocervical arthrodesis for instability secondary to various forms of dysplasia. This consists of a C1–C2 wiring with incorporation of dual corticocancellous grafts beneath the wires and extending proximally across the occiput–C1 region. The occiput is roughened to enhance fusion. A halo is used to provide immobilization until a solid fusion is achieved. The authors report seven patients with no nonunions or significant complications.

Mubarak SJ, Camp JF, Vuletich W, et al: Halo application in the infant. *J Pediatr Orthop* 1989;9:612–614.

The authors present a multiple pin technique for halo application in children less than 2 years of age. Less torque is required to provide stability because of the greater range of pin placement sites. Halo applications in three children 2 years of age or younger are described.

Nicholson JT, Sherk HH: Anomalies of the occipitocervical articulation. *J Bone Joint Surg* 1968;50A:295-304.

This article reviews the embryology, anomalies, and routine radiography of the occiput and upper cervical spine. Three types of anomalies are described: congenital occipitoatlantal fusion, accessory vertebral elements between the occiput and the atlas, and anomalies of the apex of the odontoid process. Signs and symptoms of these anomalies become evident most often in young adults who present with weakness, ataxia, suboccipital and neck pain, torticollis, and progressive quadriparesis. Surgical treatment often is needed.

Parfenchuck TA, Bertrand SL, Powers MJ, et al: Posterior occipitoatlantal hypermobility in Down syndrome: An analysis of 199 patients. *J Pediatr Orthop* 1994;14:304-308.

In a radiographic comparison of patients with Down syndrome to a matched group of normal individuals, 8.5% of patients with Down syndrome had Powers ratios of less than 0.55, indicative of posterior occipitoatlantal hypermobility. Of these, 66% had positive neurologic findings on physical examination.

Tredwell SJ, Newman DE, Lockitch G: Instability of the upper cervical spine in Down syndrome. *J Pediatr Orthop* 1990;10:602-606.

Posterior occipitoatlantal subluxation of 4 mm or more was demonstrated on extension lateral radiographs of the cervical spine in 43 of 64 children with Down syndrome. This entity, as well as atlantoaxial instability, must be considered in Down syndrome. Both are due to ligamentous laxity. Treatment is based on the space available for the spinal cord.

Atlantoaxial Instability

American Academy of Pediatrics: Atlantoaxial instability in Down syndrome. *Pediatrics* 1984;4:152-154.

This is an excellent review from the American Academy of Pediatrics regarding preparticipation sports screening for atlantoaxial instability in children and adolescents with Down syndrome. It demonstrates that radiographic assessment probably is not beneficial in asymptomatic patients and should be reserved for patients with complaints or physical findings consistent with spinal cord injury. It is an excellent reference source.

Cattell HS, Filtzer DL: Pseudosubluxation and other normal variations in the cervical spine in children: A study of one hundred and sixty children. *J Bone Joint Surg* 1965;47A:1295–1309.

This study of 160 normal lateral spine radiographs in children 1 to 16 years of age (ten radiographs per year of age) is an excellent description of the normal variations of the pediatric cervical spine, including C2–C3 pseudosubluxation. It also describes variations of curvature that may resemble muscle spasms or ligamentous injury and variations related to skeletal growth centers that may resemble fractures.

Davidson RG: Atlantoaxial instability in individuals with Down syndrome: A fresh look at the evidence. Pediatrics 1988;81:857–865.

A review of published cases reveals no evidence that the current radiographic criteria are predictive of atlantoaxial instability leading to dislocation. Those who suffered dislocation had preceding neurologic signs for at least several weeks. No atlantoaxial dislocations while participating in competitive sports were reported in 500,000 individuals with Down syndrome. The authors recommended that longitudinal studies be performed, and they suggested that a preparticipation physical examination with a careful neurologic assessment is more important than radiographic evaluation.

Goldberg MJ: Spine instability and the Special Olympics. *Clin Sports Med* 1993;12:507–515.

This is an excellent review of the current status of Down syndrome, atlantoaxial instability, and sports participation. The author recommends periodic radiographic evaluation and regular preparticipation physical examination with a careful neurologic assessment. Patients with atlantoaxial instability and a normal neurologic examination can have limited sports participation avoiding activities with stressful weightbearing to the head. Instability with myelopathy requires fusion.

Higo M, Sakou T, Taketomi E, et al: Occipitocervical fusion by Luque loop instrumentation in Down syndrome. *J Pediatr Orthop* 1995;15: 539–542.

Four children with Down syndrome who developed atlantoaxial dislocation and myelopathy had occipitocervical fusion and decompressive laminectomy of C1. The authors suggest that this method has advantages over conventional procedures because postoperative management is simplified in these patients.

Jauregui N, Lincoln T, Mubarak S, et al: Surgically related upper cervical spine canal anatomy in children. *Spine* 1993;18:1939–1944.

The normal sagittal diameter of the upper cervical spine changes with growth. In a study of 121 pediatric patients ranging in age from 1 month to 17 years the sagittal diameter of C1 measured 18.2 mm at birth, 31.2 mm by age 6 years, and was relatively constant thereafter. The space available for the spinal cord at C1 was 12.4 mm at birth and gradually increased to 19 mm by 6 years.

Locke GR, Gardner JI, Van Epps EF: Atlas-dens interval (ADI) in children: A survey based on 200 normal cervical spines. *Am J Roentgenol* 1966;97:135–140.

This is the classic article demonstrating the normal atlas-dens interval (ADI). The ADI was measured in 200 normal children 3 to 15 years of age. The tube-to-film distance was found to make a potential difference in evaluating this interval. At a 40-inch tube-to-film distance (100 patients) with the neck in the neutral position, no measurement was greater than 4 mm. At 72 inches (100 patients), there was 5 mm of ADI in only one normal patient. There were no age or sex differences.

Pueschel SM, Findley TW, Furia J, et al: Atlantoaxial instability in Down syndrome: Roentgenographic, neurologic, and somatosensory evoked potential studies. *J Pediatr* 1987;110:515–521.

A combined approach using radiographic, computed tomography (CT), neurologic, and neurophysiologic investigations provides information about the risk status of patients with Down syndrome and atlantoaxial instability.

Rizzolo S, Lemos MJ, Mason DE: Posterior spinal arthrodesis for atlantoaxial instability in Down syndrome. *J Pediatr Orthop* 1995;15:543–548.

Nine children with Down syndrome and atlantoaxial instability were treated with posterior spinal fusion. At follow-up all had stabilization or improvement of their neurologic symptoms. The authors recommend posterior spinal fusion in situ with external immobilization as the safest and most effective treatment of this condition.

Segal LS, Drummond DS, Zanotti RM, et al: Complications of posterior arthrodesis of the cervical spine in patients who have Down's syndrome. *J Bone Joint Surg* 1991;73A:1547–1554.

Complications, which occurred in all 10 patients with Down syndrome who had posterior arthrodesis of the upper cervical spine, included infection, dehiscence at the site of the wound, incomplete reduction of the atlantoaxial joint, instability of the adjacent motion segment, neurologic sequelae, resorption of the autogenous bone graft, and death. The authors recommend nonsurgical treatment for atlantoaxial instability without neurologic symptoms.

Sullivan CR, Bruwer AJ, Harris LE: Hypermobility of the cervical spine in children: A pitfall in the diagnosis of cervical dislocation. *Am J Surg* 1958;95:636–640.

This is a classic article regarding pseudosubluxation of the pediatric upper cervical spine. The authors evaluated flexion and extension lateral radiographs of the cervical spine from 100 normal children between 2 and 14 years of age to determine the incidence of hypermobility between C2 and C3 and between C3 and C4. They determined that the normal distance can be up to 4 mm. Only 15% of the children studied had distances between 3.5 and 4 mm.

Yousefzadeh DK, El-Khoury GY, Smith WL: Normal sagittal diameter and variation in the pediatric cervical spine. *Radiology* 1982;144:319–325.

The normal sagittal diameter of the cervical spine gradually decreases from C1 to C7. However, approximately 30% of children younger than 10 years of age have widening of the lower cervical canal or ballooning at the midlevel. Thus, asymptomatic children with relative widening of the lower cervical canal should not be investigated for a spinal cord lesion. However, such widening in an adolescent requires further evaluation.

Os Odontoideum

Bhatnagar M, Sponsellor PD, Carroll C IV, et al: Pediatric atlantoaxial instability presenting as cerebral and cerebellar infarcts. *J Pediatr Orthop* 1991;11:103–107.

This case report suggests that a vascular etiology may contribute the variable signs and symptoms seen in symptomatic atlantoaxial instability and os odontoideum. A 5-year-old child with an os odontoideum and 10 mm atlantoaxial instability developed infarcts in the cerebellum and occipital parietal lobes due to vertebral artery narrowing at the level of the axis and subsequent low blood flow. Neurologic recovery occurred after a posterior C1–C2 arthrodesis and halo-body cast immobilization.

Blaw ME, Langer LO: Spinal cord compression in Morquio-Brailsford's disease. *J Pediatr* 1969;74:593–600.

The authors present the distribution of spinal deformities in patients with Morquio's disease. Eight patients had radiographic evidence of hypoplasia or absence of the odontoid as well as thoracic gibbus formation. Four patients had cervical spinal cord compression due to atlantoaxial dislocation or subluxation, and two had thoracic spinal cord compression at the gibbus deformity. Periodic spinal evaluation is recommended, especially before other procedures are performed.

Fielding JW, Hensinger RN, Hawkins RJ: Os odontoideum. *J Bone Joint Surg* 1980;62A:376–383.

One of the largest series of patients (35) with os odontoideum is reviewed. A traumatic etiology is suggested. Nine patients had normal odontoids before the development of os odontoideum, and 11 others had lesions attributable to injuries before 4 years of age. Twenty-two patients had anterior instability (average 1.03 cm), five had posterior instability (average 0.84 cm), and eight had combined instability (average 1.37 cm). Twenty-five patients were symptomatic. Twenty-six patients underwent posterior C1–C2 arthrodesis, usually with wire fixation. Surgical stabilization was effective in relieving symptoms.

Schiff DC, Parke WW: The arterial supply of the odontoid process. *J Bone Joint Surg* 1973;55A:1450–1456.

This is a detailed description of the blood supply to the odontoid, which is important with respect to the etiology of os odontoideum.

Schuler TC, Kurz L, Thompson DE, et al: Natural history of os odontoideum. *J Pediatr Orthop* 1991;11:222–225.

This case report documents the natural progression of the formation of os odontoideum in a 2-year-old and correlates it with a traumatic event.

Spierings EL, Braakman R: The management of os odontoideum: Analysis of 37 cases. *J Bone Joint Surg* 1982;64B:422–428.

Twenty of 37 patients with os odontoideum were treated conservatively and 17 surgically. Two surgical patients died in the immediate postoperative period. The authors found that when the space available for the spinal cord is less than 13 mm there is a significant risk for spinal cord injury. They recommended conservative treatment for patients with local symptoms and an available space of 13 mm or more and surgery for patients with progressive spinal cord signs and those with transient signs who have less than 13 mm of space available for the spinal cord.

Klippel-Feil Syndrome

Dietz F: Congenital abnormalities of the cervical spine, in Weinstein SL (ed): *The Pediatric Spine: Principles and Practice*. New York, NY, Raven Press, 1994, pp 323–342.

This is an in depth review of the current concepts regarding Klippel-Feil syndrome. The majority of this chapter deals with this disorder. The author discusses incidence, etiology, clinical features, radiographic features, associated anomalies, natural history, and treatment. It is an excellent reference source.

Guille JT, Miller A, Bowen JR, et al: The natural history of Klippel-Feil syndrome: Clinical, roentgenographic, and magnetic resonance imaging findings at adulthood. *J Pediatr Orthop* 1995;15:617–626.

Of 22 adult patients with Klippel-Feil syndrome, 10 (45%) had abnormal findings on clinical examination and 15 (68%) had at least one complaint that could be related to the syndrome. MRI showed degenerative disk changes in all; 16 had disk protrusions.

Pizzutillo PD, Woods M, Nicholson L, et al: Risk factors in Klippel-Feil syndrome. *Spine* 1994;19:2110–2116.

Patients with Klippel-Feil syndrome with hypermobility in the upper cervical spine are at risk for neurologic sequelae whereas alterations in motion in the lower cervical spine predispose to degenerative osteoarthritis. The authors studied 111 patients with Klippel-Feil syndrome with flexion and extension lateral radiographs of the cervical spine to assess motion at each open interspace and to compare motion in 25 control patients. They found increased motion per open segment in the upper cervical spine compared to decreased motion in the lower cervical spine.

Ritterbusch JF, McGinty LD, Spar J, et al: Magnetic resonance imaging for stenosis and subluxation in Klippel-Feil syndrome. *Spine* 1991; 16(suppl 10):S539–S541.

Increased incidences of cervical spine and spinal cord anomalies in Klippel-Feil syndrome are reported. Magnetic resonance imaging (MRI) was performed in 20 patients with this syndrome. There was a 25% incidence of subluxation and stenosis and a 12% incidence of spinal cord abnormalities (diplomyelia and Arnold-Chiari malformation). The authors recommend MRI for the evaluation of spinal cord abnormalities and compression in patients with Klippel-Feil syndrome.

Torticollis

Canale ST, Griffin DW, Hubbard CN: Congenital muscular torticollis: A long-term follow-up. *J Bone Joint Surg* 1982;64A:810–816.

The authors review 57 patients followed up for a mean of 18.9 years (range, 3 to 35 years). If the contracture persists beyond 1 year of age, it will not resolve spontaneously and nonsurgical therapy rarely is successful. Children treated during the first year of life had better results than those treated later. Established facial asymmetry and limitation of motion of more than 30° usually precludes a good result, even with surgery.

Cheng JC, Au AW: Infantile torticollis: A review of 624 cases. *J Pediatr Orthop* 1994;14:802–808.

In these patients, the types of torticollis were almost evenly distributed between postural torticollis, torticollis with sternomastoid tumors, and muscular torticollis. Patients with cord-like muscular torticollis and rotation deficit of more than 30° were more likely to need surgery. Sequelae after resolution of the torticollis included intermittent head tilt and persistence of mild craniofacial asymmetry.

Davids JR, Wenger DR, Mubarak SJ: Congenital muscular torticollis: Sequela of intrauterine or perinatal compartment syndrome. *J Pediatr Orthop* 1993;13:141–147.

Because of the association of congenital muscular torticollis (CMT) with other intrauterine positioning disorders, the authors postulate, based on MRI findings in ten involved infants, that head positioning in utero can selectively injure the sternocleidomastoid muscle, leading to development of a compartment syndrome, the sequela of which is CMT.

Dubousset J: Torticollis in children caused by congenital anomalies of the atlas. *J Bone Joint Surg* 1986;68A:178–188.

Congenital hemiaplasia or hypoplasia of the atlas can result in severe and progressive torticollis. Congenital anomalies of the vertebral arteries on the side of the aplasia and the presence of other congenital spinal abnormalities are common. Observation is indicated except in the presence of severe torticollis or instability, in which case surgical fusion becomes the appropriate treatment. Orthotic management is ineffective. Seven of 17 patients required fusion with gradual correction being obtained in a halo cast.

Ferkel RD, Westin GW, Dawson EG, et al: Muscular torticollis: A modified surgical approach. *J Bone Joint Surg* 1983;65A:894–900.

A modified bipolar release of the sternocleidomastoid muscle was performed in 12 children. The muscle was divided at the mastoid process proximally and the clavicular portion distally and Z-lengthened at the sternal attachment. These patients had a greater percentage of good or excellent results than did ten patients who underwent other surgical procedures and 14 patients, most younger than 1 year of age, treated conservatively.

Fielding JW, Hawkins RJ: Atlanto-axial rotatory fixation (fixed rotatory subluxation of the atlanto-axial joint). *J Bone Joint Surg* 1977;59A:37–44.

This is the classic description of this disorder. The authors present the commonly used four group classification of rotatory fixation with or without anterior and posterior displacement. They describe the treatment, including skull traction and atlantoaxial arthrodesis, when conservative treatment fails or is followed by a recurrent deformity.

Hummer CD, MacEwen GD: The coexistence of torticollis and congenital dysplasia of the hip. *J Bone Joint Surg* 1972;54A:1255–1256.

This is a brief report describing an association between congenital muscular torticollis and hip dysplasia. It was found that 20% of 70 children with congenital muscular torticollis seen over 10 years had either developmental hip dislocation or subluxation. The authors recommend that all children with congenital muscular torticollis undergo a careful clinical and possible radiographic examination of the hips.

Ling CM: The influence of age on the results of open sternomastoid tenotomy in muscular torticollis. *Clin Orthop* 1976;116:142–148.

The author reports 60 patients who underwent sternocleidomastoid release for congenital muscular torticollis and were followed up 4.1 years (range, 1.5 to 9.8 years). The best time for surgery was between 1 and 4 years of age. Complications with scarring occurred in patients younger than 1 year and in those over 5 years of age. The latter also had more residual facial asymmetry, as well as loss of the sternocleidomastoid column and the presence of lateral bands.

Minamitani K, Inoue A, Okuno T: Results of surgical treatment of muscular torticollis for patients greater than 6 years of age. *J Pediatr Orthop* 1990;10:754–759.

Nineteen patients older than 6 years of age were treated with partial resection of the distal portion of the sternocleidomastoid muscle. Function and cosmesis were improved, but scoliosis was a residual deformity in some, especially girls.

Phillips WA, Hensinger RN: The management of rotatory atlanto-axial subluxation in children. *J Bone Joint Surg* 1989;71A:664–668.

The authors present the results of treatment of rotatory atlantoaxial subluxation (fixation) in 23 children. If symptoms were present less than 1 month, the subluxation reduced either spontaneously or after a brief period of cervical traction. Three of seven children who were seen more than a month after the onset of symptoms required posterior C1–C2 arthrodesis. Dynamic CT with the head rotated maximally to each side proved the most satisfactory method of documenting this disorder.

Ramenofsky ML, Buyse M, Goldberg MJ, et al: Gastroesophageal reflux and torticollis. *J Bone Joint Surg* 1978;60A:1140–1141.

This is the first orthopaedic description of Sandifer's syndrome, a combination of hiatal hernia and abnormal posturing of the head and neck. The abnormal posturing is attributed to an attempt to decrease the pain of esophagitis resulting from gastroesophageal reflux and hiatal hernia. The authors describe five cases, one in detail. In this syndrome the torticollis is a physical finding, not a diagnosis.

Sonnabend DH, Taylor TKF, Chapman GK: Intervertebral disc calcification syndromes in children. *J Bone Joint Surg* 1982;64B:25–31.

This is a review of 127 children with intervertebral disk calcification. Cervical (C2–C3) involvement is most common, followed by lumbar involvement. There is an abrupt onset of symptoms, such as pain in the neck, torticollis, and reduced range of motion. Neurologic symptoms are rare. Rapid clinical and gradual radiographic resolution is expected. Treatment is conservative, and the long-term prognosis is excellent.

Wirth CJ, Hagena F-W, Wuelker N, et al: Biterminal tenotomy for the treatment of congenital muscular torticollis: Long-term results. *J Bone Joint Surg* 1992;74A:427–434.

At an average 15-year follow-up, 55 patients had no functional or cosmetic impairment after biterminal tenotomy. The rate of recurrence was 2%. The authors recommend this procedure between the ages of 3 and 5 years in all patients who do not respond to nonsurgical treatment.

Miscellaneous

Aronsson DD, Kahn RH, Canady A, et al: Instability of the cervical spine after decompression in patients who have Arnold-Chiari malformation. *J Bone Joint Surg* 1991;73A:898–906.

The authors describe increased mobility and translation between C2–C3 and C3–C4 as well as angulation in children with myelodysplasia who had a partial craniectomy and upper cervical laminectomy for decompression of an Arnold-Chiari type II malfunction as compared to a similar group who did not require decompression. The authors questioned whether this increased mobility may contribute to brainstem dysfunction. They recommend anterior fusion when substantial instability occurs.

Bell DF, Walker JL, O'Connor G, et al: Spinal deformity after multiple-level cervical laminectomy in children. *Spine* 1994;19:406–411.

A review of 89 children undergoing multiple-level cervical laminectomy followed up for a mean of 5.1 years postoperatively (range, 2 to 9 years) demonstrated that 46 patients (53%) developed a significant cervical deformity. These included 33 patients with a mean kyphosis of 30° (range, 5° to 105°) and 13 patients with a mean hyperlordosis of 62° (range, 40° to 95°). The peak age at surgery was 10.5 years for the development of kyphosis and 4.2 years for development of hyperlordosis. There was no correlation between diagnosis, sex, location, the number of laminectomies, and the subsequent development of a deformity. Children who undergo cervical laminectomy require serial radiographs for assessment of late spinal deformity.

Smith MD: Congenital scoliosis of the cervical or cervicothoracic spine. *Orthop Clin North Am* 1994;25:301–310.

This excellent review article covers current concepts of etiology, clinical presentation, radiographic assessment, and treatment, and provides pertinent references regarding congenital scoliosis involving the cervical or cervicothoracic spine. It briefly describes the results of surgical treatment of 21 patients.

Yong-Hing K, Kalamachi A, MacEwen GD: Cervical spine abnormalities in neurofibromatosis. *J Bone Joint Surg* 1979;61A:695–699.

Seventeen of 56 neurofibromatosis patients (30%) had abnormal cervical spines: absent cervical lordosis, kyphosis, rotatory function, and C2–C3 subluxation. Instability was not a major problem. Ten of the 17 patients were symptomatic and four had neurologic deficits. There was a high association with scoliosis or kyphoscoliosis of the thoracic and lumbar spine. Only four patients required fusion and the others were observed. Children with neurofibromatosis require periodic radiographic evaluation of the cervical spine, especially if they are about to undergo general anesthesia.

Section 5

Vertebral Column

Stuart L. Weinstein, MD

Adolescent Idiopathic Scoliosis

Bradford DS, Moe JH, Lonstein JE, et al (eds): *Moe's Textbook of Scoliosis and Other Spinal Deformities*, ed 3. Philadelphia, PA, WB Saunders, 1995.

This is the classic textbook on all aspects of scoliosis. It has an extensive bibliography and is well illustrated.

Bridwell KH, Dewald RL (eds): *The Textbook of Spinal Surgery*. Philadelphia, PA, JB Lippincott, 1991.

This two-volume text with 60 contributors covers spinal problems. It is illustrated and provides case examples.

Weinstein SL (ed): *The Pediatric Spine: Principles and Practice*. New York, NY, Raven Press, 1994.

This comprehensive two-volume text (85 chapters, 126 international authors) provides the reader with in-depth study of all spinal disorders, related conditions, and their management. Each chapter has a comprehensive bibliography and illustrations.

Prevalence and Natural History

Bunnell WP: The natural history of idiopathic scoliosis before skeletal maturity. *Spine* 1986;11:773–776.

This is a study of the natural history in 326 patients with assessment of risk factors in progression.

Hoffman DA, Lonstein JE, Morin MM, et al: Breast cancer in women with scoliosis exposed to multiple diagnostic x-rays. *J Natl Cancer Inst* 1989; 81:1307–1312.

This excellent study documents the risk of breast cancer induction in women exposed to multiple radiographs in the management of scoliosis.

Lonstein JE, Carlson JM: The prediction of curve progression in untreated idiopathic scoliosis during growth. *J Bone Joint Surg* 1984;66A: 1061–1071.

The risk of progression is studied in 727 patients; a curve of 20° to 29° in a Risser 0-1 patient has a 68% chance of progression, whereas a curve less than 20° in a Risser 2-4 patient has only 1.6% risk of progression. Other risk factors in progression are discussed.

Pehrsson K, Larsson S, Oden A, et al: Long-term follow-up of patients with untreated scoliosis: A study of mortality, causes of death, and symptoms. *Spine* 1992;17:1091–1096.

Results of this study demonstrate that there is no increased mortality associated with adolescent idiopathic scoliosis.

Weinstein SL: Idiopathic scoliosis: Natural history. *Spine* 1986;11: 780–783.

This is a review of 54 patients with complete radiographs from initial presentation through skeletal maturity, with 30- and 40-year follow-up. Radiographic factors leading to curve progression at maturity also apply to skeletally immature patients.

Weinstein SL, Ponseti IV: Curve progression in idiopathic scoliosis. *J Bone Joint Surg* 1983;65A:447–455.

After skeletal maturity, 68% of curves progressed. Factors leading to curve progression after maturity are presented.

Weinstein SL, Zavala DC, Ponseti IV: Idiopathic scoliosis: Long-term follow-up and prognosis in untreated patients. *J Bone Joint Surg* 1981; 63A:702–712.

One hundred ninety-four patients with untreated adolescent idiopathic scoliosis reviewed with a follow-up of 39.3 years showed an incidence of backache slightly less than that in the general population. In some patients, progression occured during adulthood, especially in thoracic curves that measured between 50° and 80° at the end of growth; pulmonary function, psychosocial effects, mortality, and morbidity are discussed.

School Screening

Ashworth MA: Symposium on school screening for the Scoliosis Research Society and British Scoliosis Society. *Spine* 1988;13:1117–1200.

This excellent series of papers defines screening and evaluates results to date. Pros and cons of school screening are effectively discussed.

Lonstein JE, Bjorklund S, Wanninger MH, et al: Voluntary school screening for scoliosis in Minnesota. *J Bone Joint Surg* 1982;64A:481–488.

Of 250,000 children examined each year, 3.4% were referred for evaluation and 1.2% were found to have scoliosis. Because of screening, a marked decrease in patients needing surgery is noted.

Torell G, Nordwall A, Nachemson A: The changing pattern of scoliosis treatment due to effective screening. *J Bone Joint Surg* 1981;63A: 337–341.

A 10-year program was evaluated. A threefold increase in the number of patients treated is noted with a significant decrease in the curve severity at diagnosis. Most patients needing treatment do not require surgery due to the early diagnosis.

U.S. Preventive Services Task Force: Policy statement: Screening for adolescent idiopathic scoliosis. *JAMA* 1993;269:2664–2666.

This summary article on literature to date on school screening is a good review with controversial conclusions.

Etiology

Carr AJ, Ogilvie DJ, Wordsworth BP, et al: Segregation of structural collagen genes in adolescent idiopathic scoliosis. *Clin Orthop* 1992;274: 305–310.

Segregation analysis was done of genetic markers linked to the structural genes encoding types I and II collagen to test these candidate loci in four pedigrees with dominantly inherited adolescent idiopathic scoliosis. The authors present evidence against idiopathic scoliosis generally being caused by mutations in the types I and II collagen genes.

Charry O, Koop S, Winter R, et al: Syringomyelia and scoliosis: A review of twenty-five pediatric patients. *J Pediatr Orthop* 1994;14:309–317.

This is a retrospective review of 25 patients with scoliosis secondary to syringomyelia. Only ten of these patients had abnormal neurologic findings despite large syrinxes.

Dickson RA, Lawton JO, Archer IA, et al: The pathogenesis of idiopathic scoliosis: Biplanar spinal asymmetry. *J Bone Joint Surg* 1984;66B:8–15.

Evidence is presented that when flattening or reversal of normal thoracic kyphosis at the apex of a scoliosis is superimposed during growth, a progressive idiopathic scoliosis results. Clinical, cadaveric, biomechanical, and radiographic material is presented to support this theory of pathogenesis.

Kindsfater K, Lowe T, Lawellin D, et al: Levels of platelet calmodulin for the prediction of progression and severity of adolescent idiopathic scoliosis. *J Bone Joint Surg* 1994;76A:1186–1192.

Calmodulin is a calcium-binding receptor protein that regulates contractile proteins of muscle and platelets. The level of platelet calmodulin may be a useful predictor of curve progression.

Machida M, Dubousset J, Imamura Y, et al: An experimental study in chickens for the pathogenesis of idiopathic scoliosis. *Spine* 1993;18:1609–1615.

A pinealized chicken model is presented. All pinealized chickens developed scoliosis. Only 10% of pinealized chickens who subsequently underwent pineal autografting developed scoliosis. Authors implicate neurotransmitters or neurohormonal systems in this type of experimental scoliosis.

Muhonen MG, Menezes AH, Sawin PD, et al: Scoliosis in pediatric Chiari malformations without myelodysplasia. *J Neurosurg* 1992;77:69–77.

The authors report a prospective study of 11 patients with scoliosis and Chiari malformation (not associated with mmc) treated surgically. All patients under age 10 years had resolution of scoliosis despite preoperative curves of more than 40°. The issue of hydrosyringomyelia and Chiari malformation with reference to presenting symptoms and scoliosis management is discussed.

Schwend RM, Hennrikus W, Hall JE, et al: Childhood scoliosis: Clinical indications for magnetic resonance imaging. *J Bone Joint Surg* 1995; 77A:46–53.

This is a retrospective review of 95 patients who had idiopathic scoliosis and magnetic resonance imaging (MRI). The authors tried to identify any criteria that should be met before these studies are performed and determined primary and secondary indications for MRI.

Nonsurgical Treatment

Drummond D, Ranallo F, Lonstein J, et al: Radiation hazards in scoliosis management. *Spine* 1983;8:741–748.

The authors review risks of radiation in diagnosis and management of scoliosis. Recommendations are given for reducing radiation risks while obtaining necessary diagnostic information.

Green NE: Part-time bracing of adolescent idiopathic scoliosis. *J Bone Joint Surg* 1986;68A:738–742.

This is a 55-month average follow-up of 44 skeletally immature patients treated by 16 hour/day brace wear. The author reports improved compliance and demonstrated that curve progression could be prevented with this program.

Lonstein JE, Winter RB: The Milwaukee brace for the treatment of adolescent idiopathic scoliosis: A review of one thousand and twenty patients. *J Bone Joint Surg* 1994;76A:1207–1221.

The authors review 1,022 patients who had been managed for adolescent idiopathic scoliosis with a Milwaukee brace. The rate of failure for curves between 20° and 39° was lower in the current series of patients who had been managed with the brace than in an earlier series. Authors recommend that immature adolescents who have a curve of more than 25° and a Risser sign of 0 be managed with a brace immediately rather than after progression has been documented.

O'Donnell CS, Bunnell WP, Betz RR, et al: Electrical stimulation in the treatment of idiopathic scoliosis. *Clin Orthop* 1988;229:107–113.

This is a report of 62 patients treated with an electrospinal orthosis and evaluated at average 2.3-year follow-up. Curve progression exceeded the expected risk of curve progression of untreated curves. The results demonstrate that electrical stimulation is unsuccessful in altering the natural history of idiopathic scoliosis

Price CT, Scott DS, Reed FE Jr, et al: Nighttime bracing for adolescent idiopathic scoliosis with the Charleston bending brace: Preliminary report. *Spine* 1990;15:1294–1299.

The authors give preliminary short-term results for the Charleston bending brace worn only at night.

Surgical Treatment

Barrett DS, MacLean JG, Bettany J, et al: Costoplasty in adolescent idiopathic scoliosis: Objective results in 55 patients. *J Bone Joint Surg* 1993;75B:881–885.

The authors report a new classification of rib morphology that helps in planning the site and extent of costoplasty and in predicting the possible correction.

Bridwell KH, Betz R, Capelli AM, et al: Sagittal plane analysis in idiopathic scoliosis patients treated with Cotrel-Dubousset instrumentation. *Spine* 1990;15:921–926.

The authors demonstrate that when crossing the thoracolumbar junction, reversal of rod bend and reversal of hooks on the derotation rod appear to provide the most physiologic sagittal contour.

Bridwell KH, McAllister JW, Betz RR, et al: Coronal decompensation produced by Cotrel-Dubousset "derotation" maneuver for idiopathic right thoracic scoliosis. *Spine* 1991;16:769–777.

This is one of many good articles highlighting problems with posterior derotation systems.

Cotrel Y, Dubousset J, Guillavmat M: New universal instrumentation in spinal surgery. *Clin Orthop* 1988;227:10–23.

The authors describe the instrumentation and principles of application of this system to correct the three-dimensional aspects of spinal deformity.

The authors also present their preliminary results in 250 patients.

Dickson JH: An eleven-year clinical investigation of Harrington instrumentation: A preliminary report on 578 cases. *Clin Orthop* 1973;93: 113–130.

This is a historic overview of the development of Harrington instrumentation, fusion technique, and postoperative regimen. Results of various groups of patients treated during the evolution of techniques and management are presented.

Doubousset J, Herring JA, Shufflebarger H: The crankshaft phenomenon. *J Pediatr Orthop* 1989;9:541–550.

This article demonstrates that continued anterior spinal growth in the face of the tethering effect of a posterior fusion causes the continuing development of deformity in very immature patients.

Harvey CJ Jr, Betz RR, Clements DH, et al: Are there indications for partial rib resection in patients with adolescent idiopathic scoiliosis treated with Cotrel-Dubousset instrumentation? *Spine* 1993;18:1593–1598.

Patients with a rib prominence of more than 15° preoperatively had or should have had a rib resection. Patients with a higher chance of needing rib resection included those with a curve of more than 60°, curve flexibility of less than 20%, a preoperative rib prominence of more than 10°, or intraoperative curve correction of less than 50%.

Jeng CL, Sponseller PD, Tolo VT: Outcome of Wisconsin instrumentation in idiopathic scoliosis: Minimum 5-year follow-up. *Spine* 1993;18: 1584–1590.

The authors report 35 patients with adolescent idiopathic scoliosis with an average 6.3-year follow-up. Thoracic kyphosis was not increased. There was slight lumbar flattening in long fusion. Ninety-two percent had a successful outcome.

King HA, Moe JH, Bradford DS, et al: The selection of fusion levels in thoracic idiopathic scoliosis. *J Bone Joint Surg* 1983;65A:1302–1313.

Patients are analyzed as to the proper selection of fusion levels. The authors discuss the issue of when to fuse a lumbar curve.

LaGrone MO, Bradford DS, Moe JH, et al: Treatment of symptomatic flatback after spinal fusion. *J Bone Joint Surg* 1988;70A:569–580.

This is a classic article on treatment of flatback induced by distraction of the lumbar spine in treating deformity.

Lenke LG, Bridwell KH, Baldus C, et al: Ability of Cotrel-Dubousset instrumentation to preserve distal lumbar motion segments in adolescent idiopathic scoliosis. *J Spinal Disord* 1993;6:339–350.

In patients selected by outlined preoperative criteria, Cotrel-Dubousset instrumentation (versus traditional Harrington instrumentation) allows distal lumbar fusion levels to be saved while maintaining acceptable coronal and sagittal balance.

Lenke LG, Bridwell KH, O'Brien MF, et al: Recognition and treatment of proximal thoracic curve in adolescent idiopathic scoliosis treated with Cotrel-Dubousset instrumentation. *Spine* 1994;19:1589–1597.

This is a retrospective radiographic and clinical review of a consecutive series of patients with adolescent idiopathic scoliosis. The authors determined criteria for when the upper thoracic curve should be instrumented/fused in adolescent idiopathic scoliosis treated with Cotrel-Dubousset instrumentation and assessed the results of surgical treatment.

Lovallo JL, Banta JV, Renshaw TS: Adolescent idiopathic scoliosis treated by Harrington-rod distraction and fusion. *J Bone Joint Surg* 1986;68A:1326–1330.

In a 44-month mean follow-up of 133 surgically treated patients, the authors demonstrated that a single Harrington distraction rod and fusion followed by 6 months in a postoperative cast is a safe and effective treatment for adolescent idiopathic scoliosis. There were no neurologic injuries.

McCall RE, Bronson W: Criteria for selective fusion in idiopathic scoliosis using Cotrel-Dubousset instrumentation. *J Pediatr Orthop* 1992;12:475–479.

The authors evaluated King type II curves treated by selective posterior fusion with Cotrel-Dubousset instrumentation. In lumbar curves of more than 45° associated with a low flexibility index, the King criteria for selective thoracic fusion may not be appropriate.

McMaster MJ: Luque rod instrumentation in the treatment of adolescent idiopathic scoliosis: A comparative study with Harrington instrumentation. *J Bone Joint Surg* 1991;73B;982–989.

This is a study of 152 patients with adolescent idiopathic scoliosis treated by Luque rod instrumentation and early mobilization without external support. This series was compared with a matched group of 156 patients treated by Harrington instrumentation and immobilized in an underarm jacket for 9 months. All the operations in both groups were performed by one surgeon, and the patients were followed up for more than 2 years.

Mielke CH, Lonstein JE, Denis F, et al: Surgical treatment of adolescent idiopathic scoliosis: A comparative analysis. *J Bone Joint Surg* 1989;71A:1170–1177.

This is a detailed review of 352 patients with single right or double thoracic curves undergoing posterior arthrodesis with one of four different instrumentation systems: Harrington distraction rod, Harrington distraction plus compression rod, Harrington distraction and compression rods and a device for transverse traction and Harrington distraction rod with sublaminar wires.

Puno RM, Grossfeld SL, Johnson JR, et al: Cotrel-Dubousset instrumentation in idiopathic scoliosis. *Spine* 1992;17(suppl 8):S258–S262.

The authors present results in 64 patients with types II and III curves. There was no significant relationship between choice of distal fusion level and amount of decompensation, thereby indicating that the use of King's criteria for selection of the fusion levels may not be useful.

Richards BS, Birch JG, Herring JA, et al: Frontal plane and sagittal plane balance following Cotrel-Dubousset instrumentation for idiopathic scoliosis. *Spine* 1989;14:733–737.

The authors evaluated frontal and sagittal plane balance in 53 patients to determine optimum levels for fusion. This is one of several reports that point out problems with postoperative decompensation using the Cotrel-Dubousset instrumentation and demonstrate that the rules for selection of the fusion area outlined by King and associates may not apply when using Cotrel-Dubousset instrumentation.

Richards BS, Herring JA, Johnston CE, et al: Treatment of adolescent idiopathic scoliosis using Texas Scottish Rite Hospital instrumentation. *Spine* 1994;19:1598–1605.

To determine the effectiveness of posterior Texas Scottish Rite Hospital (TSRH) instrumentation for the treatment of adolescent idiopathic scoliosis, 103 patients were studied with a 2-year minimum follow-up. Delayed deep infections developed in ten patients between 11 and 45 months postoperatively. Two patients had pseudarthroses. The authors conclude that frontal and sagittal thoracic curve correction can be satisfactorily obtained using TSRH instrumentation.

Sanders JO, Herring JA, Browne RH: Posterior arthrodesis and instrumentation in the immature (Risser-grade-0) spine in idiopathic scoliosis. *J Bone Joint Surg* 1995;77A:39–45.

Open triradiate cartilages and a younger age at the time of surgery were predictive of the amount of progression as a result of the crankshaft phenomenon.

Tello CA: Harrington instrumentation without arthrodesis and consecutive distraction program for young children with severe spinal deformities: Experience and technical details. *Orthop Clin North Am* 1994;25:333–351.

This review article is based on the author's extensive experience.

Winter RB, Denis F: The King V curve pattern: Its analysis and surgical treatment. *Orthop Clin North Am* 1994;25:353–362.

This is an excellent review article on this topic.

Wood KB, Transfeldt EE, Ogilvie JW, et al: Rotational changes of the vertebral-pelvic axis following Cotrel-Dubousset instrumentation. *Spine* 1991;16(suppl 8):S404–S408.

The authors demonstrate that Cotrel-Dubousset instrumentation does not consistently or predictably derotate the thoracic apex relative to the pelvis, and coronal plane correction may only be apparent, because of transmitted torque and rotation of the entire spinal-pelvic axis.

Juvenile Idiopathic Scoliosis

Figueiredo UM, James JI: Juvenile idiopathic scoliosis. *J Bone Joint Surg* 1981;63B:61–66.

In this review of 98 patients with juvenile idiopathic scoliosis, curve patterns are analyzed and results of treatment by observation, bracing, and surgery are presented.

Tolo VT, Gillespie R: The characteristics of juvenile idiopathic scioliosis and results of its treatment. *J Bone Joint Surg* 1978;60B:181–188.

In this review of 59 patients with juvenile idiopathic scoliosis, the prognostic value of the rib vertebral angle difference is discussed.

Infantile Idiopathic Scoliosis

Ceballos T, Ferrer-Torrelles M, Castillo F, et al: Prognosis in infantile idiopathic scoliosis. *J Bone Joint Surg* 1980;62A:863–875.

This review of 113 patients with infantile scoliosis covers prognosis relative to sex, age at onset, and Mehta angle. Mehta's prognostic criteria are confirmed.

Mehta MH, Morel G: The nonoperative treatment of infanile idiopathic scoliosis, in Zorab PA, Siegler D (eds): *Scoliosis 1979*. London, England, Academic Press, 1980, pp 71–84.

This summary article covers the approach to the patient with infantile scoliosis and the results of nonsurgical treatment.

Congenital Scoliosis and Kyphosis

General

McMaster MJ: Occult intraspinal anomalies and congenital scoliosis. *J Bone Joint Surg* 1984;66A:588–601.

This is an excellent review of the incidence and pathology of occult intraspinal congenital abnormalities associated with congenital scoliosis. Of the 251 patients with congenital scoliosis in this series, 18% had occult intraspinal abnormalities. Diastematomyelia was the most common lesion and was most commonly associated with unilateral unsegmented bars with contralateral hemivertebrae in the lower thoracic or thoracolumbar region.

McMaster MJ, David CV: Hemivertebrae as a cause of scoliosis: A review of 104 patients. *J Bone Joint Surg* 1986;68B:588–595.

This is a review of the natural history of 154 hemivertebrae (65% fully segmented and nonincarcerated, 22% semisegmented, and 12% incarcerated) in 104 patients. Risk factors include type of hemivertebrae, location, age of patient, and number of hemivertebrae and their relationship to each other. Fully segmented, nonincarcerated hemivertebrae may require prophylactic treatment to prevent significant deformity, while semisegmented and incarcerated hemivertebrae usually do not require treatment.

Miller A, Guille JT, Bowen JR: Evaluation and treatment of diastematomyelia. *J Bone Joint Surg* 1993;75A:1308–1317.

The authors reviewed the results for 43 patients who had diastematomyelia. All of the patients had been skeletally immature when the diagnosis was made, the mean age being 6 years. They recommend resection of the spur in patients who have progressive neurologic manifestations. Patients who do not have progressive neurologic manifestations should be observed; if progression is noted, a resection should then be performed.

Winter RB (ed): *Congenital Deformities of the Spine*. New York, NY, Thieme-Stratton, 1983.

This comprehensive look at all aspects of congenital spinal deformities is based on the author's extensive experience.

Natural History

McMaster MJ, Ohtsuka K: The natural history of congenital scoliosis: A study of 251 patients. *J Bone Joint Surg* 1982;64A:1128–1147.

In this review of the natural history of 251 patients with congenital scoliosis, abnormalities are classified as regards prognosis for each pattern and curve location.

Nasca RJ, Stelling FH III, Steel HH: Progression of congenital scoliosis due to hemivertebrae and hemivertebrae with bars. *J Bone Joint Surg* 1975;57A:456–466.

The authors classify 60 cases of congenital scoliosis and kyphoscoliosis due to hemivertebrae or unilateral bar associated with hemivertebrae into six types; prognostic factors include location of hemivertebrae and presence of unilateral bars. Rates of progression are discussed.

Winter RB, Moe JH, Eilers VE: Congenital scoliosis: A study of 234 patients treated and untreated. *J Bone Joint Surg* 1968;50A:1–47.

This is a natural history and treatment study of a large group of patients with congenital scoliosis. Indications for treatment are based on the natural history of the pathologic lesion and its location in the spine.

Etiology

Ehrenhaft JL: Development of the vertebral column as related to certain congenital and pathological changes. *Surg Gynecol Obstet* 1943;76:282–292.

This is a classic embryologic study on spinal development.

Morin B, Poitras B, Duhaime M, et al: Congenital kyphosis by segmentation defect: Etiologic and pathogenic studies. *J Pediatr Orthop* 1985;5:309–314.

The authors present clinical and research evidence to support the theory that kyphosis resulting from segmentation defect represents a developmetal defect of the perivertebral structures, including the annulus fibrosus, the ring apophysis, and the anterior longitudinal ligament, rather than an intervertebral bar.

Rivard C, Narbaitz R, Uhtoff H: Congenital vertebral malformations: Time of induction in human and mouse embryos. *Orthop Rev* 1979;8:135.

The authors present experimental evidence for the role of hypoxia in etiology of congenital spinal deformities.

Tsou PM, Yau A, Hodgson AR: Embryogenesis and prenatal development of congenital vertebral anomalies and their classification. *Clin Orthop* 1980;152:211–231.

Anomalies in 144 patients are reviewed and 15 embryos and fetuses evaluated. Classification of anomalies is based on specific defects, pathogenesis, and time of origin in embryonetic or fetal development.

Treatment

Holte DC, Winter RB, Lonstein JE, et al: Excision of hemivertebrae and wedge resection in the treatment of congenital scoliosis. *J Bone Joint Surg* 1995;77A:159–171.

The authors present a retrospective review of 37 patients treated by anterior and posterior excision or wedge resection of a hemivertebrae and arthrodesis of the spine. The authors discuss the degree of correction obtained and maintained, the balance and alignment of the trunk, change in pelvic obliquity, and associated complications.

Keller PM, Lindseth RE, DeRosa GP: Progressive congenital scoliosis treatment using a transpedicular anterior and posterior convex hemiepiphysiodesis and hemiarthrodesis: A preliminary report. *Spine* 1994; 19:1933–1939.

The authors present a series of patients treated with a transpedicular anterior and posterior convex hemiepiphysiodesis and hemiarthrodesis for progressive congenital scoliosis. The average follow-up period was 4.8 years. This procedure appears to be most effective in arresting growth in the young patient who has an isolated hemivertebrae and no excessive kyphosis. The epiphysiodesis effect is less predictable.

Winter RB, Moe JH: The results of spinal arthrodesis for congenital spine deformity in patients younger than five years old. *J Bone Joint Surg* 1982;64A:419–432.

In this follow-up review of 49 patients treated surgically at less than 5 years of age, the role for early posterior fusion is outlined.

Winter RB, Moe JH, Lonstein JE: The surgical treatment of congenital kyphosis: A review of 94 patients age 5 years or older with 2 years or more follow-up in 77 patients. *Spine* 1985;10:224–231.

This is a 7-year average follow-up of 94 patients with congenital kyphosis (27 were treated by posterior fusion alone and 48 were treated by combined anterior and posterior fusion). Curve correction and maintenance were better in the combined group; pseudarthroses occurred in 31% of the posterior fusions alone compared to 8% of the combined group. Posterior fusion alone may have limited value in children and adolescents with kyphosis less than 55°.

Winter RB, Moe JH, Lonstein JE: Posterior spinal arthrodesis for congenital scoliosis: An analysis of the cases of two hundred and ninety patients, five to nineteen years old. *J Bone Joint Surg* 1984;66A:1188–1197.

This is a 6-year follow-up of 290 patients between the ages of 5 and 19 years treated by posterior spinal arthrodesis with or without Harrington instrumentation. The authors report that the most common problem was bending of the fusion mass, occurring in 40 patients (14%). Use of distraction instrumentation gave only slightly better correction but was associated with the only case of paraplegia. Bending of the fusion is probably a function of growth discrepancy between the concave and convex sides.

Scheuermann's Disease and Postural Roundback

Blumenthal SL, Roach J, Herring JA: Lumbar Scheuermann's: A clinical series and classification. *Spine* 1987;12:929–932.

The authors present 13 cases of lumbar Scheuermann's disease (T10–L4). Six patients had classic changes (Sorenson criteria) with only one having back pain. Six patients had atypical changes of end plate irregularity, anterior Schmorl's node, and disk space narrowing, and all had back pain. Based on these findings the authors propose a new classification for lumbar Scheuermann's disease.

Bradford DS, Ahmed KB, Moe JH, et al: The surgical management of patients with Scheuermann's disease: A review of twenty-four cases managed by combined anterior and posterior spine fusion. *J Bone Joint Surg* 1980;62A:705–712.

Results of combined anterior and posterior surgery in 24 patients are reported. Complications and pitfalls in treatment are discussed.

Farsetti P, Tudisco C, Caterini R, et al: Juvenile and idiopathic kyphosis: Long-term follow-up of 20 cases. *Arch Orthop Trauma Surg* 1991;110: 165–168.

Twelve patients with juvenile kyphosis and eight with idiopathic kyphosis were reviewed at an average follow-up of 19 years. At follow-up, all patients had lost the correction obtained, and the curves had become worse than originally, those in idiopathic kyphosis more so than those in juvenile kyphosis. Despite the increase in their angular deformity, all the patients managed well and only two complained of distressing back pain.

Ippolito E, Bellocci M, Montanaro A, et al: Juvenile kyphosis: An ultrastructural study. *J Pediatr Orthop* 1985;5:315–322.

Histologic and histochemical studies of the intervertebral disk, vertebral plate, physis, and part of the vertebral body in seven patients are presented. The paper confirms the previously presented findings of the author based on a single case.

Lowe TG, Kasten MD: An analysis of sagittal curves and balance after Cotrel-Dubousset instrumentation for kyphosis secondary to Scheuermann's disease: A review of 32 patients. *Spine* 1994;19: 1680–1685.

In this study preoperative and postoperative saggittal curves and spinal balance were compared in patients undergoing spinal fusion with Cotrel-Dubousset instrumentation for severe kyphosis secondary to Scheuermann's disease. This procedure appeared to yield good results when proper levels of fusion were selected and correction of more than 50% was not attempted.

Mandell GA, Morales RW, Harcke HT, et al: Bone scintigraphy in patients with atypical lumbar Scheuermann disease. *J Pediatr Orthop* 1993;13: 622–627.

During an 8-year period, 14 patients who presented with radiographic change suggestive of atypical lumbar Scheuermann's disease (ALSD) involving one or more vertebral levels and low-back pain symptoms were referred for bone scintigraphy. The authors report that these scintigraphic findings should be distinguished from the more intense radiotracer uptake patterns of infection and trauma.

Montgomery SP, Erwin WE: Scheuermann's kyphosis: Long-term results of Milwaukee brace treatment. *Spine* 1981;6:5–8.

Correction of curvature is demonstrated in this follow-up study of 39 patients. However, later follow-up at 15 months out of brace shows relapse, indicating that lasting results require brace treatment for longer than 18 months.

Murray PM, Weinstein SL, Spratt KF: The natural history and long-term follow-up of Scheuermann kyphosis. *J Bone Joint Surg* 1993;75A: 236–248.

Sixty-seven patients with a mean Scheuermann's kyphosis of 71° were followed up for an average of 32 years after diagnosis. The authors present detailed analysis of questionnaire, physical examination, pulmonary function testing, and radiographs to provide the reader with the "natural history" of this condition.

Sachs B, Bradford D, Winter R, et al: Scheuermann kyphosis: Follow-up of Milwaukee brace treatment. *J Bone Joint Surg* 1987;69A:50–57.

In this long-term follow-up (at least 5 years) of 120 patients treated for Scheuermann's disease with a Milwaukee brace, the authors found the Milwaukee brace to be an effective method of treatment for patients with Scheuermann's kyphosis, with 69% of patients showing improvement. However, with an initial kyphosis of more than 74°, a higher percentage of unsatisfactory results were seen.

Stagnara P, deMauroy JC, Dran G, et al: Reciprocal angulation of vertebral bodies in the sagittal plane: Approach to references for the evaluation of kyphosis and lordosis. *Spine* 1982;7:335–342.

The authors discuss values, based on radiographs in 100 patients, of normal thoracic kyphosis and lumbar lordosis.

Miscellaneous Spine Deformities

Cerebral Palsy and Neuromuscular Scoliosis

Boachie-Adjei O, Lonstein JE, Winter RB, et al: Management of neuromuscular spinal deformities with Luque segmental instrumentation. *J Bone Joint Surg* 1989;71A:548–562.

The authors report an average 3-year follow-up of 46 patients with neuromuscular scoliosis; 22 of the 46 patients (48%) had cerebral palsy. The authors discuss the indications for surgery, the need for pelvic extension of the instrumentation and fusion, the role of postoperative immobilization, the role of two-stage procedures, and complications in this most difficult group of patients.

Broom MJ, Banta JV, Renshaw TS: Spinal fusion augmented by Luque-rod segmental instrumentation for neuromuscular scoliosis. *J Bone Joint Surg* 1989;71A:32–44.

Although fewer than half of the patients in the series had cerebral palsy, this diagnosis accounted for the largest group in the paper. With a mean follow-up of 42 months, the authors demonstrate that Luque rod segmental instrumentation with posterior spinal instrumentation is an effective treatment for patients with neuromuscular scoliosis. Failure rates were higher when 3/16th-inch rods were used, and functional kyphosis occurred above the fusion when it did not extend to the upper thoracic spine.

Cassidy C, Craig CL, Perry A, et al: A reassessment of spinal stabilization in severe cerebral palsy. *J Pediatr Orthop* 1994;14:731–739.

Through a prospective care-burden study, a 34-month retrospective analysis, and a healthcare questionnaire, 17 institutionalized fused patients with a mean current scoliosis of 35° were compared with 20 nonfused patients with a mean scoliosis of 76°. No clinically significant differences were noted in pain or pulmonary medical utilization or therapy, decubiti, function, or time for daily care. Nevertheless, the majority of healthcare workers believed that the fused patients were more comfortable.

Gau YL, Lonstein JE, Winter RB, et al: Luque-Galveston procedure for correction and stabilization of neuromuscular scoliosis and pelvic obliquity: A review of 68 patients. *J Spinal Disord* 1991;4:399–410.

The minimum follow-up was 4 years. Diagnoses included cerebral palsy in 34 patients and other neuromuscular diseases in another 34 patients. The average age was 14. Twenty patients also had anterior spine fusion without instrumentation. Although the complication rate was 62%, most were minor. Instrumentation problems occurred in 14 patients (21%), four of which involved broken rods. Pseudarthoses occurred in seven patients (10%). Twenty-six patients had a "windshield wiper" sign at follow-up, and this group had a higher percentage of complications, but the existence of this sign did not necessarily indicate a problem.

Gersoff WK, Renshaw TS: The treatment of scoliosis in cerebral palsy by posterior spinal fusion with Luque-rod segmental instrumentation. *J Bone Joint Surg* 1988;70A:41–44.

This is a review of 33 patients with cerebral palsy who underwent posterior spinal fusion and Luque rod instrumentation at a mean follow-up of 40 months. Luque rodding accompanying posterior spinal fusion allows safe correction of the deformity, maintenance of correction, and achievement of a solid spinal fusion with minimal complications.

Shufflebarger HL, Grim JO, Bui V, et al: Anterior and posterior spinal fusion: Staged versus same day surgery. *Spine* 1991;16:930–933.

The authors present evidence to support same day surgery versus staged procedures when anterior and posterior surgical procedures are indicated.

Postlaminectomy Spinal Deformity

Dietrich U, Schirmer M, Veltrup K, et al: Postlaminectomy kyphosis and scoliosis in children with spinal tumors. *Neurol Orthop* 1989;7:36–42.

Nineteen of 22 patients treated by laminectomy in infancy and childhood for spinal tumors developed spinal deformity. Kyphosis developed in 14 patients and scoliosis in 15. The incidence of kyphosis depended on the site of laminectomy and was highest in the cervical spine and lowest in the lumbar spine. Resection of facet joints increased the risk of spinal deformity. Careful follow-up and early treatment is indicated for these patients.

Lonstein JE: Post-laminectomy kyphosis. *Clin Orthop* 1977;128:93–100.

This excellent review article covers all aspects of postlaminectomy kyphotic deformity and emphasizes the importance of facet joint integrity.

Yasuoka S, Peterson HA, McCarty CS: The incidence of spinal deformity and instability after multiple level laminectomy: Its difference in children and adults. *Orthop Trans* 1981;5:11.

The authors discuss the problem of postlaminectomy spinal deformity in a review of 58 patients.

Skeletal Dysplasia

Bethem D, Winter RB, Lutter L, et al: Spinal disorders of dwarfism: Review of the literature and report of eighty cases. *J Bone Joint Surg* 1981;63A;1412–1425.

In this review of spinal deformities in patients with osteochondrodystrophies, the authors discuss diagnosis and management.

Herniated Nucleus Pulposus

DeLuca PF, Mason DE, Weiand R, et al: Excision of herniated nucleus pulposus in children and adolescents. *J Pediatr Orthop* 1994;14:318–322.

Forty-eight patients underwent diskectomy at a mean age of 16 years. Thirteen patients at an average age of 15 who had radiographic documentation of disk disease were treated nonsurgically. The authors rated the results of surgery as excellent or good in 91% of the patients, and poor in 9% at follow-up, while only 25% of the nonsurgical group showed excellent or good results.

Savini R, Martucci E, Nardi S, et al: The herniated lumbar intervertebral disc in children and adolescents: Long-term follow-up of 101 cases treated by surgery. *Ital J Orthop Trauma* 1991;17:505–511.

The authors report that in all patients diagnosed correctly with the aid of appropriate imaging studies, diskectomy by conservative hemilaminectomy achieved satisfactory results, except in two patients with concomitant spinal instability due to spondylolysis and in one with recurrence.

Spondylolysis and Spondylolisthesis

Boxall D, Bradford DS, Winter RB, et al: Management of severe spondylolisthesis in children and adolescents. *J Bone Joint Surg* 1979;61A:479–495.

This is a review of 43 patients with 50% or greater slips. The authors discuss the importance of slip angle in addition to percent slip. The results of fusion are presented.

Bradford DS: Closed reduction of spondylolisthesis: An experience in 22 patients. *Spine* 1988;13:580–587.

This is a review of 22 patients with spondylolisthesis treated by closed reduction and posterolateral arthrodesis and followed up for an average of 40 months. The author discusses methods, results, complications, and indications.

Fredrickson BE, Baker D, McHolick WJ, et al: The natural history of spondylolysis and spondylolisthesis. *J Bone Joint Surg* 1984;66A:699–707.

This is a prospective study of 500 unselected first grade children (1955 to 1957) and their families, discussing incidence, relationship of listhesis to lysis, and etiology.

Freeman BL III, Donati NL: Spinal arthrodesis for severe spondylolisthesis in children and adolescents: A long-term follow-up study. *J Bone Joint Surg* 1989;71A:594–598.

This 12-year follow-up of 12 patients with grade III or IV spondylolisthesis demonstrated that posterior in situ arthrodesis is effective, reliable, and safe for treatment of severe spondylolisthesis.

Frennered AK, Danielson BI, Nachemson AL: Natural history of symptomatic isthmic low-grade spondylolisthesis in children and adolescents: A seven-year follow-up study. *J Pediatr Orthop* 1991;11:209–213.

Of 47 patients followed up for an average of 7 years, two (4%) had a progression of slip and 30% required surgery after an average of 3.7 years. Of the nonsurgically treated patients, 83% were rated excellent or good at follow-up. They found no factors that were prognostic of slip progression or that indicated the need for future surgery.

Harris IE, Weinstein SL: Long term follow-up of patients with grade III and IV spondylolisthesis: Treatment with and without posterior fusion. *J Bone Joint Surg* 1987;69A:960–969.

An 18-year follow-up of 11 patients with grade III and IV spondylolisthesis treated nonsurgically is compared to a 24-year follow-up of 21 surgically treated patients. The surgical group were less symptomatic and were less restricted in their activity than the nonsurgical group. In situ fusion gave good functional long-term results in grade III and IV spondylolisthesis.

Hensinger RN: Spondylolysis and spondylolisthesis in children and adolescents. *J Bone Joint Surg* 1989;71A:1098–1107.

This excellent review article covers all aspects of the topic and has an extensive bibliography.

Ishikawa S, Kumar SJ, Torres BC: Surgical treatment of dysplastic spondylolisthesis: Results after in situ fusion. *Spine* 1994;19:1691–1696.

Fourteen patients with symptomatic dysplastic spondylolisthesis with an intact pars interarticularis underwent posterolateral spinal fusion. The authors report all had a solid fusion at follow-up. A pseudarthrosis in one patient healed after a second operation.

Nicol RO, Scott JH: Lytic spondylolysis: Repair by wiring. *Spine* 1986;11:1027–1030.

This is a description of technique and early results with a technique of defect repair without facet joint sacrifice.

Pizzutillo PD, Hummer CD III: Non-operative treatment for painful adolescent spondylolysis or spondylolisthesis. *J Pediatr Orthop* 1989;9: 538–540.

The authors report symptomatic relief of pain in two thirds of patients with spondylolysis and grade I and II spondylolisthesis treated nonsurgically. Adolescents with symptomatic grade III and IV spondylolisthesis are more appropriately treated surgically.

Read MT: Single photon emission computed tomography (SPECT) scanning for adolescent back pain: A sine qua non? *Br J Sports Med* 1994; 28:56–57.

The authors argue that because management of spondylolysis differs from that of other lumbar dysfunction, SPECT scanning in children should be a sine qua non in extension-related back pain with a normal radiograph and planar bone scintigraphy.

Saraste H: Long-term clinical and radiological follow-up of spondylolysis and spondylolisthesis. *J Pediatr Orthop* 1987;7:631–638.

In this long-term (mean 29 years) clinical and radiographic follow-up of 255 patients with spondylolisthesis and spondylolysis (13% were less than 15 years of age at diagnosis), 70% of patients had been treated for low back symptoms.

Schwend RM, Waters PM, Hey LA, et al: Treatment of severe spondylolisthesis in children by reduction and L4-S4 posterior segmental hyperextension fixation. *J Pediatr Orthop* 1992;12:703–711.

Twenty children with severe lumbosacral sponylolisthesis underwent reduction, posterolateral fusion, and posterior fixation with an L4 to S2, S3, and S4 sublaminar wired rectangular rod to lessen lumbosacral kyphosis, allow early ambulation, and maintain correction. All patients reportedly had solid fusions and no progression at 43-month follow-up.

Seitsalo S, Osterman K, Hyvarinen H, et al: Progression of spondylolisthesis in children and adolescents: A long-term follow-up of 272 patients. *Spine* 1991;16:417–421.

The authors found the only radiologic parameter predictive of progression was the percentage amount of the original slip.

Seitsalo S, Osterman K, Poussa M, et al: Spondylolisthesis in children under 12 years of age: Long-term results of 56 patients treated conservatively or operatively. *J Pediatr Orthop* 1988;8:516–521.

This is a review of 32 surgically-treated and 24 nonsurgically-treated patients with spondylolisthesis. Risk factors include female sex and dysplastic olisthesis. Lumbosacral fusions in situ give good results long term (average follow-up 14.5 years) despite 16% nonunions and 19% postoperative slip progression.

Spinal Cord Monitoring

Ashkenaze D, Mudiyam R, Boachie-Adjei O, et al: Efficacy of spinal cord monitoring in neuromuscular scoliosis. *Spine* 1993;18:1627–1633.

The authors report somatosensory cortical evoked potentials are unreliable and nonspecific in neuromuscular scoliosis surgery and are not efficacious in preventing or detecting spinal cord injury when used alone, and they recommend that adjunctive techniques using epidural and motor-evoked potentials must be studied in these patients.

Forbes HJ, Allen PW, Waller CS, et al: Spinal cord monitoring in scoliosis surgery: Experience with 1168 cases. *J Bone Joint Surg* 1991;73B:487–491.

The authors present electrophysiologic monitoring of the spinal cord by the epidural measurement of somatosensory-evoked potentials (SSEPs) in response to stimulation of the posterior tibial nerve in 1,168 consecutive patients.

Loder RT, Thomson GJ, LaMont RL: Spinal cord monitoring in patients with nonidiopathic spinal deformities using somatosensory evoked potentials. *Spine* 1991;16:1359–1364.

The authors state that the predictive accuracy of intraoperative spinal cord monitoring in this patient population is not high, but the sensitivity to potentially harmful surgical events is high.

Nash CL Jr, Brown RH: Spinal cord monitoring. *J Bone Joint Surg* 1989;71A:627–630.

This good review article outlines the various types of spinal cord monitoring currently in use and their advantages and disadvantages.

Miscellaneous

Jackson RP, McManus AC: The iliac buttress: A computed tomographic study of sacral anatomy. *Spine* 1993;18:1318–1328.

This anatomic study documents a possible point of sacral fixation (lateral sacral masses) to help resist flexural loads.

Kawakami N, Winter RB, Lonstein JE, et al: Scoliosis secondary to rib resection. *J Spinal Disord* 1994;7:522–527.

The authors describe 11 patients with scoliosis after multiple rib resections. The convexity is toward the side of resection and progression relates to younger age at resection.

Sacral Agenesis

Phillips WA, Cooperman DR, Lindquist TC, et al: Orthopaedic management of lumbosacral agenesis: Long-term follow-up. *J Bone Joint Surg* 1982;64A:1282–1294.

This is a review of orthopaedic problems and management of 22 patients.

Renshaw TS: Sacral agenesis: A classification and review of twenty-three cases. *J Bone Joint Surg* 1978;60A:373–383.

This review of 23 patients at Newington Children's Hospital provides a practical classification system and discussion of management.

Section 6

Upper Extremity Deformities

Peter Waters, MD

Shoulder

Congenital Pseudarthrosis of the Clavicle

Grogan D, Love S, Guidera K, et al: Operative treatment of congenital pseudarthrosis of the clavicle. *J Pediatr Orthop* 1991;11:176–180.

The authors describe surgical treatment of eight patients with a surgical technique that provided careful preservation of the periosteum, resection of the pseudarthrosis, approximation of the freshened ends of the clavicle with a suture, use of the resected bone as morselized graft, and repair of the periosteum. Six of the eight patients were less than 29 months of age. All healed by 8 weeks with no recurrence.

Lloyd-Roberts G, Apley A, Owen R: Reflections upon the aetiology of congenital pseudarthrosis of the clavicle: With a note on cranio-cleido dysostosis. *J Bone Joint Surg* 1975;57B:24–29.

The authors propose that congenital pseudarthrosis of the clavicle is secondary to pressure on the developing clavicle from the subclavian artery. They cite this as the reason for the predominant right-sided lesion and the presence of a left-sided lesion in dextrocardia.

Schnall S, King J, Marrero G: Congenital pseudarthrosis of the clavicle: A review of the literature and surgical results of six cases. *J Pediatr Orthop* 1988;8:316–321.

Six patients were treated with resection of the pseudarthrosis, bone grafting, and internal fixation with plating. All patients were older than 4 years and symptomatic. All healed between 3 and 6 months after surgery.

Cleidocranial Dysplasia

Brueton L, Reeve A, Ellis R, et al: Apparent cleidocranial dysplasia associated with abnormalities of 8q22 in three individuals. *Am J Med Genet* 1992;43:612–618.

The authors review the clinical manifestations of this autosomal dominant disorder including frontal and parietal bossing, short stature, delayed eruption of the teeth, failure of midline ossification with a persistent open anterior fontanelle and aplasia or hypoplasia of the clavicles, and multiple wormian bones. They describe three individuals with manifestations of cleidocranial dysplasia with rearrangements of the 8q22 chromosome.

Sprengel's Deformity

Borgs JLP, Shah A, Tores BC, et al: Modified Woodward procedure for Sprengel deformity of the shoulder: Long-term results. *J Pediatr Orthop* 1996;16:508–515.

In 15 patients, shoulder abduction was improved from an average of 115° to an average of 150°. All patients except one had marked improvement in appearance, and 86% were satisfied with their results

Carson WG, Lovell WW, Whitesides TE Jr: Congenital elevation of the scapula: Surgical correction by the Woodward procedure. *J Bone Joint Surg* 1981;63A:1199–1207.

The authors discuss characteristic clinical findings, associated congenital anomalies, indications for operation, and surgical technique of the Woodward procedure, including the importance of a clavicular osteotomy. They stress the importance of the rotational component of Sprengel deformity. The results of 11 patients and 13 Woodward procedures (two bilateral) are reported. Nine of 11 patients achieved excellent or good cosmetic improvement. The mean improvement in shoulder abduction was 29° (range zero to 60°).

Greitemann B, Rondhuis JJ, Karbowski A: Treatment of congenital elevation of the scapula: Ten (2-18) year follow-up of 37 cases of Sprengel's deformity. *Acta Orthop Scand* 1993;64:365–368.

The authors describe 37 patients with Sprengel's deformity, 23 of whom had surgery. Long-term functional deficits were related to limited shoulder abduction. Resection of the superior angle of the scapula for cosmetic deformity and a Woodward procedure for patients with impaired function are recommended.

Leibovic S, Ehrlich M, Zaleske D: Sprengel deformity. *J Bone Joint Surg* 1990;72A:192–197.

Eighteen patients with Sprengel's deformity were treated with a modification of the Green procedure. In 11 of 15 patients available for follow-up, appearance improved moderately or dramatically, and abduction increased an average of 57°. The malrotation of the scapula was corrected initially but usually recurred after 2 years; this did not compromise the increase in abduction. The authors describe a useful radiographic method for measuring scapular rotation and elevation.

Woodward JW: Congenital elevation of the scapula: Correction by release and transplantation of muscle origins. A preliminary report. *J Bone Joint Surg* 1961;43A:219–228.

This original description of Woodward's surgical procedure to correct congenital elevation of the scapula (Sprengel's deformity) describes the results in nine patients. There was improvement in cosmesis and shoulder abduction ranging from 20° to 70° in those with limited function postoperatively. Brachial plexus palsy that developed postoperatively in one patient resolved over 6 months.

Obstetric Brachial Plexopathy

Goddard NJ, Fixsen J: Rotation osteotomy of the humerus for birth injuries of the brachial plexus. *J Bone Joint Surg* 1984;66B:257–259.

The authors present results of ten derotation osteotomies in patients with internal rotation contractures and functional disability. The surgical technique is outlined. It is best indicated for patients with an abnormal glenohumeral joint and functional loss of external rotation.

Hentz V, Meyer R: Brachial plexus microsurgery in children. *Microsurgery* 1991;12:175–185.

This is a thorough summary of the results of both spontaneous recovery and microsurgical reconstruction in obstetrical brachial plexopathy. It outlines the rationale for microsurgery, defines the pathologic anatomy of upper trunk rupture outside of the spinal cord and lower root avulsion, and describes intra- and postoperative management.

Hoffer MM, Wickenden R, Roper B: Brachial plexus birth palsies: Results of tendon transfers to the rotator cuff. *J Bone Joint Surg* 1978;60A:691–695.

This is a description of latissimus dorsi and teres major tendon transfer to correct internal rotation contracture and to provide external rotation and forward flexion active use.

Michelow B, Clarke H, Curtis C, et al: The natural history of obstetrical brachial plexus palsy. *Plast Reconstr Surg* 1994;93:675–680.

Sixty-six infants with upper trunk involvement (42%) or total plexopathy (58%) were in the study group. The presence of elbow flexion at 3 months was an accurate predictor of good recovery at 12 months in all but 12.8% of the infants. When combined with the presence of elbow, wrist, thumb, and finger extension, the rate of inaccurate prediction dropped to 5.2%.

Elbow and Forearm

Radioulnar Synostosis

Lin HH, Strecker WB, Manske PR, et al: A surgical technique of radioulnar osteoclasis to correct severe forearm rotation deformities. *J Pediatr Orthop* 1995;15:53–58.

Osteoclasis of 26 forearms with marked pronation or supination deformities resulted in an arc of motion in a more functional hand position, although range of motion was not significantly changed. Functional improvement was obtained in 25.

Ogino T, Hikino K: Congenital radio-ulnar synostosis: Compensatory rotation around the wrist and rotation osteotomy. *J Hand Surg* 1987;12B:173–178.

This paper describes the clinical features in 40 patients with radioulnar synostosis. The authors define compensatory wrist rotation (average 119°) and provide a method for planning the derotation osteotomy, taking into account the compensatory wrist rotation in each patient.

Simmons B, Southmayd W, Riseborough E: Congenital radioulnar synostosis. *J Hand Surg* 1983;8:829–838.

The authors review the results of derotation osteotomy in 20 patients. They cite a complication rate of 36%, mainly loss of correction in a cast and neurovascular compromise, and they recommend the use of percutaneous fixation to prevent loss of correction and to allow for easy derotation in the presence of a compartment syndrome.

Congenital Radial Head Dislocation

Agnew DK, Davis RJ: Congenital unilateral dislocation of the radial head. *J Pediatr Orthop* 1993;13:526–528.

The identification of unilateral dislocations in 6 patients confirms the existence of this entity.

Bell S, Morrey B, Bianco A: Chronic posterior subluxation and dislocation of the radial head. *J Bone Joint Surg* 1991;73A:392–396.

This article covers classification of three types of congenital subluxation or dislocation. Type I (subluxation) was most likely to cause pain, clicking, and late degenerative arthritis. Loss of rotation was the most significant functional problem. Prominence of the radial head was a cosmetic problem and was considered an indication for excision.

Campbell C, Waters P, Emans J: Excision of the radial head for congenital dislocation. *J Bone Joint Surg* 1992;74A:726–733.

Eight radial heads in six patients were excised because of congenital dislocation with persistent elbow pain or recurrent loose osteochondral fragments. Forearm rotation improved an average 53° and elbow pain was decreased. There was associated minor wrist pain. There were no significant complications at an average follow-up of 7 years.

Congenital Pseudarthrosis of the Forearm

Bell D: Congenital forearm pseudarthrosis: Report of six cases and review of the literature *J Pediatr Orthop* 1989;9:438–443.

The author reviews the characteristics of 27 patients described in the literature and reports six additional patients. Conventional bone grafting was successful in only 35% of 20 patients reported in the literature and in one of three patients reported by the author. Union was obtained in two patients with vascularized fibular grafting.

Mathoulin C, Gilbert A, Azze R: Congenital pseudarthrosis of the forearm: Treatment of six cases with vascularized fibular graft and review of the literature. *Microsurgery* 1993;14:252–259.

Wide resection of the pseudarthrosis and free vascularized fibular grafts were used for the treatment of six children with congenital pseudarthrosis of the forearm, five of whom had neurofibromatosis. In two of the four children with pseudarthroses of both the radius and ulna, a one-bone forearm was created. All pseudarthroses healed with moderate forearm shortening. Tibial corticoperiosteal flaps used to reconstruct the fibula reportedly prevented valgus deformity at the ankle.

Wrist

Radial Club Hand

Buck-Gramcko D: Radialization as a new treatment for radial club hand. *J Hand Surg* 1985;10A:964–968.

This now is a classic description of dynamic rebalancing of the hand on the distal ulna without carpal resection.

Lamb D: Radial club hand: A continuing study of sixty-eight patients with one hundred and seventeen club hands. *J Bone Joint Surg* 1977;59A:1–13.

This is a classic description of the technique of centralization of the carpus on the ulna, including carpal resection and ulnar osteotomy as necessary.

Urban M, Osterman AL: Management of radial dysplasia. *Hand Clin* 1990;6:589–605.

This is a comprehensive review of the classification, associated anomalies, and surgical treatment of radial dysplasia. It includes a thorough review of the literature and complete bibliography.

Ulnar Club Hand

Broudy A, Smith R: Deformities of the hand and wrist with ulnar deficiency. *J Hand Surg* 1979;4:304–315.

This classic review includes description of the hand, wrist, and elbow deformities as well as the results of surgical treatment.

Madelung's Deformity

Ranawat C, DeFiore J, Straub L: Madelung's deformity: An end result study of surgical treatment. *J Bone Joint Surg* 1975;57:772–780.

The authors describe typical deformities of the forearm and wrist and outline wrist realignment by corrective osteotomies, including ulnar shortening and radial closing wedge osteotomy.

Hand

Polydactyly

Simmons B: Polydactyly. *Hand Clin* 1985;1:545–565.

This is a summary of the incidence, classification, associated anomalies, and treatment of polydactyly.

Syndactyly

Eaton C, Lister G: Syndactyly. *Hand Clin* 1990;6:555–575.

This is a comprehensive review of the incidence, pathologic anatomy, principles of surgical reconstruction, and complications of syndactyly. It includes a section on difficult problems.

Lundkvist L, Barfred T: A double pulp technique for creating nail-folds in syndactyly release. *J Hand Surg* 1991;16B:32–34.

The authors describe improved nail folds and epinychia by reconstruction with pulp flaps in complete and complex syndactylies.

Sommerkamp T, Ezaki M, Carter P, et al: The pulp plasty: A composite graft for complete syndactyly fingertip separations. *J Hand Surg* 1992;17A:15–20.

Composite skin and subcutaneous tissue grafts from glabrous areas of the foot were used in complex syndactyly reconstruction to reconstitute an epinychium. Patient satisfaction was high.

van der Biezen J, Bloem JJ: Dividing the fingers in congenital syndactyly release: A review of more than 200 years of surgical experience. *Ann Plast Surg* 1994;3:225–230.

This is a historic review of the techniques of syndactyly release with illustrations of the multiple options for Z-plasties and web space flaps.

Camptodactyly

Benson LS, Waters PM, Kamil NI, et al: Camptodactyly: Classification and results of nonoperative treatment. *J Pediatr Orthop* 1994;14:814–819.

Splinting and occupational therapy are recommended for types I, II, and III camptodactyly, with operative treatment reserved for patients in whom nonoperative management is unsuccessful.

Cleft Hand

Ogino T: Cleft hand. *Hand Clin* 1990;6:661–671.

This is a summary article on the classification, incidence, and surgical options in this difficult problem. It presents the author's method of flaps but does not include the more classic options for reconstruction.

Constriction Band Syndrome

Foulkes G, Reinker K: Congenital constriction band syndrome: A seventy-year experience. *J Pediatr Orthop* 1994;14:242–248.

This is a review of 71 patients, 60% of whom had abnormal gestational histories. The distal, central digits of the upper extremity were most commonly involved (98%). Associated problems were present in 50%; the most common was clubfeet. The authors recommend that the term "early amnion rupture sequence" be used to more accurately reflect the pathology.

Thumb

Buck-Gramcko D: Pollicization of the index finger: Methods and results in aplasia and hypoplasia of the thumb. *J Bone Joint Surg* 1971;53:1605–1617.

This is a classic description of what has become the standard operation for most hand surgeons throughout the world.

Goldner JL, Koman LA, Gelberman R, et al: Arthrodesis of the metacarpophalangeal joint of the thumb in children and adults: Adjunctive treatment of thumb-in-palm deformity in cerebral palsy. *Clin Orthop* 1990; 253:75–89.

In 68 pediatric patients, joint fusion was a predictable procedure to establish stability of the joint without disturbing longitudinal or circumferential growth. Measurable function was improved to a mild or moderate degree in 44 of 50 children followed to maturity.

Jennings JF, Peimer CA, Sherwin FS: Reduction osteotomy for triphalangeal thumb: An 11 year review. *J Hand Surg* 1992;17A:8–14.

The authors present the results of excision of excess bone with maintenance of a metacarpophalangeal (MCP) and interphalangeal (IP) joint in 13 triphalangeal thumbs in nine patients. With average follow-up of 5.4 years there was no malalignment or instability and active IP and MCP motion was preserved.

Kawabata H, Tada K, Masada K, et al: Revision of residual deformities after operations for duplication of thumb. *J Bone Joint Surg* 1990; 72A:988–998.

Results are presented of revision surgery for 38 thumbs with IP (eight), MCP (16), or zigzag (14) deformity. The indication for surgery was cosmetic, because only eight had functional deficits before surgery. It was difficult to correct the zigzag deformity.

Manske P, McCarroll H: Reconstruction of the congenitally deficient thumb. *Hand Clin* 1992;8:177–196.

This is a review article on the classification of thumb hypoplasia, surgical options for each subgroup, and rationale for treatment decisions.

Naasan A, Page R: Duplication of the thumb: A 20-year retrospective review. *J Hand Surg* 1994;19B:355–360.

The authors provide data on 43 duplicated thumbs treated surgically with an average follow-up of 5.2 years. Residual deformity, most commonly malangulation and instability at the IP or MCP joints, was present in 49%.

Rodgers W, Waters P: Incidence of trigger digits in newborns. *J Hand Surg* 1994;19A:364–368.

In this prospective study of 1,046 neonates, no trigger digits were found, correlating to an incidence of zero to three per 1,000 live births. The article includes a retrospective review of 73 children with 89 trigger finger releases. Only seven presented at less than 6 months of age and none at less than 3 months. Trigger digits may be acquired, not congenital.

Seidman GD, Wenner SM: Surgical treatment of the duplicated thumb. *J Pediatr Orthop* 1993;13:660–662.

The authors compared the results of ablation alone with ablation and radial collateral ligament reconstruction. Recurrent deformity and instability were present in the ablation alone group, reinforcing the axiom that ablation alone of a thumb polydactyly will not be adequate treatment.

Wood VE, Sicilia M: Congenital trigger digit. *Clin Orthop* 1992;285: 205–209.

Release of the sheath of the flexor tendon was successful in 33 trigger digits and the authors recommend it as simple and effective.

Syndromes

Apert's Syndrome

Upton J: Apert syndrome: Classification and pathologic anatomy of limb anomalies. *Clin Plast Surg* 1991;18:321–355.

This is a thorough review of all extremity anomalies in patients with Apert's syndrome, including a review of the literature and the results of care for 68 patients. It has an exhaustive bibliography.

Arthrogryposis

Bennett J, Hansen P, Granberry W, et al: Surgical management of arthrogryposis in the upper extremity. *J Pediatr Orthop* 1985;5:281–286.

This is a summary of conservative and surgical treatment options in the upper extremity.

Mennen U: Early corrective surgery of the wrist and elbow in arthrogryposis multiplex congenita. *J Hand Surg* 1993;18B:304–307.

The author describes the use of a single-stage procedure that included proximal row carpectomy, wrist palmarflexion to dorsiflexion tendon transfer, and triceps to biceps tendon transfer in 47 limbs of 25 patients. The best results were obtained in children operated on between 3 and 6 months of age. Average follow-up was 7.5 years.

Section 7

The Hip

George T. Rab, MD

Developmental Dysplasia of the Hip

Greene WB, Dias LS, Lindseth RE, et al: Musculoskeletal problems in association with cloacal exstrophy. *J Bone Joint Surg* 1991;73A: 551–560.

All 13 patients with cloacal exstrophy had spina bifida, four had congenital scoliosis, two had congenital kyphosis, and three had noncongenital scoliosis. All had lipomeningocele, and 11 had paralysis of the lower extremities. Mild dysplasia was present in six of the 26 hips, and foot deformities were common.

Vascular Supply

Brougham DI, Broughton NS, Cole WG, et al: Avascular necrosis following closed reduction of congenital dislocation of the hip: Review of influencing factors and long-term follow-up. *J Bone Joint Surg* 1990;72B: 557–562.

Of 210 hips, 99 (47%) had some evidence of osteonecrosis. The incidence was not influenced by the age at reduction, the use of traction, or the use of adductor tenotomy. Patients with closed reduction without preliminary traction did not have a higher incidence of osteonecrosis.

Chung SM: The arterial supply of the developing proximal end of the human femur. *J Bone Joint Surg* 1976;58A:961–970.

Perfusion studies on 150 autopsy specimens from children 26 weeks gestation to 14 years of age revealed two anastomotic rings formed by the medial and lateral circumflex vessels, which ascend to the capital epiphysis via the perichondral ring. Major vessels to the head and neck of the femur came from the lateral ascending cervical branches of the extracap-sular ring, which is supplied predominantly by the medial circumflex femoral artery. The physis was an absolute barrier to blood vessels in all but two cases. Arteries in the ligamentum teres were inconsistently present.

Ogden JA: Changing patterns of proximal femoral vascularity. *J Bone Joint Surg* 1974;56A:941–950.

Thirty-six autopsy specimens from children 7 months gestation to 3 years of age were studied. Initially, the proximal femoral chondroepiphysis and physis are supplied approximately equally by the medial and lateral circumflex systems, but the lateral system later regresses, and the medial circumflex system becomes the dominant source. Differential growth of the proximal femur was a significant factor in changing this distribution.

Trueta J: The normal vascular anatomy of the human femoral head during growth. *J Bone Joint Surg* 1957;39B:358–394.

This is a classic article on the blood supply of the developing proximal femur.

Screening, Evaluation, and Detection

Ando M, Gotoh E: Significance of inguinal folds for the diagnosis of congenital dislocation of the hip in infants aged three to four months. *J Pediatr Orthop* 1990;10:331–334.

Abnormal inguinal folds were present in all patients with complete dislocation among a screening population of 2,111 infants. They also were present in some infants with subluxation. Abnormal inguinal folds are asymmetric; or, if symmetric, they extend posteriorly beyond the anus.

Beoree NR, Clarke NM: Ultrasound imaging and secondary screening for congenital dislocation of the hip. *J Bone Joint Surg* 1994;76B:525–533.

Hernandez RJ, Cornell RG, Hensinger RN: Ultrasound diagnosis of neonatal congenital dislocation of the hip: A decision analysis assessment. *J Bone Joint Surg* 1994;76B:539–543.

These articles present opposing views on the value of ultrasound evaluation. The first found that routine ultrasound evaluation of high-risk patients was not advantageous, while the second recommends delayed secondary ultrasound screening.

Bialik V, Fishman J, Katzir J, et al: Clinical assessment of hip instability in the newborn by an orthopaedic surgeon and a pediatrician. *J Pediatr Orthop* 1986;6:703–705.

A pediatric orthopaedic surgeon, neonatal pediatrician, and general pediatrician, each working independently, examined babies for hip stability. All three detected 51 babies with instability. Twenty-five babies with instability were not recognized by at least one physician, and 36 babies thought to be stable at birth eventually required orthopaedic treatment. This study emphasizes the ease of missing unstable hips with a clinical examination and the need to continue screening examinations throughout the first year of life.

Davids JR, Benson LJ, Mubarak SJ, et al: Ultrasonography and developmental dysplasia of the hip: A cost-benefit analysis of three delivery systems. *J Pediatr Orthop* 1995;15:325–329.

Of three delivery systems: radiology-based, combined radiology/orthopaedic-based, and orthopaedic office-based, the third was most convenient, efficient, and cost-effective.

Garvey M, Donoghue VB, Gorman WA, et al: Radiographic screening at four months of infants at risk for congenital hip dislocation. *J Bone Joint Surg* 1992;74B:704–707.

In this large series of over 13,000 infants, radiographic screening at 4 months of age was successful in detecting dysplasia. None of the infants who had normal radiographs developed late dysplasia. Radiography provides an alternative when ultrasound is not convenient or available.

Graf R: Fundamentals of sonographic diagnosis of infant hip dysplasia. *J Pediatr Orthop* 1984;4:735–740.

The author describes classification and interpretation of ultasound in newborns and reports experience with 3,500 infants.

Greenhill BJ, Hugosson C, Jacobsson B, et al: Magnetic resonance imaging study of acetabular morphology in developmental dysplasia of the hip. *J Pediatr Orthop* 1993;13:314–317.

This article describes the pathoanatomy of older children with untreated developmental dysplasia of the hip (DDH) as revealed by MRI studies.

Hangen DH, Kasser JR, Emans JB, et al: The Pavlik harness and development dysplasia of the hip: Has ultrasound changed treatment patterns? *J Pediatr Orthop* 1995;15:729–735.

In a comparison of Pavlik harness treatment with and without ultrasound monitoring, treatment failure was recognized earlier with ultrasound monitoring, and the total number of radiographs was decreased.

Harcke HT, Kumar SJ: The role of ultrasound in the diagnosis and management of congenital dislocation and dysplasia of the hip. *J Bone Joint Surg* 1991;73A:622–628.

This is a general review of the use of ultrasound.

Hoaglund FT, Healey JH: Osteoarthrosis and congenital dysplasia of the hip in family members of children who have congenital dysplasia of the hip. *J Bone Joint Surg* 1990;72A:1510–1518.

This is the report of a large epidemiologic study of 408 relatives of 78 children with DDH. Some families had higher incidences of dysplasia, but many normal relatives were encountered. Evidence suggests a multifactorial cause.

Ilfeld W, Westin GW, Makin M: Missed or developmental dislocation of the hip. *Clin Orthop* 1986;203:276–281.

This important article documents discovery of subluxation and dislocation in hips that had been repeatedly examined by knowledgeable physicians (pediatric orthopaedists). Delay in diagnosis is not necessarily evidence of an inadequate examination.

Kahle WK, Coleman SS: The value of the acetabular teardrop figure in assessing pediatric hip disorders. *J Pediatr Orthop* 1992;12:586–591.

This is a good description of the "teardrop," its interpretation, and relationship to acetabular development. This issue is not yet well-described in standard orthopaedic texts, but has been a long-term interest of the senior author.

Lee DY, Choi IH, Lee CK, et al: Assessment of complex hip deformity using three-dimensional CT image. *J Pediatr Orthop* 1991;11:13–19.

The authors provide a persuasive argument that certain patients (previous osteotomy, complex dysplasia) benefit from a three-dimensional computed tomography scan as a preoperative planning tool.

Nonsurgical Treatment

Harris IE, Dickens R, Menelaus MB: Use of the Pavlik harness for hip displacements: When to abandon treatment. *Clin Orthop* 1992;281:29–33.

The authors describe guidelines developed in treatment of 720 hips with the Pavlik harness. They suggest abandoning the device if failure persists after 2 to 4 weeks of appropriate use. This is a large, well-documented study.

Jones GT, Schoenecker PL, Dias LS: Developmental hip dysplasia potentiated by inappropriate use of the Pavlik harness. *J Pediatr Orthop* 1992; 12:722–726.

Overzealous and prolonged use of the Pavlik harness when early failure was unrecognized led to posterolateral acetabular dysplasia and difficulty maintaining stability after closed reduction. This article contains guidelines for appropriate use of the device.

Mubarak S, Garfin S, Vance R, et al: Pitfalls in the use of the use of the Pavlik harness for treatment of congenital dysplasia, subluxation, and dislocation of the hip. *J Bone Joint Surg* 1981;63A:1239–1248.

This clear, practical, and readable article outlines proper indications and application of the Pavlik harness. It contains a specific management protocol and recommendations for adjustment. The most common difficulties were failure to achieve reduction and failure to recognize that it had not been achieved.

Suzuki S, Yamamuro T: Avascular necrosis in patients treated with the Pavlik harness for congenital dislocation of the hip. *J Bone Joint Surg* 1990;72A:1048–1055.

In this large, well-supervised study, 6% failed and 16% developed osteonecrosis during treatment with the Pavlik harness. The results provide some reason for caution in a treatment often lauded for its safety.

Viere RG, Birch JG, Herring JA, et al: Use of the Pavlik harness in congenital dislocation of the hip: An analysis of failures of treatment. *J Bone Joint Surg* 1990;72A:238–244.

Statistically significant risk factors for failure of the harness included an absent Ortolani sign at initial evaluation, bilateral dislocation, and age of more than 7 weeks before harness treatment was begun.

Closed Reduction and Traction

Brougham DI, Broughton NS, Cole WG, et al: Avascular necrosis following closed reduction of congenital dislocation of the hip: Review of influencing factors and long-term follow-up. *J Bone Joint Surg* 1990;72B:557–562.

In this study of 210 hips treated with closed reduction, osteonecrosis was not related to age at reduction, use of preliminary traction, or adductor tenotomy. Osteonecrosis was detected in 99 hips (47%); 81 hips (39%) had total involvement and 18 (9%) had partial involvement.

Camp J, Herring JA, Dworezynski C: Comparison of inpatient and outpatient traction in developmental dislocation of the hip. *J Pediatr Orthop* 1994;14:9–12.

After either inpatient (40 hips) or outpatient (home) Bryant's skin traction (43 hips), closed reduction was obtained in 55 hips (66%). The rate of severe osteonecrosis was low in both groups.

Daoud A, Saighi-Bououina A: Congenital dislocation of the hip in the older child: The effectiveness of overhead traction. *J Bone Joint Surg* 1996;78A:30–40.

Of 50 hips treated with overhead traction, 20 needed no additional treatment, 16 had innominate osteotomies, two had femoral derotation and innominate osteotomies, and 12 required open reduction after failed closed reduction. Osteonecrosis developed in two hips treated with closed reduction followed by Salter osteotomy and in three treated with primary open reduction. The authors suggest that preliminary overhead traction facilitated closed reduction of untreated congenitally dislocated hips in children 18 to 72 months old.

Fish DN, Herzenberg JE, Hensinger RN: Current practice in the use of prereduction traction for congenital dislocation of the hip. *J Pediatr Orthop* 1991;11:149–153.

This survey of members of the Pediatric Orthopaedic Society of North America gives guidelines of current practices in the use of traction. Ninety-five percent used it at least sometimes, most commonly in 12- to 18-month-old children; 28% rarely or never used it for children under 6 months; and 31% used home traction. Use of preliminary traction is controversial.

Kahle WK, Anderson MB, Alpert J, et al: The value of preliminary traction in the treatment of congenital dislocation of the hip. *J Bone Joint Surg* 1990;72A:1043–1047.

Forty-seven hips were treated by closed or open reduction without the use of preliminary traction. All were immobilized in the "human" position with marked flexion and slight abduction. The osteonecrosis rate was 4% at 2-year minimum follow-up, and was believed to be more likely after 1 year of age. The authors do not recommend traction, challenging a practice that has been almost universal for 20 years.

Malvitz TA, Weinstein SL: Closed reduction for congenital dysplasia of the hip: Functional and radiographic results after an average of thirty years. *J Bone Joint Surg* 1994;76A:1777–1792.

At latest follow-up of 152 hips in 119 patients, the Iowa hip rating averaged 91 points and the Harris hip scored 90 points. Disturbance of growth in the proximal femur occurred in 91 (60%). Twelve patients (17 hips) had total replacements at an average age of 35 years, and 65 hips (43%) had evidence of degenerative joint disease. Function tended to deteriorate with time in all patients.

Noritake K, Yoshihashi Y, Hattori T, et al: Acetabular development after closed reduction of congenital dislocation of the hip. *J Bone Joint Surg* 1993;75B:737–743.

Serial radiographs of 47 children (54 hips) followed until at least age 14 years revealed that acetabular development after the age of 11 or 12 years was significantly worse in Severin group III hips than in Severin group I hips on the affected side or Severin group III in unaffected control hips. One of the causes of acetabular dysplasia at maturity was impairment of acetabular development after the age of 11 or 12 years. The authors emphasize the importance of continuing follow-up of these patients until full skeletal maturity.

Quinn RH, Renshaw TS, DeLuca PA: Preliminary traction in the treatment of developmental dislocation of the hip. *J Pediatr Orthop* 1994; 14:636–642.

Ninety dislocated hips in 72 patients underwent attempted closed reduction after 3 weeks of traction: 52 (58%) had successful closed reduction and 38 (42%) required open reduction. No significant difference was found in either the rate of successful closed reduction or the incidence of osteonecrosis compared to recently published series in which preliminary traction was not used.

Schoenecker PL, Dollard PA, Sheridan JJ, et al: Closed reduction of developmental dislocation of the hip in children older than 18 months. *J Pediatr Orthop* 1995;15:763–767.

Of 38 attempted closed reductions, 26 (68%) were initially successful; three of these required open reduction during cast treatment. Of the 23 remaining hips, 11 required no further treatment at an average follow-up of 8 years and 8 months, and 12 required femoral or pelvic osteotomy for failure to remodel. Younger age (less than 22 months) at the time of reduction and lower grade dislocation were favorable prognostic indicators.

Zionts LE, MacEwen GD: Treatment of congenital dislocation of the hip in children between the ages of one and three years. *J Bone Joint Surg* 1986;68A:829–846.

This article reports 51 hips treated by preoperative traction, adductor tenotomy where appropriate, and closed reduction under anesthesia. Twenty-five percent required open reduction because of failure to achieve satisfactory reduction closed. Results were excellent in 90% of hips, with significant osteonecrosis in three hips, only one of which was treated by closed reduction. The authors suggest that treatment by closed reduction

Open Reduction

Castillo R, Sherman FC: Medial adductor open reduction for congenital dislocation of the hip. *J Pediatr Orthop* 1990;10:335–340.

At 7-year follow-up of 26 hips, 73% were Severin classification grade I or II; 88% of patients treated between the ages of 5 and 14 months had grade I or II results. Osteonecrosis occurred in 15% and correlated positively with increased age at surgery.

Galpin RD, Roach JW, Wenger DR, et al: One-stage treatment of congenital dislocation of the hip in older children, including femoral shortening. *J Bone Joint Surg* 1989;71A:734–741.

The authors describe results of 33 hips (25 patients) treated by open reduction and femoral shortening combined. No traction was used, and three hips (10%) developed osteonecrosis. Leg length discrepancy resolved with time and required no treatment.

Imatani J, Miyake Y, Nakatsuka Y, et al: Coxa magna after open reduction for developmental dislocation of the hip. *J Pediatr Orthop* 1995;15:337–341.

Coxa magna was identified in 34% of hips treated with open reduction. Causes were overwidening of the acetabular capacity by excision of the limbus and surgical invasion and synovitis of the hip joint.

Mankey MG, Arntz GT, Staheli LT: Open reduction through a medial approach for congenital dislocation of the hip. *J Bone Joint Surg* 1993;75A:1334–1345.

This is a review of 66 hips in 63 patients (average age 12 months) treated by open reduction through a medial approach. Osteonecrosis occurred in 11% of hips, and residual acetabular dysplasia required pelvic osteotomy in 33%.

Simons GW: A comparative evaluation of the current methods for open reduction of the congenitally displaced hip. *Orthop Clin North Am* 1980;11:161–181.

This is an exhaustive comparative review of the five basic forms of open reduction. The author presents his indications for the use of each.

Weinstein SL, Ponseti IV: Congenital dislocation of the hip: Open reduction through a medial approach. *J Bone Joint Surg* 1979;61A:119–124.

The authors report the use of a medial approach for open reduction of 20 congenital hip dislocations in 17 patients; at an average follow-up of 42.2 months, two (10%) had developed osteonecrosis. The authors recommend the medial approach as a safe, effective method of reduction in infants; for children more than 24 months old, they recommend an anterior approach.

Pelvic and Femoral Osteotomy

Chiari K: Medial displacement osteotomy of the pelvis. *Clin Orthop* 1974;98:55–71.

Pemberton PA: Pericapsular osteotomy of the ilium for treatment of congenital subluxation and dislocation of the hip. *J Bone Joint Surg* 1965;47A:65–86.

Salter RB: Innominate osteotomy in the treatment of congenital dislocation and subluxation of the hip. *J Bone Joint Surg* 1961;43B:518–539.

Salter RB, Dubos J-P: The first fifteen years' personal experience with innominate osteotomy in the treatment of congenital dislocation and subluxation of the hip. *Clin Orthop* 1974;98:72–103.

Steel HH: Triple osteotomy of the innominate bone. *J Bone Joint Surg* 1973;55A:343–350.

Sutherland DH, Greenfield R: Double innominate osteotomy. *J Bone Joint Surg* 1977;59A:1082–1091.

These six classic articles describe specific procedures.

Faciszewski T, Kiefer GN, Coleman SS: Pemberton osteotomy for residual acetabular dysplasia in children who have congenital dislocation of the hip. *J Bone Joint Surg* 1993;75A:643–649.

This large (52 hips), long-term study of the commonly used Pemberton osteotomy indicated that it yielded excellent results unless there was pre-existing osteonecrosis. Average age at surgery was 4 years. Average follow-up was 10 years.

Guille JT, Forlin E, Kumar SJ, et al: Triple osteotomy of the innominate bone in treatment of developmental dysplasia of the hip. *J Pediatr Orthop* 1992;12:718–721.

In this long-term (12-year) study, ten of 11 hips improved radiographically and Iowa hip scores were improved in eight of 11 after triple innominate osteotomy.

Staheli LT, Chew DE: Slotted acetabular augmentation in childhood and adolescence. *J Pediatr Orthop* 1992;12:569–580.

This long-term study of a large series of hips treated with the acetabular augmentation technique reproted generally satisfactory results. The authors describe the operation as a simpler alternative to Chiari osteotomy, and they analyze technical reasons for failure.

Suda H, Hattori T, Iwata H: Varus derotation osteotomy for persistent dysplasia in congenital dislocation of the hip: Proximal femoral growth and alignment changes in the leg. *J Bone Joint Surg* 1995;77B:756–761.

In a study of the morphologic changes after varus derotation osteotomy in 42 hips, the authors found that postoperative femoral neck-shaft angle was not related to the final result but that the center-edge angle obtained at surgery influenced the outcome.

Wenger DR, Lee CS, Kolman B: Derotational femoral shortening for developmental dislocation of the hip: Special indications and results in the child younger than 2 years. *J Pediatr Orthop* 1995;15:768–779.

Femoral shortening was combined with open reduction in 15 children (20 hips) ranging in age from 5 to 23 months; 14 hips required concurrent pelvic osteotomy. Complications included partial osteonecrosis in two hips, residual subluxation requiring acetabular osteotomy in two, and residual dysplasia in two. Radiographic evaluation (Severin method) revealed 15 good or excellent results and five fair or poor results.

Osteonecrosis

Bucholz RW, Ogden JA: Patterns of ischemic necrosis of the proximal femur in nonoperatively treated congenital hip disease, in *The Hip: Proceedings of the Sixth Open Scientific Meeting of The Hip Society*. St. Louis, MO, CV Mosby, 1978, pp 43–63.

This classic article describes the modes of vascular injury resulting in four types of ischemic necrosis of the femoral head and emphasizes its iatrogenic etiology.

Gage JR, Winter RB: Avascular necrosis of the capital femoral epiphysis as a complication of closed reduction of congenital dislocation of the hip: A critical review of twenty years' experience at Gillette Children's Hospital. *J Bone Joint Surg* 1972;54A:373–388.

This classic article describes the risks of osteonecrosis and the use of preliminary traction in an attempt to reduce the incidence. Specific traction guidelines are given. The era described also saw advances in use of the "human" position for immobilization. This article was a major factor in the past 20 years' use of preliminary traction, which is now being challenged.

Kalamchi A, MacEwen GD: Avascular necrosis following treatment of congenital dislocation of the hip. *J Bone Joint Surg* 1980;62A:876–888.

This review of 119 patients with DDH complicated by osteonecrosis classified the vascular disturbances into four types; this classification was accurate in predicting the natural history of osteonecrosis. Severe osteonecrosis was most frequent in patients who were initially treated before the age of 6 months, and the authors suggest that the use of preliminary traction and general anesthesia reduce the frequency of severe osteonecrosis.

Robinson HJ Jr, Shannon MA: Avascular necrosis in congenital hip dysplasia: The effect of treatment. *J Pediatr Orthop* 1989;9:293–303.

Thirty-nine patients with 50 involved hips were evaluated at a mean follow-up of 25 years. Nonsurgical maintenance of reduction carried the best prognosis, followed by pelvic or femoral osteotomy if reduction could not otherwise be obtained. The combination of osteonecrosis and persistent subluxation carried a poor prognosis.

Thomas IH, Dunin AJ, Cole WG, et al: Avascular necrosis after open reduction for congenital dislocation of the hip: Analysis of causative factors and natural history. *J Pediatr Orthop* 1989;9:525–531.

Osteonecrosis occurred in 37% of 87 hips undergoing open reduction. Apparent causative factors are reviewed. The authors believe that open reduction itself was not a causative factor. Eighty-five percent of hips with osteonecrosis had satisfactory late results. Traction did not reduce the incidence of osteonecrosis.

Long-term Results

Campbell P, Tarlow SD: Lateral tethering of the proximal femoral physis complicating the treatment of congenital hip dysplasia. *J Pediatr Orthop* 1990;10:6–8.

Lateral physeal tethers, seen in 10% of patients treated for DDH, could lead to coxa valga. The lesion often presented late (average 8 years), and occurred after all forms of treatment.

Malvitz TA, Weinstein SL: Closed reduction for congenital dysplasia of the hip: Functional and radiographic results after an average of thirty years. *J Bone Joint Surg* 1994;76A:1777–1792.

This article is a comprehensive review of 119 patients with DDH treated by closed reduction and casting, with average age at follow-up of 31 years. Sixty percent of hips had at least partial evidence of proximal growth arrest, which wasn't evident for many years, and 43% had degenerative changes. This is an excellent baseline study for current treatment methods.

Noritake K, Yoshihashi Y, Hattori T, et al: Acetabular development after closed reduction of congenital dislocation of the hip. *J Bone Joint Surg* 1993;75B:737–743.

This long-term radiographic study emphasizes the potential for remodeling and dysplasia related to the secondary ossification centers after 12 years of age, and underscores the need for long follow-up of DDH patients.

O'Brien T, Millis MB, Griffin PP: The early identification and classification of growth disturbances of the proximal end of the femur. *J Bone Joint Surg* 1986;68A:970–980.

Sixty-eight patients undergoing treatment for congenital dislocation of the hip were analyzed by serial radiographs. A line appearing in the proximal femur within the first year after treatment is an indicator of future growth disturbance. This line also can be used to predict which of two different patterns of growth disturbance will occur.

Tucci JJ, Kumar SJ, Guille JT, et al: Late acetabular dysplasia following early successful Pavlik harness treatment of congenital dislocation of the hip. *J Pediatr Orthop* 1991;11:502–505.

The appearance of radiographic dysplasia in 17% of 74 hips treated for DDH with an average follow-up age of 12 years suggests caution and need for long-term follow-up of treated patients. This group had normal radiographic appearance at age 5 years, which subsequently deteriorated.

Slipped Capital Femoral Epiphysis

Detection and Pathoanatomy

Kallio PE, Foster BK, LeQuesne GW, et al: Remodeling in slipped capital femoral epiphysis: Sonographic assessment after pinning. *J Pediatr Orthop* 1992;12:438–443.

This unique sonographic assessment of anterior metaphyseal remodeling after slipped capital femoral epiphysis (SCFE) fixation suggests that rapid remodeling begins as early as 3 weeks postoperatively. The authors did not control for femoral rotation.

Loder RT: The demographics of slipped capital femoral epiphysis: An international study. *Clin Orthop* 1996;322:8–27.

In a study of 1,630 children with 1,993 slips, 41.2% were girls and 58.8% were boys. The diseased hip was unilateral in 77.7% and bilateral in 22.3%. Slips were chronic in 85.5% and acute in 14.5%. The child's weight was greater than or equal to the 90th percentile in 63.2%. The average age at diagnosis was 12 years in girls and 13.5 years in boys; the age at diagnosis decreased with increasing obesity. Other demographic data are presented.

Loder RT, Aronson DD, Greenfield ML: The epidemiology of bilateral slipped capital femoral epiphysis: A study of children in Michigan. *J Bone Joint Surg* 1993;75A:1141–1147.

This well-documented, careful study of the epidemiology of SCFE documents bilaterality in 37% and suggests that most contralateral slips occur within 18 months of initial presentation.

Loder RT, Wittenberg B, DeSilva G: Slipped capital femoral epiphysis associated with endocrine disorders. *J Pediatr Orthop* 1995;15:349–356.

Of 85 patients with endocrine disorders and SCFE, 40% had hypothyroidism, 25% had growth hormone deficiency, and 35% had other disorders. Because the prevalence of bilaterality was 61%, prophylactic treatment of the opposite hip should be considered.

Wells D, King JD, Roe TF, et al: Review of slipped capital femoral epiphysis associated with endocrine disease. *J Pediatr Orthop* 1993; 13:610–614.

This review article discusses the detection and work-up of endocrinopathies that are associated with SCFE. The most common abnormality is hypothyroidism. The authors recommend bilateral (prophylactic, if necessary) pinning because 100% of their patients eventually had bilateral slips.

Treatment

Abraham E, Garst J, Barmada R: Treatment of moderate to severe slipped capital femoral epiphysis with extracapsular base-of-neck osteotomy. *J Pediatr Orthop* 1993;13:294–302.

At average follow-up of 9 years, 90% of 36 hips had excellent or good results; none had osteonecrosis. This osteotomy is recommended as a safe and effective way to prevent further slipping and improve hip range of motion in severe chronic slips.

Aronson DD, Carlson WE: Slipped capital femoral epiphysis: A prospective study of fixation with a single screw. *J Bone Joint Surg* 1992;74A: 810–819.

This prospective study of in situ fixation of 58 hips with SCFE documents the absence of chondrolysis. One patient with an acute slip developed osteonecrosis. This is one of several papers that outline a safe, straightforward surgical approach to SCFE using a single cannulated screw.

Aronson DD, Peterson DA, Miller DV: Slipped capital femoral epiphysis: The case for internal fixation in situ. *Clin Orthop* 1992;281:115–122.

This is a clinical and radiographic review of 80 hips with 3.3-year (average) follow-up after in situ fixation. Results were best in mild cases, but osteonecrosis occurred in only two hips. Poor pin position was seen in 60% of the 20 hips with poor results; these data emphasize the need for careful technical execution of the operation.

Blanco JS, Taylor B, Johnston CE II: Comparison of single pin versus multiple pin fixation in treatment of slipped capital femoral epiphysis. *J Pediatr Orthop* 1992;12:384–389.

In this study of 114 hips with SCFE, a single central screw was found to provide adequate fixation and was associated with few complications.

Crandall DG, Gabriel KR, Akbarnia BA: Second operation for slipped capital femoral epiphysis: Pin removal. *J Pediatr Orthop* 1992;12: 434–437.

Documentation of "routine" pin/screw removal in 43 hips suggests that the complication rate is significant. The authors question the value of routine removal in asymptomatic patients.

Herman MJ, Dormans JP, Davidson RS, et al: Screw fixation of grade III slipped capital femoral epiphysis. *Clin Orthop* 1996;322:77–85.

At 2.8-year follow-up of 21 grade III slips fixed with one or two screws, four had major complications, three had osteonecrosis of the femoral head, and one had chrondrolysis. The mean Harris hip score for these four patients was 85 points, compared to a mean score of 94 points for all 21 patients.

Jerre R, Billing L, Hansson G, et al: The contralateral hip in patients primarily treated for unilateral slipped upper femoral epiphysis: Long-term follow-up of 61 hips. *J Bone Joint Surg* 1994;76B:563–567.

The authors point out the issues of slipping, osteoarthritis, and need for contralateral surgery in the "unaffected" hip in SCFE. They stop short of recommending prophylactic pinning of uninvolved hips, but give guidelines for clinical follow-up.

Kibiloski LJ, Doane RM, Karol LA, et al: Biomechanical analysis of single- versus double-screw fixation in slipped capital femoral epiphysis at physiological load levels. *J Pediatr Orthop* 1994;14:627–630.

Authors of this biomechanical study using bovine hips suggest that single-screw fixation of SCFE is adequate in most clinical situations.

Laplaza FJ, Burke SW: Epiphyseal growth after pinning of slipped capital femoral epiphysis. *J Pediatr Orthop* 1995;15:357–361.

Of 77 hips, evidence of the epiphysis "growing off" the pins was seen in 29% of those fixed with Steinmann pins, in 18% with Knowles pins, and in one fixed with cannulated screws.

Lindaman LM, Canale ST, Beaty JH, et al: A fluoroscopic technique for determining the incision site for percutaneous fixation of slipped capital femoral epiphysis. *J Pediatr Orthop* 1991;11:397–401.

A very practical method for estimation of the screw insertion site during in situ fixation of SCFE is described.

Zionts LE, Simonian PT, Harvey JP Jr: Transient penetration of the hip joint during in situ cannulated-screw fixation of slipped capital femoral epiphysis. *J Bone Joint Surg* 1991;73A:1054–1060.

Fourteen hips with documented intraoperative penetration of fixation devices during surgery for SCFE were treated with repositioning of the device. No complications occurred. This study documents the clinically benign event of transient penetration and suggests that chronic pin penetration is the etiologic culprit for major articular complications of SCFE.

Acute Slips

Aronsson DD, Loder RT: Treatment of the unstable (acute) slipped capital femoral epiphysis. *Clin Orthop* 1996;322:99–110.

The authors recommend preoperative bed rest to decrease synovitis and intra-articular effusion. Their surgical technique for single-screw fixation is described.

Dietz FR: Traction reduction of acute and acute-on-chronic slipped capital femoral epiphysis. *Clin Orthop* 1994;302:101–110.

This study of 30 patients with acute-on-chronic or acute SCFE documents that those undergoing longitudinal traction with internal rotation often (> 50%) failed to achieve detectable reduction, and they had rates of osteonecrosis similar to or greater than patients with acute slips pinned in situ.

Loder RT, Richards BS, Shapiro PS, et al: Acute slipped capital femoral epiphysis: The importance of physeal stability. *J Bone Joint Surg* 1993; 75A:1134–1140.

The authors describe a simple, two-part classification of acute SCFE: In their report of 55 acute slips, satisfactory results were obtained in 96% of stable slips and in only 47% of unstable slips. The complication rate in unstable slips (particularly osteonecrosis) was nearly 50%.

Long-term Results

Abraham E, Garst J, Barmada R: Treatment of moderate to severe slipped capital femoral epiphysis with extracapsular base-of-neck osteotomy. *J Pediatr Orthop* 1993;13:294–302.

The authors used an anterior closing wedge, obliquely oriented osteotomy at the base of the neck to achieve early correction of impingement in moderate to high-grade SCFE. This study documents the high (90%) clinical success rate and absence of osteonecrosis in a series of 36 consecutive patients.

Canale ST, Azar F, Young J, et al: Subtrochanteric fracture after fixation of slipped capital femoral epiphysis: A complication of unused drill holes. *J Pediatr Orthop* 1994;14:623–626.

Four subtrochanteric fractures (1.4% of patients) occurred through unused drill holes. Avoiding extraneous screw holes seems to be the best way to prevent this complication.

Carney BT, Weinstein SL, Noble J: Long-term follow-up of slipped capital femoral epiphysis. *J Bone Joint Surg* 1991;73A:667–674.

This article reports an exhaustive study of 155 hips with SCFE followed up an average of 41 years. Regardless of the severity of the slip, pinning in situ provided the best long-term function and delay of degenerative arthritis, with a low risk of complications.

Carney BT, Weinstein SL: Natural history of untreated chronic slipped capital femoral epiphysis. *Clin Orthop* 1996;322:43–47.

A review of patients with a mean age of 54 years at a mean follow-up of 41 years found degenerative arthritis in hips with displaced slips, but the authors concluded that the natural history of chronic SCFE is favorable provided that displacement is minimal and remains so.

DeRosa GP, Mullins RC, Kling TF Jr: Cuneiform osteotomy of the femoral neck in severe slipped capital femoral epiphysis. *Clin Orthop* 1996;322:48–60.

At an average follow-up of 8 years and 5 months, 19 of 27 severe slips had good results, four had fair, and four poor results. Osteonecrosis occurred in 15%. All patients, including those with osteonecrosis, had improved joint flexion and internal rotation.

Fish JB: Cuneiform osteotomy of the femoral neck in the treatment of slipped capital femoral epiphysis: A follow-up note. *J Bone Joint Surg* 1994;76A:46–59.

This article documents the relatively favorable long-term results of salvage of the high-grade SCFE with cuneiform osteotomy, an operation that has engendered a lot of controversy. Osteonecrosis developed in two of 66, and all six of the 66 patients with osteoarthrosis had pin penetration.

Hansson G, Jerre R, Sanders SM, et al: Radiographic assessment of coxarthrosis following slipped capital femoral epiphysis: A 32-year follow-up study of 151 hips. *Acta Radiol* 1993;34:117–123.

In this retrospective radiographic review of SCFE in patients at an average age of 47 years, 42% had joint space narrowing in at least one view. Not all the individual radiographs were abnormal in patients with obvious abnormalities in at least one view, demonstrating the need for several studies of the hip when attempting evaluation or follow-up of SCFE.

Krahn TH, Canale ST, Beaty JH, et al: Long-term follow-up of patients with avascular necrosis after treatment of slipped capital femoral epiphysis. *J Pediatr Orthop* 1993;13:154–158.

Twenty-four of 264 patients with SCFE who developed osteonecrosis are reported in this study. The authors suggest that a conservative regimen can sometimes allow delay of definitive treatment of problems until adulthood.

Legg-Calvé-Perthes Disease

Etiology

Glueck CJ, Crawford A, Roy D, et al: Association of antithrombotic factor deficiencies and hypofibrinolysis with Legg-Perthes disease. *J Bone Joint Surg* 1996;78A:3–13.

Thirty-three (75%) of 44 unselected children with Legg-Perthes disease had coagulation abnormalities. Protein-C or S deficiency, hypofibrinolysis, or a high level of lipoprotein(a) may result in thrombotic venous occlusion of the femur, which leads to the venous hypertension and osteonecrosis of the femoral head characteristic of Legg-Perthes disease. These levels should be measured in children diagnosed with Legg-Perthes disease. Early diagnosis of the coagulation abnormality may open avenues for pharmacological preventive therapy.

Glueck CJ, Glueck HI, Greenfield D, et al: Protein C and S deficiency, thrombophilia, and hypofibrinolysis: Pathophysiologic causes of Legg-Perthes disease. *Pediatr Res* 1994;35:383–388.

Of eight patients with Legg-Calvé-Perthes (LCP) disease, three had protein C deficiency, one had protein S deficiency, and one had fibrinolysis; all of these problems are associated with hypercoagulation or thrombotic complications. Statistical chances of this are extremely rare, offering a suggestion about the etiology of LCP.

Loder RT, Schwartz EM, Hensinger RN: Behavioral characteristics of children with Legg-Calve-Perthes disease. *J Pediatr Orthop* 1993;13: 598–601.

Further evidence (in addition to delayed bone age) is presented in this article to suggest that certain children are more susceptible to LCP.

Evaluation

Conway JJ: A scintigraphic classification of Legg-Calve-Perthes disease. *Semin Nucl Med* 1993;23:274–295.

Although scintigraphy is now rarely used for LCP (either diagnosis or follow-up), this review offers good guidelines for interpretation.

Herring JA, Neustadt JB, Williams JJ, et al: The lateral pillar classification of Legg-Calvé-Perthes disease. *J Pediatr Orthop* 1992;12:143–150.
Ritterbusch JF, Shantharam SS, Gelinas C: Comparison of lateral pillar classification and Catterall classification of Legg-Calve-Perthes' disease. *J Pediatr Orthop* 1993;13:200–202.

The "lateral pillar" classification is being used in some centers and is still undergoing evaluation in others. Physicians seeing patients with LCP should be aware of it, and these two articles are the place to start.

Loder RT, Farley FA, Herring JA, et al: Bone age determination in children with Legg-Calvé-Perthes disease: A comparison of two methods. *J Pediatr Orthop* 1995;15:90–94.

In 100 children, the average chronological age, pelvic bone age, and hand-wrist bone age were significantly different for girls and for boys. For girls, the chronological age was greater than the other two, but there was no difference between the pelvis and hand-wrist bone ages. For boys, chronological age was greatest, pelvis bone age was greater than hand-wrist bone age and less than chronological age. The acromelic growth in Legg-Calvé-Perthes disease may explain why the more proximal pelvis bone age in boys was less delayed than that of the more distal hand-wrist.

Simmons ED, Graham HK, Szalai JP: Interobserver variability in grading Perthes' disease. *J Bone Joint Surg* 1990;72B:202–204.

The authors point out the recognized difficulties of achieving uniform opinions about the classification and extent of LCP. Less interobserver variability was seen with the simpler Salter-Thompson classification than with Catterall's classification.

Terjesen T: Ultrasonography in the primary evaluation of patients with Perthes disease. *J Pediatr Orthop* 1993;13:437–443.

The authors used noninvasive ultrasound to quantify femoral coverage and fragmentation in LCP and correlated it with radiographic findings. Synovitis was also detectable. This method offers an alternative for imaging LCP hips.

Treatment

Coates CJ, Paterson JM, Woods KR, et al: Femoral osteotomy in Perthes' disease: Results at maturity. *J Bone Joint Surg* 1990;72B:581–585.

In this series from Great Britain of 48 hips treated by femoral osteotomy, results were better than in historic nonsurgical controls (in patients older than 5 years). Clinical ratings as well as radiographic assessment were used.

Doudoulakis JK: Trochanteric advancement for premature arrest of the femoral-head growth plate: 6-year review of 30 hips. *Acta Orthop Scand* 1991;62:92–94.

Macnicol MF, Makris D: Distal transfer of the greater trochanter. *J Bone Joint Surg* 1991;73B:838–841.

These two articles document the method, indications, and results of distal or lateral transfer of the greater trochanter for residuals of LCP (or DDH). Short-term results were generally favorable, but late osteoarthrosis was an issue, which is not surprising, considering the diseases that are generally treated by this operation.

Martinez AG, Weinstein SL, Deitz FR: The weight-bearing abduction brace for the treatment of Legg-Perthes disease. *J Bone Joint Surg* 1992;74A:12–21.

Meehan PL, Angel D, Nelson JM: The Scottish Rite abduction orthosis for the treatment of Legg-Perthes disease: A radiographic analysis. *J Bone Joint Surg* 1992;74A:2–12.

Neither of these articles suggests any advantage of abduction orthosis treatment over other methods of management or no treatment.

Fulford GE, Lunn PG, Macnicol MF: A prospective study of nonoperative and operative management for Perthes' disease. *J Pediatr Orthop* 1993; 13:281–285.

This prospective study included a brace group and an osteotomy group, which had equal results. Arthrogram and age were the best predictors of outcome.

Herring JA: The treatment of Legg-Calve-Perthes disease: A critical review of the literature. *J Bone Joint Surg* 1994;76A:448–458.

This comprehensive review includes outcomes of and comparison between various methods of treatment and recommendations for treatment.

Hoikka V, Poussa M, Yrjonen T, et al: Intertrochanteric varus osteotomy for Perthes' disease: Radiographic changes after 2-16-year follow-up of 126 hips. *Acta Orthop Scand* 1991;62:549–553.

The authors reporting this Scandinavian series of femoral osteotomies failed to confirm the prognostic value of Catterall classification or head-at-risk signs, but did document better results in children who were younger at onset. Achievement of centralization of the femoral head was important to the final result.

Kiepurska A: Late results of treatment in Perthes' disease by a functional method. *Clin Orthop* 1991;272:76–81.

Two hundred and ninety-six children (334 hips)with LCP were treated by broomstick plaster casts in abduction and rotation, with overall favorable results. Age at onset was important to prognosis, as was subluxation.

Leitch JM, Paterson DC, Foster BK: Growth disturbance in Legg-Calvé-Perthes disease and the consequences of surgical treatment. *Clin Orthop* 1991;262:178–184.

Seventy-two patients with LCPD were studied to evaluate the interference with proximal femoral growth resulting from the disease or from surgical treatment. Overall, 6% of patients had leg-length discrepancies of more than 2 cm after both surgical (47) and nonsurgical (25) treatment. The articulotrochanteric distance (ATD) was less than 5 mm in 23%, of whom 43% had positive Trendelenburg signs. Because the mean ATD was significantly lower in patients treated by femoral varus osteotomy, the authors suggest that this should be avoided in patients older than 8 years of age.

Martinez AG, Weinstein SL, Dietz FR: The weight-bearing abduction brace for the treatment of Legg-Perthes disease. *J Bone Joint Surg* 1992;74A:12–21.

Meehan PL, Angel D, Nelson JM: The Scottish Rite abduction orthosis for the treatment of Legg-Perthes disease: A radiographic analysis. *J Bone Joint Surg* 1992;74A:2–12.

These two important articles from well-respected centers throw doubt on the value of ambulatory containment treatment in general and the Atlanta Scottish Rite brace in particular for Catterall III and IV LCP.

Paterson DC, Leitch JM, Foster BK: Results of innominate osteotomy in the treatment of Legg-Calvé-Perthes disease. *Clin Orthop* 1991;266:96–103.

Satisfactory results were obtained in 96% of 27 patients treated with innominate osteotomy. The presence or absence of subchondral fracture before and at time of surgery was not found to significantly influence long-term results.

Poussa M, Yrjonen T, Hoikka V, et al: Prognosis after conservative and operative treatment in Perthes' disease. *Clin Orthop* 1993;297:82–86.

A large series of LCP patients were treated surgically and conservatively. The authors make a case for containment treatment (osteotomy) and point out the difficulty in determining prognosis early. Diverse patient selection may affect results.

Wang L, Bowen JR, Puniak MA, et al: An evaluation of various methods of treatment for Legg-Calvé-Perthes disease. *Clin Orthop* 1995;314:225–233.

Five methods were analyzed; Scottish Rite orthosis, nonweightbearing and exercises, Petrie cast, femoral varus osteotomy, and Salter osteotomy. Hips treated by the Scottish Rite orthosis had a significantly worse Mose measurement than those treated by other methods. There was, however, no significant difference in the distribution of hips according to the Stulberg et al classification at last follow-up.

Weiner SD, Weiner DS, Riley PM: Pitfalls in treatment of Legg-Calvé-Perthes disease using proximal femoral varus osteotomy. *J Pediatr Orthop* 1991;11:20–24.

In this review of 79 femoral varus osteotomies, the authors warn of the dangers of overcorrection. Trochanteric overgrowth should also be anticipated.

Willett K, Hudson I, Catterall A: Lateral shelf acetabuloplasty: An operation for older children with Perthes' disease. *J Pediatr Orthop* 1992;12: 563–568.

Results in 20 children older than 8 years of age treated with lateral shelf acetabuloplasty were compared to those in 14 children with no treatment. Acetabuloplasty improved early outcome.

Remodeling and Long-term Prognosis

Bennett JT, Mazurek RT, Cash JD: Chiari's osteotomy in the treatment of Perthes' disease. *J Bone Joint Surg* 1991;73B:225–228.

Crutcher JP, Staheli LT: Combined osteotomy as a salvage procedure for severe Legg-Calvé-Perthes disease. *J Pediatr Orthop* 1992;12:151–156.

These two articles outline indications for and clinical results of salvage pelvic osteotomy or shelf osteotomy in the patient with severe LCP. The first article also included combined femoral osteotomy.

Herring JA, Williams JJ, Neustadt JN, et al: Evolution of femoral head deformity during the healing phase of Legg-Calvé-Perthes disease. *J Pediatr Orthop* 1993;13:41–45.

Forty-nine of 136 hips became progressively rounder, and 15 hips became progressively flatter after onset of reossification of the femoral head. The femoral head was more likely to undergo progressive flattening in older patients, in those with more severe lateral pillar involvement, and in those with prolonged reossification.

Kamegaya M, Shinada Y, Moriya H, et al: Acetabular remodelling in Perthes' disease after primary healing. *J Pediatr Orthop* 1992;12: 308–314.

The authors of this article link subluxation during LCP (a real but incompletely understood phenomenon) with long-term outcome and acetabular remodeling. They point out the transient nature of subluxation in some patients and make a case for delaying treatment until the position of the femoral head at "primary healing" has been established.

Kurse RW, Guille JT, Bowen JR: Shelf arthroplasty in patients who have Legg-Calvé-Perthes disease: A study of long-term results. *J Bone Joint Surg* 1991;73A:1338–1347.

Twenty hips treated with shelf arthroplasty were compared to 18 hips with nonsurgical treatment. In the operated group the center-edge (CE) angle was significantly improved and the average Iowa hip score was 91 points; in the nonsurgical group, no significant improvement in the CE angle occurred and the average Iowa hip score was 81 points. Shelf arthroplasty is recommended when additional bone is needed at the lateral aspect of the acetabulum to cover the extruded portion of the femoral head, to prevent additional incongruity and delay onset of degenerative changes.

Yrjonen T: Prognosis in Perthes' disease after noncontainment treatment: 106 hips followed for 28-47 years. *Acta Orthop Scand* 1992;63:523–526.

This long-term follow-up of 106 hips with LCP documents the prognostic value of age at onset and femoral head sphericity at maturity. So-called "head at risk" signs were not helpful in determining long-term outcome. Many patients developed osteoarthrosis.

Transient Synovitis of the Hip

Briggs RD, Baird KS, Gibson PH: Transient synovitis of the hip joint. *J Roy Col Surg* 1990;35:48–50.

LCP was eventually diagnosed in only one of 286 children with classic transient synovitis of the hip. The authors believed that extensive diagnostic work-up and follow-up for the typical patient was not indicated.

Erken EH, Katz K: Irritable hip and Perthes' disease. *J Pediatr Orthop* 1990;10:322–326.

Comparison of two large groups of patients—one with transient synovitis, the other with synovitis associated with LCP—highlights the differences in the diseases. Irritable hip patients were younger (3 years old). Intra-articular pressure was correlated with hip position. Pressure tamponade in the irritable hip syndrome was not believed to be responsible for LCP.

Arthrodesis of the Hip

Blasier RB, Holmes JR: Intraoperative positioning for arthrodesis of the hip with the double beanbag technique. *J Bone Joint Surg* 1990;72A:766–769.

The authors present a useful method for achieving proper positioning for arthrodesis of the hip using the cobra plate technique. Two beanbags are used; one holds the patient in a lateral decubitus position, and the second (between the legs) forms a trough to hold the surgical side in the optimum position for fusion. The leg can be moved during surgery and dropped back into the trough for correct alignment at any point.

Lipscomb PR, McCaslin FE Jr: Arthrodesis of the hip: Review of 371 cases. *J Bone Joint Surg* 1961;43A:923–938.

This classic article reporting hip fusion in a large series gives advice about positioning the joint, technique, and indications. The authors' preference is combined intra- and extra-articular type fusion with intertrochanteric osteotomy. There is an excellent discussion about the method of assuring proper degree of hip flexion when applying the postoperative spica cast.

Müller ME, Allgöwer M, Schneider R, et al (eds): *Manual of Internal Fixation: Techniques Recommended by the AO Group*, ed 2. Berlin, Germany, Springer-Verlag, 1979.

This book contains a review of the Schneider technique of cobra plate hip arthrodesis. A transverse pelvic osteotomy is included in the procedure to reduce intra-articular movement during healing.

Price CT, Lovell WW: Thompson arthrodesis of the hip in children. *J Bone Joint Surg* 1980;62A:1118–1123.

This is a report of 15 children and adolescents (average age 13 years) with Thompson-type intra- and extra-articular arthrodeses, which produced solid fusion in 14. Pain was resolved and function was satisfactory with the hip fused in 30° flexion. Progressive adduction with growth was not observed.

Sponseller PD, McBeath AA, Perpich M: Hip arthrodesis in young patients: A long-term follow-up study. *J Bone Joint Surg* 1984;66A: 853–859.

Long-term (20-year) follow-up of hip fusions performed before 35 years of age indicated generally satisfactory clinical results. Knee and back problems were troublesome but not disabling, and there was a high rate of employment among patients. Using modern techniques, surgeons should get as good or better results.

Section 8

The Knee

Carl L. Stanitski, MD

Knee Dislocation

Johnson E, Audell R, Oppenheim WL: Congenital dislocation of the knee. *J Pediatr Orthop* 1987;7:194–200.

Twenty-three congenital knee dislocations in 17 patients were reviewed at an average follow-up of 11 years after treatment. Eighty-eight percent of patients had significant associated musculoskeletal abnormalities: developmental dysplasia of the hip, 71%; clubfoot, 41%; congenital vertical talus, 18%. Serial casting after knee manipulation produced satisfactory results in ten knees, while open reduction and quadricepsplasty yielded satisfactory results in 13. The authors emphasize the need for treatment of knee dislocation before treatment of hip or foot deformities.

Ooishi T, Sugioka Y, Matsumoto S, et al: Congenital dislocation of the knee: Its pathologic features and treatment. *Clin Orthop* 1993;287: 187–192.

Arthrograms and operative findings in 26 congenitally dislocated knees revealed fundamental pathologic features, which included shortening of the quadriceps femoris tendon, tight anterior articular capsule, and hypoplasia of the suprapatellar bursa. The success of nonsurgical therapy depended on the extent of pathologic changes.

Parsch K, Schulz R: Ultrasonography in congenital dislocation of the knee. *J Pediatr Orthop* 1994;3B:76.

Ultrasound was used to evaluate ten congenitally hyperextended knees in seven patients shortly after birth and through the first year. Two knees had hyperextension (type I); five, subluxation (type II); and three, dislocation (type III). Ultrasound does not use ionizing radiation or need sedation/anesthesia. A posterior ultrasound approach is needed for type III knees. Verification of progress by ultrasonography provided the rationale for continued nonsurgical management.

Patella

Bourne MH, Bianco AJ Jr: Bipartite patella in the adolescent: Results of surgical excision. *J Pediatr Orthop* 1990;10:69–73.

At 7-year follow-up of 16 patients with excision of a type III fragment at an average age of 14.6 years, nine had pain after trauma and seven had insidious pain onset. Twelve had at least 6 months of a variety of treatments including immobilization, and 15 were improved postoperatively. This condition may represent a traction-type apophysis, such as Osgood-Schlatter's. All 16 patients had a complete fragment, ie, cleavage through bone and articular surface.

Fulkerson JP, Shea KP: Patello-femoral alignment. *J Bone Joint Surg* 1990;72A:1424–1429.

Classification of subluxation, tilt plus subluxation, and tilt alone is given for standard radiographs and computed tomography (CT) scans. Patients with only tilt and without chondral change do well with a lateral release. Those in the other two classes require more specific management. Imaging for patellar instability remains a static technique for a dynamic problem. Newer magnetic resonance imaging (MRI) programs may provide more kinetic (but nonweightbearing) data. Imaging should be done with the knee in less than 30° of flexion.

Gao GX, Lee EH, Bose K: Surgical management of congenital and habitual dislocation of the patella. *J Pediatr Orthop* 1990;10:255–260.

Twelve patients with congenital patellar dislocation were evaluated at an average of 5 years after surgery. Ten patellae remained centralized, full knee flexion was gained in 88%, and extensor lag took 3 to 6 months to recover. The authors recommended early surgical intervention. Patellar and quadriceps mechanism development appeared normal at follow-up in most patients.

Guidera KJ, Satterwhite Y, Ogden JA, et al: Nail patella syndrome: A review of 44 orthopaedic patients. *J Pediatr Orthop* 1991;11:737–742.

This multicenter analysis of an uncommon autosomal dominant tetrad of nail hypoplasia, patellar hypoplasia or absence, radial head subluxation/dislocation, and iliac horns found all patients to be ambulatory and foot abnormalities to be the chief presenting complaint. Twenty patients had knee surgery, including patellar realignment procedures in ten and various soft-tissue or bone procedures for knee extension or flexion deformities. Results of the knee procedures were mixed.

Guzzanti V, Gigante A, Di Lazzaro A, et al: Patellofemoral malalignment in adolescents: Computerized tomographic assessment with or without quadriceps contraction. *Am J Sports Med* 1994;22:55–60.

On CT scans of 27 adolescents with knee pain with and without minor patellar instability, measurements of various patellofemoral relationships were made with the knee in 15° of flexion and the quadriceps relaxed or contracted. Changes in type and severity of patellofemoral malalignment were seen in 52% after quadriceps contraction (more evident tilt and lateralization). This dynamic component is a helpful adjunct in difficult diagnostic circumstances and aids surgical decision-making.

Mori Y, Okumo H, Iketani H, et al: Efficacy of lateral retinacular release for painful bipartite patella. *Am J Sports Med* 1995;23:13–18.

The authors described an excisional lateral retinacular release used to treat 16 adolescent athletes' knees with symptomatic type II and III bipartite patellae. Fifteen knees had radiographic evidence of fragment union by 8 months postoperatively. Most (68%) had union and were asymptomatic within 4 months. Subjective and objective postoperative ratings showed excellent results.

Nietosvaara Y, Aalto K, Kallio PE: Acute patellar dislocation in children: Incidence and associated osteochondral fractures. *J Pediatr Orthop* 1994;14:513–515.

Seventy-two knees in 69 children (average age, 13.3 years) with acute, initial patellar dislocation were evaluated clinically, radiologically, and surgically. Forty-two percent had osteochondral fractures and an additional 13% had isolated chondral lesions. Radiologically silent osteochondral injury occurred in 20%. This study emphasizes the significant amount of articular damage done at the time of dislocation/relocation. Arthroscopy affords a more accurate diagnosis of intra-articular pathology, with simultaneous ability for surgical correction.

Safran MR, McDonough P, Seeger L, et al: Dorsal defect of the patella. *J Pediatr Orthop* 1994;14:603–607.

This report of eight superolateral patellar lesions in five patients followed up for 2 months to 9 years includes an excellent literature review. The lesion is characteristic with a sclerotic circular margin and lucent center with an average size of 9 mm. Rate of resolution of this radiographic curiosity is variable as is the final lesion morphology. The condition is self-limited, with resolution without sequelae. Hypotheses on its etiology include diminished blood flow to the patella's superior lateral corner, response to tension stress, and variant of ossification.

Stanciu C, Labelle HB, Morin B, et al: The value of computed tomography for the diagnosis of recurrent patellar subluxation in adolescents. *Can J Surg* 1994;37:319–323.

Forty adolescents with recurrent patellar subluxations were compared with a matched group of 14 normal volunteers by clinical examination and imaging (standard radiographs and CT scans). All volunteers had normal examinations and imaging. In the group with patellar subluxation, an increased lateral patellofemoral angle was seen on axial radiograph in 25% in neutral rotation and in 42% in tibial external rotation. Eighty-six percent had abnormal patellofemoral angles by CT criteria with abnormal centralization on CT in 79%. Eighty-eight percent of 25 asymptomatic knees with clinical evidence of subluxation also had imaging criteria for subluxation.

Stanitski CL: Anterior knee pain syndromes in the adolescent. *J Bone Joint Surg* 1993;75A:1407–1416.

This article reviews potential causes of anterior knee pain in adolescents (Osgood-Schlatter disease, Sinding-Larsen Johansson disease, multipartite patella, pathologic plica, and reflex sympathetic dystrophy). The need for a search for a specific diagnosis in "idiopathic" anterior knee pain is emphasized. Patellar instability, overuse conditions, and patellar lesions must be ruled out. The term "chondromalacia" applied to this condition is a misnomer, and its use should be eliminated.

Stanitski CL: Articular hypermobility and chondral injury in patients with acute patellar dislocation. *Am J Sports Med* 1995;23:146–150.

The relationship between generalized, nonpathologic articular hypermobility and chondral injury seen at arthroscopy was evaluated in 30 gender- and age-matched adolescents with initial noncontact patellar dislocations. Fifteen patients without hypermobility had 2.5 times increased frequency of articular damage. Articular lesions were radiographically "silent" in 71%. Acute patellar dislocation may cause intra-articular damage, which is unrecognized, especially in patients without ligamentous laxity.

Vainionpaa S, Laasonen E, Silvennoinen T, et al: Acute dislocation of the patella: A prospective review of operative treatment. *J Bone Joint Surg* 1990;72B:366–369.

Fifty-five patients (including 39 school children) with acute, primary patellar dislocations were prospectively studied at 3, 12, and 24 months postoperatively. Subjective results were excellent or good; 9% had redislocation within 2 years. The authors concluded that this primary surgery can improve function and diminish recurrence potential.

Menisci

Walsh ME, Tait GR, Bennett GC, et al: McMurray test in children. *J Pediatr Orthop* 1992;1B:79–80.

The knees of 513 children, 1 to 18 years of age, were tested for McMurray's sign (an audible clunk or palpable joint line click with knee hyperflexion) and generalized ligamentous laxity. One or both knees had positive McMurray tests in 30% of the patients, with lateral and medial sides equally represented. No evidence of increased laxity was found in 42% of patients; 21% met the criteria for hyperlaxity. No correlation was seen between increased ligamentous laxity and a positive McMurray test. The incidence of McMurray's sign and ligamentous laxity diminished with age; the changes were independent of gender.

General

Dietz FR, Mathews KD, Montgomery WJ: Reflex sympathetic dystrophy in children. *Clin Orthop* 1990;258:225–231.

Five new cases and 80 reported cases of reflex sympathetic dystrophy (RSD) in 3- to 17-year-old patients were reviewed. The increasing recognition of RSD in children and adolescents was emphasized. Diagnosis (as in adults) is based on prolonged pain out of proportion to injury/surgery, and skin hypersensitivity. In contrast to adults, lower extremity involvement was more common. Noninvasive, functional treatment resulted in symptom resolution without recurrence.

Henderson RC, Howes CL, Erickson KL, et al: Knee flexor-extensor strength in children. *J Orthop Sports Phys Ther* 1993;18:559–563.

The authors measured side-to-side differences in isokinetic quadriceps and hamstring strength measurements of 21 normal children 6 to 16 years old. Sixteen children were 12 years older or younger. Testing was done at angular velocities of 90° and 240°/second. A constant linear correlation for height, weight, and age was seen for maximum peak torque (MPT) values. A wide range of MPT was seen for each age group's side-to-side comparisons. The dominant leg (defined as the one used to kick a ball) did not constantly show increased strength.

Kanehisa H, Ikegawa S, Tsunoda N, et al: Strength and cross-sectional area of knee extensor muscles in childen. *Eur J Appl Physiol* 1994; 68:402–405.

The authors compared quadriceps isokinetic strength measurements and ultrasound determined knee extensor muscle cross-sectional area in 60 children 6 to 9 years old with similar measurements in 71 young adults. The ability of children to produce dynamic quadriceps peak torques was significantly lower than that of the adults, even when quadriceps mass was considered. Girls' peak torques were lower than boys'. The authors hypothesize that the age and gender differences are due to neural control (motor unit activation and recruitment) during voluntary contractions.

Kelly MA, Flock TJ, Kimmel JA, et al: MR imaging of the knee: Clarification of its role. *Arthroscopy* 1991;7:78–85.

This retrospective study compared 60 patients' MRI diagnoses with findings at arthroscopy. A wide age range included patients as young as 11 years. MRI of medial meniscal tears had 97% sensitivity and 77% specificity; MRI of lateral meniscal tears had 90% sensitivity and 87%

specificity. Seven of eight patients with anterior cruciate ligament (ACL) tears were correctly identified by MRI, but three of 52 patients without a tear were falsely diagnosed with a tear. MRI has a high negative predictive value. Advanced imaging technology and more uniform grading systems have improved MRI accuracy but limited data are present in the pediatric group. MRI should not replace a thorough history and physical examination as a screening tool.

LaPrade RF, Burnett QM II, Veenstra MA, et al: The prevalence of abnormal magnetic resonance imaging findings in asymptomatic knees: With correlation of magnetic resonance imaging to arthroscopic findings in symptomatic knees. *Am J Sports Med* 1994;22:739–745.

MRIs of 54 adult patients were studied prospectively. The subjects were asymptomatic and had normal clinical examinations. Meniscal tears were believed to be present in 5.6%: 1.9% medial and 3.7% lateral. Grade II signal changes (increased signal intensity not extending to the joint surface) were seen in 24% of medial meniscal posterior horns.

This study emphasizes the need for clinical correlation with imaging findings. Such grade II changes are believed to represent collagen degeneration and separation and are commonly reported in MRIs of knees of children and adolescents who have no clinical meniscal symptoms or findings. Caution must be taken to avoid overinterpretation and overresponse to what may be a normal physiologic variant.

Rodriquez Merchan EC, Galindo E, Ladreda JM, et al: Surgical synovectomy in haemophilic arthroscopy of the knee. *Int Orthop* 1994;18:38–41.

The authors reviewed 27 patients of similar ages who underwent surgical synovectomy to manage recurrent knee bleeds. Eighteen were treated by formal arthrotomy and nine by arthroscopy. Recurrent bleeds and replacement factor requirements were significantly diminished in both groups. In the small arthroscopically treated group, hospitalization time was 50% that of the open group. Knee range of motion was improved in seven of nine compared with loss of motion in the open group.

Safran MR, Johnston-Jones K, Kabo JM, et al: The effect of experimental hemarthrosis on joint stiffness and synovial histology in a rabbit model. *Clin Orthop* 1994;303:280–288.

The authors studied the effect of a single injection of autologous blood compared with a saline injection in the contralateral ankle in an immobilized and unimmobilized lapin model. Transient stiffness was produced in the hemarthrosis group; it was obvious at 10 days and abated by 28 days with no differences at that time in gross or microscopic appearance of either group of ankles. The authors concluded that an acute hemarthrosis in an otherwise uninjured joint does not compromise cartilage integrity or joint function.

Stanitski CL, Harvell JC, Fu F: Observations on acute knee hemarthrosis in children and adolescents. *J Pediatr Orthop* 1993;13:506–510.

The authors arthroscopically evaluated 70 patients, 15 preadolescents (7 to 12 years old) and 55 adolescents (13 to 18 years old) with acute traumatic knee hemarthroses. In preadolescents, 47% had isolated ACL tears, 47% had isolated meniscal tears, and 6% had combined meniscal and ACL tears. ACL tears were partial in 68%. In the adolescent group, 55% had isolated ACL tears, 27% had isolated meniscal tears, and 18% had a combination of meniscal and ACL tears; 62% of ACL tears were partial. Six percent had osteochondral injuries. The authors emphasize that hemarthrosis indicates a significant intra-articular injury that requires an accurate diagnosis so a specific treatment program can be prescribed.

Wilder RT, Berde CB, Wolohan M, et al: Reflex sympathetic dystrophy in children: Clinical characteristics and follow-up of seventy patients. *J Bone Joint Surg* 1992;74A:910–919.

The authors report a series of 70 patients with RSD whose average diagnostic delay was 1 year. The management algorithm presented includes functional clinical plus cognitive behavioral management techniques. Outcome in children was better than in adults.

Osteochondritis Dissecans

Crawfurd EJ, Emery RJ, Aichroth PM: Stable osteochondritis dissecans: Does the lesion unite? *J Bone Joint Surg* 1990;72B:320.

Thirty-one knees in 28 patients with arthroscopically documented stable femoral osteochondritis dissecans (OCD) were studied. Review at an average of 7.5 years after arthroscopy showed 13 of the 21 stable lesions had healed. Of the ten stable lesions in the "classical" position, only three had united. Ten of the other 11 lesions had healed. No correlation was seen with healing and lesion size, patient age, or gender.

Ligament Injuries

Angel KR, Hall DJ: Anterior cruciate ligament injury in children and adolescents. *Arthroscopy* 1989;5:197–200.

The authors reported arthroscopically documented ACL tears in 27 patients (31 knees in 2 preadolescents and 25 adolescents). Tears were partial in 59%. The authors noted correct clinical examination in only 39% of patients and strongly recommended arthroscopic assessment for any patient with an acute hemarthrosis.

Grace TG, Skipper BJ, Newberry JC, et al: Prophylactic knee braces and injury to the lower extremity. *J Bone Joint Surg* 1988;70A:422–427.

Over two football seasons, 580 high school players were prospectively studied to assess the effect of prophylactic knee braces. Two hundred forty-seven wore single and 83 wore double-hinged braces. The comparison group was 250 players of similar weight, height, and position who did not wear braces. Fifty-three knee injuries occurred and were significantly more frequent in the single-hinged brace group than in the nonbrace group. A significant increase in foot and ankle injuries was seen in the braced groups.

Graf BK, Lange RH, Fujisaki CK, et al: Anterior cruciate ligament tears in skeletally immature patients: Meniscal pathology at presentation and after attempted conservative treatment. *Arthroscopy* 1992;8:229–233.

Twelve skeletally immature patients 11 to 16 years old had arthroscopically documented complete ACL tears. Eight of 12 were treated nonsurgically with a brace and rehabilitation program and returned to high-demand sports. Knee instability symptoms developed at an average of 7 months, with seven of the eight developing meniscal tears. All eight eventually required transphyseal intra-articular reconstructions. Four patients had primary reconstruction, two intra-articular and two extra-articular. The two patients with extra-articular procedures required repeat reconstruction by intra-articular methods.

Jones RE, Henley MB, Francis P: Nonoperative management of isolated grade III collateral ligament injury in high school football players. *Clin Orthop* 1986;213:137–140.

Twenty-four scholastic (14 to 18 years old), skeletally mature football players with isolated grade III medial collateral ligament (MCL) tears were treated nonsurgically (protected motion, lower extremity muscle strengthening). All returned to play (average, 34 days) and were asymptomatic at follow-up. The authors emphasized that functional treatment, not surgery, is indicated for this isolated injury.

Liu SH, Lunsford T, Gude S, et al: Comparison of functional knee braces for control of anterior tibial displacement. *Clin Orthop* 1994;303:203–210.

The authors used a prosthetic "surrogate" knee model to evaluate the ability of ten custom functional braces to prevent anterior tibial displacement at loads from 50 to 400 N at an unspecified rate of loading. Displacement resistance was directly related to brace design, with post, bilateral hinged shell models providing the greatest translation resistance, which was still well below normal knee function.

McCarroll JR, Shelbourne KD, Porter DA, et al: Patellar tendon graft reconstruction for midsubstance anterior cruciate ligament rupture in junior high school athletes: An algorithm for management. *Am J Sports Med* 1994;22:478–484.

The authors report the results of treatment of arthroscopically documented acute midsubstance complete ACL tears in skeletally immature (by Tanner staging) patients. Follow-up ranged from 2 to 7 years (average, 4.3 years). In Tanner I to II patients, the authors recommend postponing ACL reconstruction until a more predictable adult-type reconstruction can be done. In the more mature patients, central physeal violation did not cause growth abnormalities.

Parker AW, Drez D Jr, Cooper JL: Anterior cruciate ligament injuries in patients with open physes. *Am J Sports Med* 1994;22:44–47.

The authors described the technique of physeal sparing, hamstring-incontinuity grafts for ACL reconstruction in six patients 10 to 14 years of age. At an average follow-up of 32-months, objective and functional testing showed excellent results, with no apparent effect on physeal growth.

Speer KP, Spritzer CE, Bassett FH III, et al: Osseous injury associated with acute tears of the anterior cruciate ligament. *Am J Sports Med* 1992;20:382–389.

The MRIs of 54 adolescents and young adults with arthroscopically documented acute ACL tears were retrospectively reviewed for the presence of osseous injury. A spectrum of soft and hard tissue posterolateral injury was seen. In follow-up of patients, chronic tears, such subchondral lesions, completely resolved within 90 days of the index injury.

The posterolateral tenderness often found at time of acute knee injury examination is related to the soft-tissue, articular cartilage, and subchondral bone insult and should not automatically be consigned to a lateral meniscal tear.

Stanitski CL: Anterior cruciate ligament injury in the skeletally immature patient: Diagnosis and treatment. *J Am Acad Orthop Surg* 1995;3:146–158.

This comprehensive review of ACL injury in skeletally immature patients emphasized accuracy of diagnosis and establishment of maturity state by physiologic (Tanner stages) and radiographic (bone age) criteria. Lesions were classified as acute (< 3 weeks); subacute, (3 to 12 weeks); and chronic, (> 12 weeks). Reconstruction can be by intra-articular physeal sparing, partial transphyseal techniques, or complete transphyseal techniques, depending on physeal maturity status. Extra-articular reconstructions alone have not been successful. Nonsurgical management emphasizes rehabilitation and activity modification to eliminate sports with high-demand deceleration/rotation stresses.

Wester W, Canale ST, Dutkowsky JP, et al: Prediction of angular deformity and leg-length discrepancy after anterior cruciate ligament reconstruction in skeletally immature patients. *J Pediatr Orthop* 1994;14:516–521.

The authors developed theoretic trigonometric derivatives using modifications of the Moseley graph to predict deformity magnitude after femoral and/or tibial transepiphyseal tunnels for ACL reconstruction. Peripheral bony bar formation was assumed. The incidence of such deformities after ACL surgery is unknown. Although mathematically sound on a theoretical basis, data are based on significant assumptions, eg, the 6- to 12-month range of error of bone-age determinations. Current surgical techniques use central, not peripheral tunnels, for reconstruction.

Plica

Johnson DP, Eastwood DM, Witherow PJ: Symptomatic synovial plicae of the knee. *J Bone Joint Surg* 1993;75A:1485–1496.

Forty-five knees in 30 patients (average age, 14 years) with symptomatic knee plicae were studied in this prospective, randomized, controlled double-blind study. All failed a 3-month nonsurgical treatment protocol and underwent arthroscopy. Group I (21 knees) did not have the pathologic plica excised, and group II (24 knees) had arthroscopic plica resection.

Pathologic plica formation must be evaluated as a consequence of abnormal patella tracking or recurrent overuse microtrauma. Plica resection is not indicated without specific criteria to document abnormality.

Osgood-Schlatter Disease

Krause BL, Williams JP, Catterall A: Natural history of Osgood-Schlatter disease. *J Pediatr Orthop* 1990;10:65–68.

This large series documenting the "natural" history of Osgood-Schlatter disease (OSD) provides a valuable baseline for comparison. The authors retrospectively reviewed 69 knees (62 patients) with a previous history of OSD at an average follow-up of 9 years (3 to 30 years). Twelve patients had varying periods of immobilization and 50 patients had no specific treatment. Sixty percent still complained of pain while kneeling, but 76% had no limitation of activity. Of the 12 patients who had continuing symptoms, nine had tubercle tenderness. The tubercle outline was clinically abnormal in 48 of 69 knees and more frequently noted in those with tubercle fragmentation on the initial radiographs. All 21 knees with normal profiles were completely asymptomatic. Results in patients treated with or without immobilization were the same.

Rosenberg ZS, Kawelblum M, Cheung YY, et al: Osgood-Schlatter lesion: Fracture or tendinitis? Scintigraphic, CT, and MR imaging features. *Radiology* 1992;185:853–858.

A variety of longitudinal imaging studies (other than routine radiographs) in 26 knees with OSD were retrospectively reviewed. Pre- and posttreatment and symptom resolution studies were done on 21 knees. Treatment was by knee immobilization or Lidocaine injection into the tibial tubercle. All patients had imaging evidence of tendinitis, which had almost fully resolved at time of follow-up when they were asymptomatic. Only one patient had evidence of increased bone scan activity at the tibial tubercle. The authors suggested that soft-tissue inflammation of the patellar tendon and the retrotendinous bursa and not an avulsion fracture is the source of symptoms.

Section 9

The Foot and Ankle

R. Jay Cummings, MD

Normal Feet

Ounpuu S, Gage JR, Davis RB: Three-dimensional lower extremity joint kinetics in normal pediatric gait. *J Pediatr Orthop* 1991;11:341–349.

Thirty-one normal children aged 5 to 16 years underwent complete gait analysis, including calculations of their three-dimensional joint kinematics and kinetics. Their data were similar to those for normal adults. This study establishes a normal reference to which other children's data can be compared.

Vanderwilde R, Staheli LT, Chew DE, et al: Measurements on radiographs of the foot in normal infants and children. *J Bone Joint Surg* 1988; 70A:407–415.

In this study, 74 normal infants and children aged 6 to 127 months had standing anteroposterior (AP), lateral, and maximum dorsiflexion lateral radiographs. Eleven angles were measured on their films, establishing a range of normal values for each angle for the various ages represented in the study.

Clubfoot

Pathologic Anatomy

Dimeglio A, Bensahel H, Souchet P, et al: Classification of clubfoot. *J Pediatr Orthop* 1995;4B:129–136.

A scale of 0 to 20 was established on the basis of four parameters: equinus in the sagittal plane, varus deviation in the frontal plane, derotation around the talus of the calcaneo-forefoot block, and adduction of the forefoot on the hindfoot in the horizontal plane. Using these parameters, four grades of clubfeet were identified.

Gray DH, Katz JM: A histochemical study of muscle in clubfoot. *J Bone Joint Surg* 1981;63B:417–423.

One hundred three muscle biopsies from 62 patients with clubfeet were analyzed. Thirteen patients with unilateral deformities had the normal leg sampled as a control. No significant differences were present in fiber diameter, indicating calf wasting is due to a reduction in number of fibers. Affected soleus muscles had a greater percentage of type 1 fibers than controls.

Howard CB, Benson MK: Clubfoot: Its pathological anatomy. *J Pediatr Orthop* 1993;13:654–659.

This study, based on anatomic dissection of three clubfoot specimens, confirmed the long-accepted finding of abnormal talar neck direction in clubfoot. Tibial torsion was not present and medial rotation of the talus in the ankle joint resulted from plantarflexion and was not pathologic. The subtalar joint was abnormal, leading to supination of the calcaneus with its anterior pole coming to rest beneath the talus. No abnormalities in the calcaneocuboid joint were present.

Howard CB, Benson MK: The ossific nuclei and the cartilage anlage of the talus and calcaneum. *J Bone Joint Surg* 1992;74B:620–623.

This comparison, based on anatomical dissection of two clubfoot specimens and one normal specimen, demonstrated that the hindfoot ossific nuclei are positioned differently in their anlages in clubfeet than in the hindfoot anlage of normal feet. This difference renders radiographic angular measurement comparisons between clubfeet and normal feet prone to error.

Johnston CE II, Hobatho MC, Baker KJ, et al: Three-dimensional analysis of clubfoot deformity by computed tomography. *J Pediatr Orthop* 1995;4B:39–48.

Bone pathoanatomy of clubfoot was analyzed by 3-D reconstruction of transverse CT images obtained from 27 feet in children aged 3 to 10 years. This technique shows deformity that normally cannot be analyzed on plain radiographs and shows that a variety of interosseous relationships make up the clinical entity of clubfoot.

Maffulli N, Capasso G, Testa V, et al: Histochemistry of the triceps surae muscle in idiopathic congenital clubfoot. *Foot Ankle* 1992;13:80–84.

This study, in contrast to that of Gray and Katz, found no difference in the percentage of type 1 fibers in the calf muscles between clubfeet and normal controls.

Sodre H, Bruschini S, Mestriner LA, et al: Arterial abnormalities in talipes equinovarus as assessed by angiography and the Doppler technique. *J Pediatr Orthop* 1990;10:101–104.

Preoperative angiograms of 30 clubfeet demonstrated abnormalities in all but two, with the posterior tibial artery serving as the sole blood supply in most clubfeet. Postoperative Doppler flow studies did not confirm the arteriogram findings and are, therefore, believed to be unreliable.

Genetics

Cowell HR, Wein BK: Genetic aspects of clubfoot. *J Bone Joint Surg* 1980;62A:1381–1384.

This current concepts review examines the genetics of congenital clubfoot; it describes deformity associated with extrinsic causes, syndromes with known Mendelian inheritance, and cytogenetic abnormalities. The most common type, known as the idiopathic variety, is primarily associated with a multifactorial inheritance, with the genetic influence acting in a dominant fashion.

Nonsurgical Treatment

Bensahel H, Catterall A, Dimeglio A: Practical applications in idiopathic clubfoot: A retrospective multicentric study in EPOS. *J Pediatr Orthop* 1990;10:186–188.

Survey revealed that most EPOS members treated idiopathic clubfoot at birth with plaster casts; results of this conservative treatment vary. Surgery usually is indicated at an age ranging from 4 to 15 months. A classification system for idiopathic clubfoot is proposed.

Bensahel H, Guillaume A, Czukonyi Z, et al: Results of physical therapy for idiopathic clubfoot: A long-term follow-up study. *J Pediatr Orthop* 1990;10:189–192.

These authors report that of 338 feet treated with a physical therapy program, 77% achieved good or fair results as determined by follow-up from ages 10 to 14 years. With surgery for the physical therapy failures, the percentage of good and fair results reached 96%.

Kite HJ: Principles involved in the treatment of congenital club-foot: The results of treatment. *J Bone Joint Surg* 1939;21:595–606.

This article outlines the principles of and describes a technique for non-surgical treatment of congenital clubfoot through serial manipulation and casting.

Ponseti IV: Treatment of congenital clubfoot. *J Bone Joint Surg* 1992; 74A:448–454.

This review reports an 89% success rate for treatment consisting of manipulation and serial casting. Percutaneous Achilles tenotomy was performed during the initial casting in 70% of patients. The condition recurred in 50% of patients, who required repeat casting and often anterior tendon transfer as well.

Surgical Treatment: Soft-Tissue Release

Cooper DM, Dietz FR: Treatment of idiopathic clubfoot: A thirty-year follow-up note. *J Bone Joint Surg* 1995;77A:1477–1489.

Review of 45 patients with 71 congenital clubfeet suggests that a sedentary occupation and avoidance of excessive weight gain may improve the overall long-term result. Because excessive weakening of the triceps surae may predispose patients to poor results, overlengthening of this muscle should be avoided. The outcome could not be predicted from the radiographic result of surgical treatment.

Hudson I, Catterall A: Posterolateral release for resistant club foot. *J Bone Joint Surg* 1994;76B:281–284.

Fifty-three feet that had undergone posterior lateral release were reviewed at an average follow-up of 10 years. Of 17 feet that required reoperation, only one was rated as unsatisfactory; that one had had four procedures including a bony operation. Keeping that in mind, the overall success rate for the group was 68%.

Hutchins PM, Foster BK, Paterson AC, et al: Long-term results of early surgical release in clubfeet. *J Bone Joint Surg* 1985;67B:791–799.

This article reports the results at an average follow-up of 15 years, 10 months, for 252 clubfeet that underwent posterior release. Surgery was performed after failure of manipulation and casting and generally within the first year of life. Additional procedures were done on one fourth of the patients before follow-up. Overall 81% of patients achieved a satisfactory result.

McKay DW: New concept of and approach to clubfoot treatment: Section I. Principles and morbid anatomy. *J Pediatr Orthop* 1982;2:347–356.

McKay DW: New concept of and approach to clubfoot treatment: Section II. Correction of the clubfoot. *J Pediatr Orthop* 1983;3:10–21.

McKay DW: New concept of and approach to clubfoot treatment: Section III. Evaluation and results. *J Pediatr Orthop* 1983;3:141–148.

These three classic articles describe a different concept for the pathoanatomy and treatment of clubfoot. The surgery is described and an evaluation at an average follow-up of 3 years, 2 months is included.

Simons GW: Complete subtalar release in clubfeet: Part I. A preliminary report. Part II. Comparison with less extensive procedures. *J Bone Joint Surg* 1985;67A:1044–1065.

In Section I of this article, the author describes his technique for circumferential soft-tissue release for congenital clubfoot. Section II compares the results of more limited soft-tissue releases in 26 feet to 25 feet treated by circumferential release at an average follow-up of 39 and 29 months, respectively. The limited procedures resulted in 5% clinical and 46% radiographic satisfactory results compared to 72% clinical and 64% radiographic satisfactory results for the more extensive procedure.

Stanitski CL, Ward WT, Grossman W: Noninvasive vascular studies in clubfoot. *J Pediatr Orthop* 1992;12:514–517.

Pulse oximetry and Doppler evaluation proved to be readily available, noninvasive, and reproducible means of monitoring vascular integrity in 50 clubfeet undergoing comprehensive soft-tissue releases.

Thometz JG, Simons GW: Deformity of the calcaneocuboid joint in patients who have talipes equinovarus. *J Bone Joint Surg* 1993; 75A:190–195.

A retrospective analysis of 100 postoperative clubfeet uncovered 26 with significant calcanocuboid joint deformity. Of 24 feet with this abnormality at over 2 years follow-up, 11 treated with complete release of the joint had normal alignment. All deformed joints that did not undergo complete release remained deformed.

Turco VJ: Resistant congenital clubfoot: One-stage posteromedial release with internal fixation. A follow-up report of a fifteen-year experience. *J Bone Joint Surg* 1979;61A:805–814.

The results of posterior medial release in 149 feet were evaluated at 2 to 15 years after surgery. The percentage of excellent and good results did not diminish with longer follow-up. Prolonged nonsurgical treatment and prior surgery were associated with poor results. The optimal age for surgery was between 1 and 2 years of age. Overall results were 83.8% excellent or good, 10.7% fair, and 5.3% failure.

Yngve DA, Gross RH, Sullivan JA: Clubfoot release without wide subtalar release. *J Pediatr Orthop* 1990;10:473–476.

The results of the soft-tissue release procedure popularized by Goldner were reviewed in 52 feet at a mean follow-up of 7 years. Eleven feet had undergone another procedure by the time of review. Eighty-two percent were rated good or excellent. An advantage of the procedure was believed to be that only 4% of patients were found to have overcorrection.

Surgical Treatment: Tendon Transfers

Laaveg SJ, Ponseti IV: Long-term results of treatment of congenital club foot. *J Bone Joint Surg* 1980;62A:23–31.

This review of 104 feet, conducted at a mean age of 18.8 years, found 90% of patients were satisfied and 88.5% had satisfactory objective ratings. Serial casting was supplemented by percutaneous Achilles tendon lengthening in 93%. Forty-eight feet had supplemental transfer of the anterior tibial tendon to the third cuneiform, a procedure which was found to reduce the frequency of recurrence.

Surgical Treatment: Bony Operations

Addison A, Fixsen JA, Lloyd-Roberts GC: A review of the Dillwyn Evans type collateral operation in severe club feet. *J Bone Joint Surg* 1983; 65B:12–14.

The results of posterior medial release combined with lateral column shortening at the calcaneocuboid joint were evaluated in 45 feet at an average follow-up of 9 years, 9 months. Forty-two had failed previous surgery. Thirty feet were rated as satisfactory.

Hjelmstedt A, Sahlstedt B: Role of talocalcaneal osteotomy in clubfoot surgery: Results in 31 surgically treated feet. *J Pediatr Orthop* 1990; 10:193–197.

This study reports the results of osteotomy through the talar neck to correct medial and plantar deviation in 31 feet at a mean follow-up of 11 years, 3 months. Twenty-two had undergone previous surgery. There were 19 good, six fair, and six poor results.

McHale KA, Lenhart MK: Treatment of residual clubfoot deformity—the "bean shaped" foot—by opening wedge medial cuneiform osteotomy and closing wedge cuboid osteotomy: Clinical review and cadaver correlations. *J Pediatr Orthop* 1991;11:374–381.

The procedure described in the title proved successful in six of seven feet at an average follow-up of over 2 years. This procedure was believed to correct both forefoot adduction and midfoot supination and was suitable for patients too old for soft-tissue release and too young for triple arthrodesis.

Sangeorzan BJ, Mosca V, Hansen ST Jr: Effect of calcaneal lengthening on relationships among the hindfoot, midfoot, and forefoot. *Foot Ankle* 1993;14:136–141.

In this study based on pre- and postoperative standing radiographs of seven feet, Evans' concepts of the relationship between deformity and medial versus lateral column length were confirmed. Information useful for calculating the graft size required to correct various deformities is also presented.

Miscellaneous

Grant AD, Atar D, Lehman WB: The Ilizarov technique in correction of complex foot deformities. *Clin Orthop* 1992;280:94–103.

This article presents an overview of the indications, techniques, and results of the Ilizarov technique for various complex foot deformities. This technique may occasionally be useful in clubfoot correction.

McKay DW: Dorsal bunions in children. *J Bone Joint Surg* 1983;65A: 975–980.

In this series of 24 feet, 11 dorsal bunions occurred in children with surgically treated clubfeet. The results of transferring the flexor brevis and abductor and adductor muscles of the hallux to the first metatarsal neck supplemented with capsular release and tenodesis or arthrodesis of the metatarsophalangeal joint in 17 of these feet were reviewed at a mean 5-year follow-up. All children having the complete procedures were corrected.

Metatarsus Adductus

Berg EE: A reappraisal of metatarsus adductus and skewfoot. *J Bone Joint Surg* 1986;68A:1185–1196.

This study of 84 patients with 124 involved feet establishes a radiographic classification of metatarsus adductus and skewfoot deformity. This classification proved useful in that it demonstrated that feet with deformity classified as simple metatarsus adductus all resolved whether treated or not. Feet in the other three (progressively more complex deformity) groups required correspondingly longer casting to achieve correction. The use of a Denis Browne bar holding the foot in external rotation predisposed patients to a flatfoot deformity.

Berman A, Gartland JJ: Metatarsal osteotomy for the correction of adduction of the fore part of the foot in children. *J Bone Joint Surg* 1971;53A:498–506.

Seventy-eight patients were evaluated at an average 5-year follow-up to determine the results of metatarsal osteotomies for forefoot adduction. Of 18 children with congenital metatarsus varus, all but one had excellent or good results. Of 44 children with adduction due to residual clubfoot deformity, 37 had excellent or good results, five were fair, and two were poor. All poor results were due to loss of position, and pin fixation was therefore recommended. The operation was recommended for children 6 years of age and older.

Pentz AS, Weiner DS: Management of metatarsus adductovarus. *Foot Ankle* 1993;14:241–246.

In this retrospective review of 795 patients, the incidence of the deformity was not related to birth weight or birth order, a finding inconsistent with an intrauterine molding etiology. The combination of reverse last shoes and a Denis Browne bar was associated with a 99% incidence of excellent or good results, a success rate superior to historic natural history controls.

Peterson HA: Skewfoot (forefoot adduction with heel valgus). *J Pediatr Orthop* 1986;6:24–30.

This report includes an excellent review of the literature on this topic and adds four more cases to the literature. Although one patient was successfully treated nonsurgically, three required surgical correction. The deformity was noted to recur unless hindfoot stabilization was a part of the procedure.

Smith JT, Bleck EE, Gamble JG, et al: Simple method of documenting metatarsus adductus. *J Pediatr Orthop* 1991;11:679–680.

A simple, accurate, and inexpensive method of documenting metatarsus adductus involves taking photocopies of the foot in the weightbearing position. Treatment progress can be evaluated by reviewing serial photocopies.

Stark JG, Johanson JE, Winter RB: The Heyman-Herndon tarsal-metatarsal capsulotomy for metatarsus adductus: Results in 48 feet.
J Pediatr Orthop 1987;7:305–310.

This series documents a high failure rate (41%) in patients undergoing tarsometatarsal capsulotomy procedure for simple metatarsus adduction as well as deformity related to clubfoot and other orthopaedic conditions. Half of the patients reported a painful dorsal prominence postoperatively. Age at surgery had no effect on results.

Flatfoot

Evans D: Calcaneo-valgus deformity. *J Bone Joint Surg* 1975;57B: 270–278.

This article describes the results of lengthening of the lateral column of the foot in 56 feet. The operation was found not to be reliable for spastic or spina bifida feet, but in flat feet due to polio, severe idiopathic valgus, and even rigid feet due to calcaneo-navicular bar, correction was achieved and triple arthrodesis avoided.

Forriol F, Pascual J: Footprint analysis between three and seventeen years of age. *Foot Ankle* 1990;11:101–104.

One thousand six hundred seventy-six children, aged 3 to 17 years, were evaluated by measuring their Chippaux-Smirvak Index and foot print angles. The incidence of low arches was significantly greater in the younger age groups than in the older age groups. Based on their study, the authors concluded arch development may occur up to age 5 or 6 years in normal children.

Fraser RK, Menelaus MB, Williams PF, et al: The Miller procedure for mobile flat feet. *J Bone Joint Surg* 1995;77B:369–399.

Twenty-two patients (38 feet) with persistently symptomatic mobile flat feet associated with isolated naviculocuneiform break were treated with the Miller procedure at an average age of 13 years. Satisfactory results were obtained in 84%.

MacNicol MF, Voutsinas S: Surgical treatment of the symptomatic accessory navicular. *J Bone Joint Surg* 1984;66B:218–226.

The authors compare the results of excision of the accessory navicular with posterior tibial tendon advancement (Kidner's operation) in 26 patients to results of simple excision of the accessory navicular and contouring of the remaining navicular in 21 patients. Because the results were identical in both groups, they concluded that the 6 week postoperative casting after the Kidner procedure could not be justified.

Mosca VS: Calcaneal lengthening for valgus deformity of the hindfoot: Results in children who have severe, symptomatic flatfoot and skewfoot. *J Bone Joint Surg* 1995;77A:500–512.

Severe, symptomatic valgus deformities of the hindfoot in 20 children who had flatfoot (25 feet) or skewfoot (6 feet) were corrected clinically and radiographically in all but two of the most severely deformed feet. Pain and callus were eliminated, bracewear was tolerated, and shoe wear was improved.

Pirani SP, Tredwell SJ, Beauchamp RD: Extraarticular subtalar arthrodesis: The dowel method. *J Pediatr Orthop* 1990;10:244–247.

Fifty feet in 30 children were treated with extra-articular subtalar arthrodesis for valgus deformities resulting from myelomeningocele, idiopathic flatfoot, and cerebral palsy. Results were excellent in 56%, satisfactory in 30%, and unsatisfactory in 14%. Intraoperative positioning error and simultaneous peroneal tendon lengthening in children with cerebral palsy were the major sources of unsatisfactory results.

Rao UB, Joseph B: The influence of footwear on the prevalence of flat foot: A survey of 2,300 children. *J Bone Joint Surg* 1992;74B:525–527.

Foot print analysis of 2,300 children who differed only in their frequency and type of shoewear demonstrated that children wearing closed toed shoes had the highest likelihood of flat feet. Children who did not wear shoes at all were the most likely to develop arches, and children who wore sandals had intermediate arch development.

Congenital Vertical Talus

Coleman SS, Stelling FH III, Jarett J: Pathomechanics and treatment of congenital vertical talus. *Clin Orthop* 1970;70:62–72.

These authors conclude that nonsurgical treatment, while helpful for stretching, does not correct this deformity. A two-staged surgical procedure is recommended. First, the extensor tendons are lengthened, the talo-navicular joint reduced and fixed, and if the child is 2.5 to 3 years old, a Grice procedure is performed. Six weeks later, a posterior release and advancement of the posterior tibial tendon are performed.

Jacobsen ST, Crawford AH: Congenital vertical talus. *J Pediatr Orthop* 1983;3:306–310.

The results of the Coleman-Stelling two-staged correction for congenital vertical talus are reported for nine patients with an average 2.1-year follow-up. The patients achieved an 8.89 out of a possible 10 rating postoperatively. Only one patient required further surgery.

Ogata K, Schoenecker PL, Sheridan J: Congenital vertical talus and its familial occurrence: An analysis of 36 patients. *Clin Orthop* 1979; 139:128–132.

This series of 57 feet represents the largest group of patients with this problem seen at one institution. For patients with the primary isolated type deformity, there was a 50% incidence of foot deformities in first degree relatives. Nonsurgical treatment was unsuccessful and two-stage procedures were associated with a high rate of complications, especially osteonecrosis of the talus. The authors recommended a one-stage correction.

Seimon LP: Surgical correction of congenital vertical talus under the age of two years. *J Pediatr Orthop* 1987;7:405–411.

Ten congenital vertical talus feet in seven patients were treated with simple open reduction of the talonavicular joint, lengthening of any tight extensor tendons, and percutaneous Achilles tendon lengthening as a one-stage procedure. Excellent results were obtained in seven feet and good results in the remaining three.

Walker AP, Ghali NN, Silk FF: Congenital vertical talus: The results of staged operative reduction. *J Bone Joint Surg* 1985;67B:117–121.

In 15 feet with congenital vertical talus, nonsurgical treatment could not completely correct the deformity. A two-staged release procedure without internal fixation or a Grice procedure produced satisfactory outcomes in 12 of the 15 feet at follow-up ranging from 1.5 to 21 years.

Tarsal Coalition

Gonzalez P, Kumar SJ: Calcaneonavicular coalition treated by resection and interposition of the extensor digitorum brevis muscle. *J Bone Joint Surg* 1990;72A:71–77.

In this large series of calcaneonavicular coalitions (75 feet), 77% rated good or excellent at final follow-up. Three feet with fair results initially improved to good over time. Talar beaking was not a contraindication to surgery. Best results were seen in patients between 11 and 15 years old at the time of surgery and those with cartilaginous bars. Partial reformation of the bar was seen in 23% of feet as compared to the up to 66% recurrence rate reported when no interposition is performed.

Kumar SJ, Guille JT, Lee MS, et al: Osseous and non-osseous coalition of the middle facet of the talocalcaneal joint. *J Bone Joint Surg* 1992; 74A:529–535.

Of 18 feet (16 patients) treated with resection of the coalition, 16 had excellent or good results. Three types of talocalcaneal coalition were identified, but did not influence the final result. Fibrous coalitions were the most difficult to detect.

Inglis G, Buxton RA, Macnicol MF: Symptomatic calcaneonavicular bars: The results 20 years after surgical excision. *J Bone Joint Surg* 1986; 68B:128–131.

Although this series is small (16 feet), it is important because it provides long-term (minimum 20 year, average 23 year) follow-up of the results of surgical excision of calcaneonavicular bars. Sixty-nine percent of feet had good or excellent results. Failures were more common in patients with preoperative talar beaking and responded better to triple arthrodesis than repeat bar excision.

Mosier KM, Asher M: Tarsal coalitions and peroneal spastic flatfoot: A review. *J Bone Joint Surg* 1984;66A:976–984.

This excellent review based on 60 references outlines the history, incidence, genetics, clinical presentation, radiographic findings, differential diagnosis, and pathomechanics of this condition. A trial of nonsurgical treatment is recommended initially and is reported to be effective in one third of patients. Surgical resection was believed to be a proven procedure for calcaneonavicular coalitions and possibly for talocalcaneal coalitions as well.

Moyes ST, Crawfurd EJ, Aichroth PM: The interposition of extensor digitorum brevis in the resection of calcaneonavicular bars. *J Pediatr Orthop* 1994;14:387–388.

After resection of 19 calcaneonavicular bars for peroneal spastic flatfoot, with interposition of the extensor digitorum brevis, asymptomatic mobile feet were obtained in 90% with no recurrence of the bar.

Olney BW, Asher MA: Excision of symptomatic coalition of the middle facet of the talocalcaneal joint. *J Bone Joint Surg* 1987;69A:539–544.

The results of surgical excision of middle facet talocalcaneal coalitions in ten feet at 42-month follow-up were eight excellent or good, one fair, and one poor. Age, sex, coalition type, and the presence of talar beaking did not correlate with outcome.

Takakura Y, Sugimoto K, Tanaka Y, et al: Symptomatic talocalcaneal coalition: Its clinical significance and treatment. *Clin Orthop* 1991; 269:249–256.

This is one of the largest reported series of talocalcaneal coalitions. Of 67 feet, 36 required surgery. Thirty one of 33 undergoing bar resection were rated excellent or good at follow-up. Three feet treated with arthrodesis had good results. In 23 patients, an associated tarsal tunnel syndrome was present.

Wilde PH, Torode IP, Dickens DR, et al: Resection for symptomatic talocalcaneal coalition. *J Bone Joint Surg* 1994;76B:797–801.

This study of the results of surgical resection of talocalcaneal coalitions in 20 feet found fair or poor results in half the patients. Talar beaking was not predictive of a poor result. Coalition of more than 50% of the area of the posterior facet, heel valgus of more than 16°, narrowing of the posterior talocalcaneal joint, and impingement of the lateral process of the talus on the calcaneus were all associated with poor results.

Adolescent Bunions

Canale PB, Aronsson DD, Lamont RL, et al: The Mitchell procedure for the treatment of adolescent hallux valgus: A long term study. *J Bone Joint Surg* 1993;75A:1610–1618.

From a group of 53 adolescents undergoing 88 Mitchell osteotomies, 30 were available for review at an average of 7 years after surgery. Results were excellent or good in 68%, fair in 12%, and poor in 20%. Poor fixation and failure to plantarflex the distal fragment were associated with suboptimal results.

Geissele AE, Stanton RP: Surgical treatment of adolescent hallux valgus. *J Pediatr Orthop* 1990;10:642–648.

Of 253 patients with adolescent hallux valgus, all but 39 were managed nonsurgically. Surgical results of 32 feet were evaluated at an average 9-year follow-up. Satisfactory results were obtained in 70%. The most common cause of dissatisfaction was a persistent increased intermetatarsal angle.

Groiso JA: Juvenile hallux valgus: A conservative approach to treatment. *J Bone Joint Surg* 1992;74A:1367–1374.

In this study, 56 children with hallux valgus were treated with corrective splinting. Improvement was obtained in 50% and was maintained at 2- to 6-year follow-up.

Houghton GR, Dickson RA: Hallux valgus in the younger patient: The structural abnormality. *J Bone Joint Surg* 1979;61B:176–177.

In this comparison of the radiographs of 50 patients with hallux valgus to those of 15 control patients, it was found that although the intemetatarsal angle was increased in patients with hallux valgus, the angle between the long axis of the medial cuneiform and the first metatarsal (metatarsus primus varus angle) was not increased. The authors concluded that the primary structural abnormality in this condition is valgus angulation of the second through the fifth metatarsals.

Kilmartin TE, Barrington RL, Wallace WA: Metatarsus primus varus: A statistical study. *J Bone Joint Surg* 1991;73B:937–940.

This radiographic study of 36 children with unilateral hallux valgus and 65 with bilateral hallux valgus confirmed an increased intermetatarsal angle in early juvenile hallux valgus. This increase was not the result of intercuneiform splaying, deformity of the medial cuneiform, metatarsal varus, or abnormal growth of the first metatarsal.

Kilmartin TE, Wallace WA: The significance of pes planus in juvenile hallux valgus. *Foot Ankle* 1992;13:53–56.

This study compared arch height in 32 11-year-olds with hallux valgus to that in 32 controls. No correlation between decreased arch height and the likelihood of having hallux valgus could be demonstrated.

Mann RA, Rudicel S, Graves SC: Repair of hallux valgus with a distal soft-tissue procedure and proximal metatarsal osteotomy: A long-term follow-up. *J Bone Joint Surg* 1992;74A:124–129.

Ninety-three percent of 75 patients with 109 treated feet were satisfied with this procedure at an average 34-month follow-up. This series included seven patients younger than 20 years old.

Peterson HA, Newman S: Adolescent bunion deformity treated with double osteotomy and longitudinal pin fixation of the first ray. *J Pediatr Orthop* 1993;13:80–84.

In ten patients with 15 affected feet, a closing medial wedge osteotomy of the distal first metatarsal was combined with a proximal opening medial wedge osteotomy. The combination allowed correction of deformity without metatarsal shortening. Pin fixation prevented loss of correction. Thir-teen feet were rated satisfactory at an average 32.5-month follow-up.

Congenital Short Achilles Tendon

Griffin PP, Wheelhouse WW, Shiavi R, et al: Habitual toe-walkers: A clinical and electromyographic gait analysis. *J Bone Joint Surg* 1977;59A:97–101.

In this study, six patients who habitually walked on their toes but could when asked walk with a heel-toe gait were treated with serial casts. These patients' pre- and posttreatment electromyograms (EMGs) were compared to EMGs for six control patients. Before treatment, the toe walkers demonstrated prolonged and increased anterior tibialis activity, which was thought to be a response to a shortened triceps surae. No patient required Achilles tendon lengthening and all patients responded to serial casting. Posttreatment EMGs demonstrated a return of normal tibialis anterior function.

Hall JE, Salter RB, Bhalla SK: Congenital short tendo calcaneus. *J Bone Joint Surg* 1967;49B:695–697.

This report describes 20 patients with an average age of 7.5 years who were toe walkers and demonstrated equinus deformities of 30° to 60°. After 6 to 24 months of observation, they failed to demonstrate spontaneous resolution and Achilles tendon lengthening was performed. At an average follow-up of 3 years postoperatively, all had a normal gait.

Katz MM, Mubarak SJ: Hereditary tendo Achillis contractures. *J Pediatr Orthop* 1984;4:711–714.

This study of eight patients who walked with a toe-toe pattern confirmed the effectiveness of serial casting for these patients and suggested an autosomal dominant mode of inheritance. Even though ankle dorsiflexion decreased with time after treatment and toe walking occasionally recurred, Achilles tendon lengthening was not found to be necessary.

Osteochondroses of the Foot

Canale ST, Belding RH: Osteochondral lesions of the talus. *J Bone Joint Surg* 1980;62A:97–102.

In this retrospective review of 31 ankles with osteochondral lesions, lateral lesions proved to be the result of trauma, were shallow, were prone to displacement, and were more likely to cause persistent symptoms. Medial lesions were both traumatic and atraumatic, deep, and less symptomatic. Recommendations as to conservative versus surgical treatment based on the Berndt and Harty classification are included.

Citron N, Neil M: Dorsal wedge osteotomy of the proximal phalanx for hallux rigidus: Long-term results. *J Bone Joint Surg* 1987;69B:835–837.

In this small series, eight patients with ten affected toes were evaluated at an average follow-up of 22 years after osteotomy of the proximal phalanx designed to provide more dorsiflexion. Five patients remained pain free, four had mild soreness, one required metatarsophalangeal fusion.

Falkenberg MP, Dickens DR, Menelaus MB: Osteochondritis of the first metatarsal epiphysis. *J Pediatr Orthop* 1990;10:797–799.

Two cases of osteochondritis of the epiphysis at the base of the first metatarsal are reported. Both did well with symptomatic treatment.

Ippolito E, Ricciardi Pollini PT, Falez F: Kohler's disease of the tarsal navicular: Long-term follow-up of 12 cases. *J Pediatr Orthop* 1984; 4:416–417.

This series of 12 patients, reviewed at a minimum of 30 years after presentation, represents the longest term follow-up of this problem in the literature. The average age at presentation was 6 years and all patients had unilateral symptomatic disease. Nine patients were treated with walking casts for 3 months and three patients were treated with arch supports and rest. All demonstrated complete bony restoration between 6 and 13 months after onset, and no differences were seen based on treatment regimen. No patients had problems at long-term follow-up.

Mann RA, Coughlin MJ, DuVries HL: Hallux rigidus: A review of the literature and a method of treatment. *Clin Orthop* 1979;142:57–63.

This article reports the results of cheilectomy in 20 patients with hallux rigidus at an average follow-up of 67 months. Three patients had mild residual pain. Postoperative dorsiflexion averaged 30°.

McMaster MJ: The pathogenesis of hallux rigidus. *J Bone Joint Surg* 1978;60B:82–87.

This study reports the clinical, radiographic, and pathologic features of hallux rigidus. All patients had pain on motion. Dorsiflexion was limited more than plantarflexion. Radiographs demonstrated a subchondral defect in the metatarsal head. Pathologic examination revealed a cleavage defect in the articular surface. Trauma is postulated as the etiology. Over half of the patients required arthrodesis.

Micheli LJ, Ireland ML: Prevention and management of calcaneal apophysitis in children: An overuse syndrome. *J Pediatr Orthop* 1987;7:34–38.

Eighty-five children with 137 affected heels were diagnosed as having Sever's disease. Most demonstrated heel cord tightness and 16 had forefoot pronation. Patients were treated with stretching exercises, heelcups, and/or orthotics. The average time to return of sports was two months. There were only two recurrences with this regimen.

Mubarak SJ: Osteochondrosis of the lateral cuneiform: Another cause of a limp in a child: A case report. *J Bone Joint Surg* 1992;74A:285–289.

This case report is significant in that it is the first report of osteochondrosis of the lateral cuneiform. It also reviews the literature on osteochondrosis of the medial and intermediate cuneiforms. The prognosis for all of these appears to be excellent with symptomatic treatment alone.

Smith TW, Stanley D, Rowley DI: Treatment of Freiberg's disease: A new operative technique. *J Bone Joint Surg* 1991;73B:129–130.

This relatively large series included 28 patients with this problem. Thirteen improved with shoe inserts or cast immobilization. The remaining 15 were treated with a shortening procedure (4 mm) of the involved metatarsal. Pain was relieved in all but one patient at a mean follow-up of 4.9 years.

Peroneal Tendon Instability

Andersen E: Stenosing peroneal tenosynovitis symptomatically simulating ankle instability. *Am J Sports Med* 1987;15:258–259.

This entity, which may present as a "snapping" ankle with complaints of instability, is described together with its surgical findings and treatment.

Micheli LJ, Waters PM, Sanders DP: Sliding fibular graft repair for chronic dislocation of the peroneal tendons. *Am J Sports Med* 1989;17:68–71.

Eleven patients treated for recurrent subluxation of the peroneal tendons by a sliding fibular bone graft were reviewed at an average 28-month follow-up. All but one were relieved of their symptoms and returned to sports. One patient fractured the graft but was successfully treated with cast immobilization. Two patients required reoperation for swelling and pain.

Toe Deformity

Cockin J: Butler's operation for an over-riding fifth toe. *J Bone Joint Surg* 1968;50B:78–81.

Butler's operation for this deformity and the results in 70 toes at a follow-up of from 1 to 10 years after surgery are presented. Ninety-one percent of patients had satisfactory results.

Dennyson WG, Bear JN, Bhoola KD: Macrodactyly in the foot. *J Bone Joint Surg* 1977;59B:355–359.

Seven patients with macrodactyly unrelated to neurofibromatosis or other syndromes served as the basis for this review. Overgrowth of fibro-fatty tissue was found in pathologic specimens submitted after amputation, the procedure recommended for symptomatic individuals.

Grogan DP, Bernstein RM, Habal MB, et al: Congenital lipofibromatosis associated with macrodactyly of the foot. *Foot Ankle* 1991;12:40–46.

This report presents 11 children with macrodactyly. Surgical options included debulking, ray resection, epiphysiodesis, and syndactylization.

Hamer AJ, Stanley D, Smith TW: Surgery for curly toe deformity: A double-blind, randomised, prospective trial. *J Bone Joint Surg* 1993;75B:662–663.

The results of simple flexor tenotomy were compared to those of flexor-to-extensor transfer for this deformity in 23 pairs of toes at a 4-year follow-up. There was no significant difference between the two, indicating that flexor release was the important part of the surgery and that transfer of the flexor to the extensor was unnecessary.

Lapidus PW: Transplantation of the extensor tendon for correction of the overlapping fifth toe. *J Bone Joint Surg* 1942;24:555–559.

A procedure consisting of tenotomy of the long extensor of the fifth toe at the mid metatarsal level and transfer of its distal stump underneath the fifth toe to the abductor digit minimi after capsulotomy of the metatarsophalangeal joint is described; it is recommended for this deformity.

Mills JA, Menelaus MB: Hallux varus. *J Bone Joint Surg* 1989;71B: 437–440.

Twenty feet were evaluated at an average follow-up of 12.7 years after surgical correction. Twelve of 16 feet treated by medial capsular release, lateral capsular reefing, and syndactylization to the second toe had satisfactory results. Six of nine feet treated by medial capsular release alone had satisfactory results.

Phelps DA, Grogan DP: Polydactyly of the foot. *J Pediatr Orthop* 1985;5:446–451.

Sixty-one patients with 97 duplications were reviewed at an average follow-up of 15.1 years. Results were excellent or good in 94% and poor in 6%. Most poor results were in preaxial duplications and were associated with hallux varus.

Robertson WW Jr: The bifid great toe: A surgical approach. *J Pediatr Orthop* 1987;7:25–28.

Four bifid great toes treated by a modified Bilhaut-Cloquet procedure were reviewed 4 years postoperatively. Nail abnormalities followed a nail splitting incision; therefore, this type of incision should be avoided.

Venn-Watson EA: Problems in polydactyly of the foot. *Orthop Clin North Am* 1976;7:909–927.

The results of surgical treatment of 56 patients with polydactyly of the foot were evaluated at an average follow-up of 3.2 years. In feet with duplicated border toes, excision of the lateral-most toe is favored. Completely duplicated metatarsals require excision. Resection of the redundant portion of widened metatarsal heads with the cut at 90° to the physis is recommended. Poorest results occurred in patients with shortened broad first metatarsals.

Miscellaneous Foot Deformities

Blauth W, Borisch NC: Cleft feet: Proposals for a new classification based on roentgenographic morphology. *Clin Orthop* 1990;258:41–48.

A classification of cleft foot deformity based on the authors' own 45 patients and 128 from the literature is presented in this article. A discussion of the pathogenesis of the deformity and an extensive reference list also make this a useful article.

Borges JL, Guille JT, Bowen JR: Kohler's bone disease of the tarsal navicular. *J Pediatr Orthop* 1995;15:596–598.

In 16 feet reviewed an average of 31.5 years after diagnosis, the type and length of treatment did not affect the final outcome; however, short-leg cast immobilization did decrease the duration of symptoms.

Kovalsky E, Guttmann GG: Early surgical correction of unilateral cleft foot deformity. *Orthopedics* 1990;13:347–350.

This article advocates early surgical reconstruction (less than 2 months) for patients with this deformity.

Phillips RS: Congenital split foot (lobster claw) and triphalangeal thumb. *J Bone Joint Surg* 1971;53B:247–257.

This report describes three generations of a family with five members who had split feet and triphalangeal thumbs. The results of surgical reconstruction in these patients are also presented.

Ryoppy S, Poussa M, Merikanto J, et al: Foot deformities in diastrophic dysplasia: An analysis of 102 patients. *J Bone Joint Surg* 1992;74B: 441–444.

In 102 patients with diastrophic dysplasia, the most common foot abnormality (43%) was tarsal valgus deformity and metatarsus adductus; 37% had either equinovarus adductus or equinus deformities.

Synder M, Kumar SJ, Stecyk MD: Split tibialis posterior tendon transfer and tendo-Achilles lengthening for spastic equinovarus feet. *J Pediatr Orthop* 1993;13:20–23.

This combined procedure obtained excellent or good results in 15 of 18 ambulatory patients and produced a plantigrade foot in three non-ambulatory patients. Three procedures failed because of technical errors.

Section 10

Limb-Length Discrepancy and Angular Deformity

Deborah F. Stanitski, MD

Limb-Length Discrepancy

General

Friberg O: Clinical symptoms and biomechanics of lumbar spine and hip joint in leg length inequality. *Spine* 1983;8:643–651.

A well-referenced discussion of the biomechanics of leg-length discrepancy precedes a clinical study of Finnish Army conscripts and other patients with chronic hip or back symptoms. The author describes a radiographic method for evaluation leg-length discrepancy. Shoe lifts are often recommended.

Gross RH: Leg length discrepancy: How much is too much? *Orthopedics* 1978;1:307–310.

This survey of 74 mature patients revealed that discrepancies of less than 2.0 cm were not perceived as problematic by the patients.

Kaufman KR, Miller LS, Sutherland DH: Gait asymmetry in patients with limb-length inequality. *J Pediatr Orthop* 1996;16:144–150.

In a study of 20 subjects, limb-length inequality of more than 2 cm resulted in gait asymmetry that was greater than that observed in the normal population; however, the amount of asymmetry varied for each individual. Dynamic gait findings are helpful to support static measurements of deformities.

Robertson WW Jr, Butler MS, D'Angio GJ, et al: Leg length discrepancy following irradiation for childhood tumors. *J Pediatr Orthop* 1991; 11:284–287.

Leg-length discrepancy (LLD) developed in 12 (21%) of 57 children treated with radiation therapy to the kidney. The development of LLD was related to the total dose of radiation to the pelvic area, asymmetric irradiation to the pelvis, and high-dose irradiation to the leg.

Rogalski R, Hensinger R, Loder R: Vascular abnormalities of the extremities: Clinical findings and management. *J Pediatr Orthop* 1993;13:9–14.

Of 41 patients with angiodysplastic lesions of the extremities, 22 had masses, 11 had limb-length discrepancies with or without hemihypertrophy, and two had recurrent joint effusions. Enhanced computed tomography and magnetic resonance imaging were most valuable for diagnosis and preoperative planning. Twenty-nine patients (77%) required operation.

Evaluation

Aaron A, Weinstein D, Thickman D, et al: Comparison of orthoroentgenography and computed tomography in the measurement of limb-length discrepancy. *J Bone Joint Surg* 1992;74A:897–902.

No statistically significant differences in the measurements of the length of the femur were found between the two methods; however, computed tomography (CT) was significantly more accurate in measurement of the length of the tibia and total length of the limb when the knee was flexed to 30° or more. CT is more accurate than orthoroentgenography for measurement of limb-length discrepancy in patients who have a flexion deformity of the knee.

Cundy P, Paterson D, Morris L, et al: Skeletal age estimation in leg length discrepancy. *J Pediatr Orthop* 1988;8:513–515.

This article defines the dangers of onetime, bone-age determination in the prediction of leg-length discrepancy.

Eastwood DM, Cole WG: A graphic method for timing the correction of leg-length discrepancy. *J Bone Joint Surg* 1995;77B:743–747.

This is a graphic depiction of the White/Menelaus arithmetic method for timing epiphysiodesis. Clinical examinations only are performed during early childhood. Computed tomography measurements are used in middle and late childhood. Excellent accuracy is reported.

Grayhack JJ, Carroll NC: Projected limb length inequality: Selecting patients for surgery. *Orthop Clin North Am* 1991;22:581–587.

Considerations before surgery for limb-length discrepancy should include the patient's desires, limitations of surgery, the patient's ability to tolerate surgery, the cause of the discrepancy, accompanying deformities or pathology, other medical conditions, and the predicted mature stature of the patient.

Huurman WW, Jacobsen FS, Anderson JC, et al: Limb-length discrepancy measured with computerized axial tomographic equipment. *J Bone Joint Surg* 1987;69A:699–705.

This report indicates that computerized tomography is more accurate and delivers less radiation than standard orthoroentgenograms in measurement of leg-length discrepancy.

Moseley CF: Assessment and prediction in leg-length discrepancy, in Barr JS Jr (ed): *Instructional Course Lectures XXXVIII*. Park Ridge, IL, American Academy of Orthopaedic Surgeons, 1989, pp 325–330.

Moseley CF: A straight-line graph for leg-length discrepancies. *J Bone Joint Surg* 1977;59A:174–179.

These classic articles present in detail the concept and usage of the straight-line graph.

Shapiro F: Developmental patterns in lower-extremity length discrepancies. *J Bone Joint Surg* 1982;64A:639–651.

Five patterns of growth inhibition were noted in patients of the Growth Study Unit established by Green and Anderson. The author believes the straight-line graph of growth inhibition method may lead to inaccurate projections in some of these patterns.

Shortening/Epiphysiodesis

Blair VP III, Schoenecker PL, Sheridan JJ, et al: Closed shortening of the femur. *J Bone Joint Surg* 1989;71A:1440–1447.

The technical difficulty of performing closed shortening is emphasized in this review of 20 skeletally mature patients. Results were generally excellent, but complications were reported.

Broughton NS, Olney BW, Menelaus MB: Tibial shortening for leg length discrepancy. *J Bone Joint Surg* 1989;71B:242–245.

The authors report long-term follow-up of 12 patients with tibial shortening. This procedure should be performed with caution.

Canale ST, Russell TA, Holcomb RL: Percutaneous epiphysiodesis: Experimental study and preliminary clinical results. *J Pediatr Orthop* 1986;6:150–156.

Ogilvie JW: Epiphysiodesis: Evaluation of a new technique. *J Pediatr Orthop* 1986;6:147–149.

These two articles, published together, illustrate an approach to epiphysiodesis.

Horton GA, Olney BW: Epiphysiodesis of the lower extremity: Results of the percutaneous technique. *J Pediatr Orthop* 1996;16:180–182.

Physeal arrest was obtained by all 42 percutaneous epiphysiodeses in 26 patients, with no angular deformity, neurovascular complications, or fractures. Advantages of this technique include cosmetic scar, short hospital stay, low incidence of complications, and reliable physeal arrest.

Liotta FJ, Ambrose TA II, Eilert RE: Fluoroscopic technique versus Phemister technique for epiphysiodesis. *J Pediatr Orthop* 1992;12:248–251.

In this comparison of the fluoroscopic technique (26 patients) and the Phemister technique (44 patients), both obtained physeal arrest in 100% of patients with similar complication rates. Because the fluoroscopic technique results in a much smaller scar, less postoperative knee stiffness, and shorter hospital stay, it is recommended over the Phemister technique.

Little DG, Nigo L, Aiona MD: Deficiencies of current methods for the timing of epiphysiodesis. *J Pediatr Orthop* 1996;16:173–179.

Seventy-one epiphysiodeses were reviewed to compare the methods of Anderson and Green, Menelaus, and Moseley. Differing the methodology did not have a meaningful effect on their similar but limited accuracy. The routine use of serial Gruelich and Pyle skeletal age data was not shown to increase the accuracy in predicting outcome. The authors prefer the Menelaus method.

Sasso RC, Urquhart BA, Cain TE: Closed femoral shortening. *J Pediatr Orthop* 1993;13:51–56.

This is an excellent description of technique, complications, and management of these patients.

Lengthening

Aaron AD, Eilert RE: Results of the Wagner and Ilizarov methods of limb-lengthening. *J Bone Joint Surg* 1996;78A:20–29.

In a comparison of the Wagner (20 extremities) and Ilizarov (21 extremities) methods, those with the Wagner technique had 30 major complications and those with the Ilizarov technique had only 13. Forty complications (major and minor) were associated with the use of the uniaxial Wagner external apparatus and 16 with the multiaxial Ilizarov fixator.

Aronson J: Section I: Symposium. Biological and clinical evaluation of distraction histogenesis. *Clin Orthop* 1994;301:1–164.

Green SA (ed): Limb lengthening. *Orthop Clin North Am* 1991;22:555–734.

Paley D: Section I: Symposium. Modern techniques in limb lengthening. *Clin Orthop* 1990;250:1–159.

These well-referenced articles include classics, basic science, several surgical techniques, and a discussion of complications.

Glorion C, Pouliquen JC, Langlais J, et al: Femoral lengthening using the callotasis method: Study of the complications in a series of 70 cases in children and adolescents. *J Pediatr Orthop* 1996;16:161–167.

In 70 femoral lengthenings using either the Judet lengthener or the Orthofix external fixator, 83 complications occurred. Bony consolidation was obtained without additional surgery in 88%.

Hope PG, Crawfurd EJ, Catterall A: Bone growth following lengthening for congenital shortening of the lower limb. *J Pediatr Orthop* 1994; 14:339–342.

Twelve patients were reviewed who had undergone femoral or tibial lengthening for congenital shortening of the leg. None of the patients exhibited significant stimulation or reduction in their growth velocity rate in lengthenings performed after the age of 9 years.

Murray DW, Kambouroglou G, Kenwright J: One-stage lengthening for femoral shortening with associated deformity. *J Bone Joint Surg* 1993; 75B:566–571.
Sanders R, Anglen JO, Mark JB: Oblique osteotomy for the correction of tibial malunion. *J Bone Joint Surg* 1995;77A:240–246.

These two papers describe acute correction and lengthening with immediate gain averaging 4.0 cm in the femur and 1.3 cm in the tibia. This treatment is contrary to conventional wisdom but may be considered for small discrepancies with deformity.

Price CT, Cole JD: Limb lengthening by callotasis for children and adolescents: Early experience. *Clin Orthop* 1990;250:105–111.

The technique of De Bastiani, used for 11 lower extremity lengthenings, obtained desired length in all but one patient, who lacked 1.1 cm. The average gain in length was 5 cm per segment (15% of original bone length). The method is recommended for moderate limb-length discrepancies.

Shapiro F: Longitudinal growth of the femur and tibia after diaphyseal lengthening. *J Bone Joint Surg* 1987;69A:684–690.

Eighteen patients were followed to maturity to assess the effect of subsequent growth on lengthening. Femurs grew faster and tibias slower.

Stanitski DF: The effect of limb lengthening on articular cartilage: An experimental study. *Clin Orthop* 1994;301:68–72.

Findings in a canine study confirm direct evidence of cartilage injury during limb lengthening, including gross cartilage fibrillation and frank cartilage necrosis.

Stanitski DF, Bullard M, Armstrong P, et al: Results of femoral lengthening using the Ilizarov technique. *J Pediatr Orthop* 1995;15:224–231.

An average lengthening of 8.3 cm (range, 3.5 to 12 cm) was obtained in 30 patients. Complications included premature consolidation in four patients, malunion of more than 10° in two patients, and residual limb-length inequality of less than 2 cm in two patients.

Young N, Bell DF, Anthony A: Pediatric pain patterns during Ilizarov treatment of limb length discrepancy and angular deformity. *J Pediatr Orthop* 1994;14:352–357.

In a prospective study, measurement of pain in 23 patients indicated high levels of pain extending over several months, in sharp contrast to the general orthopaedic pain experience. The prolongation of pain throughout the entire correction and consolidation process must be recognized to ensure appropriate management, especially in an outpatient setting.

Angular Deformity

General

Heath CH, Staheli LT: Normal limits of knee angle in white children: Genu varum and genu valgum. *J Pediatr Orthop* 1993;13:259–262.

Measurements of 196 children determined that children were maximally bowlegged at age 6 months and progressed toward approximately neutral knee angles by 18 months of age. Knock-knee was greatest (8°) at 4 years of age, followed by gradual decrease to a mean of less than 6° at 11 years. Normal children aged 2 to 11 years had knock-knee up to 12° and intermalleolar distance up to 8 cm; the existence of bowlegs after 2 years of age was abnormal.

Oppenheim WL, Shayestehfar S, Saluksy IB: Tibial physeal changes in renal osteodystrophy: Lateral Blount's disease. *J Pediatr Orthop* 1992;12:774–779.

In a group of 17 children with chronic renal failure and renal osteodystrophy, eight (15 knees) had significant involvement of the proximal tibial physis with radiographic changes analogous to those in Blount disease but involving the lateral physis rather than the medial physis. The authors suggest that this is further evidence that such changes are related to eccentric weightbearing rather than to trauma, infection, or heredity.

Paley D, Tetsworth K (eds): Malalignment and realignment of the lower extremity. *Orthop Clin North Am* 1994;25.

This symposium volume contains excellent papers that discuss normal alignment, mechanics of malalignment, deformity analysis, and management techniques. It is a "must read" for understanding lower extremity deformity.

Paley D, Tetsworth K: Mechanical axis deviation of the lower limbs: Preoperative planning of uniapical angular deformities of the tibia or femur. *Clin Orthop* 1992;280:48–64.

Paley D, Tetsworth K: Mechanical axis deviation of the lower limbs: Preoperative planning of multiapical frontal plane angular and bowing deformities of the femur and tibia. *Clin Orthop* 1992;280:65–71.

These two detailed articles cover deformity analysis and preoperative planning for deformity correction.

Tuncay IC, Johnston CE II, Birch JG: Spontaneous resolution of congenital anterolateral bowing of the tibia. *J Pediatr Orthop* 1994;14: 599–602.

Of 43 patients with congenital pseudarthrosis of the tibia, the deformities corrected spontaneously in five patients who had no other congenital anomalies or evidence of neurofibromatosis. In patients with subperiosteal callus formation on the posteromedial concavity of the deformity and an uninvolved fibula, no treatment appears necessary, as this deformity will spontaneously resolve.

Evaluation

Bylander B, Hansson LI, Selvik G: Pattern of growth retardation after Blount stapling: A roentgen stereophotogrammetric analysis. *J Pediatr Orthop* 1983;3:63–72.

Thirty-one stapled and 25 intact growth regions of distal femur or proximal tibia were studied longitudinally. A uniform pattern of growth retardation was noted after stapling; the retardation was more pronounced and rapid with more advanced skeletal age. Five of 31 had significant asymmetric growth.

Davids JR, Fisher R, Lumb G, et al: Angular deformity of the lower extremity in children with renal osteodystrophy. *J Pediatr Orthop* 1992;12:291–299.

The authors determined that periods of metabolic instability, best characterized as an alkaline phosphatase of 500 U for at least 10 months, were associated with progression of deformity. Complications of corrective osteotomy also were related to perioperative metabolic instability. A surgical treatment protocol is described, emphasizing preoperative assessment by histomorphometric bone biopsy and multimodal medical management to maintain metabolic stability perioperatively.

Doyle BS, Volk AG, Smith CF: Infantile Blount disease: Long-term follow-up of surgically treated patients at skeletal maturity. *J Pediatr Orthop* 1996;16:469–476.

In 17 patients followed for an average of 15 years, recurrence of the deformity requiring repeat osteotomy occurred more frequently in children who underwent initial osteotomy at more than 4 years of age or who had Langenskiöld stage III or more involvement.

Feldman MD, Schoenecker PL: Use of the metaphyseal-diaphyseal angle in the evaluation of bowed legs. *J Bone Joint Surg* 1993;75A:1602–1609.

The metaphyseal-diaphyseal angle described by Levine and Drennan was found to be helpful in the identification of Blount disease, but it should not be the sole criterion.

Gilbert A, Brockman R: Congenital pseudarthrosis of the tibia: Long-term followup of 29 cases treated by microvascular bone transfer. *Clin Orthop* 1995;314:37–44.

Results in 29 patients reveal that rate and speed of healing were superior to those obtained by other published methods. Final outcome at maturity was generally acceptable. Age at first fracture, age at operation, gender, and type of fixation did not appear to significantly influence outcome.

Timperlake RW, Bowen JR, Guille JT, et al: Prospective evaluation of fifty-three consecutive percutaneous epiphysiodeses of the distal femur and proximal tibia and fibula. *J Pediatr Orthop* 1991;11:350–357.

At follow-up of approximately 3 years, no statistically significant difference was found in the actual discrepancy and that calculated by standard growth charts.

Treatment

Anderson DJ, Schoenecker PL, Sheridan JJ, et al: Use of an intramedullary rod for the treatment of congenital pseudarthrosis of the tibia. *J Bone Joint Surg* 1992;74A:161–168.

Baker JK, Cain TE, Tullos HS: Intramedullary fixation for congenital pseudarthrosis of the tibia. *J Bone Joint Surg* 1992;74A:169–178.

Both of these articles report good results with intramedullary rod fixation.

Bell DF, Boyer MI, Armstrong PF: The use of the Ilizarov technique in the correction of limb deformities associated with skeletal dysplasia. *J Pediatr Orthop* 1992;12:283–290.

This technique was used in 15 patients for correction of angular deformities or limb-length discrepancies. Patients undergoing extended limb lengthening had the most complications, but all patients obtained their preoperative goals.

Bowen JR, Leahey JL, Zhang ZH, et al: Partial epiphysiodesis at the knee to correct angular deformity. *Clin Orthop* 1985;198:184–190.

This article clarifies the timing and technique of hemiepiphysiodesis.

Coogan PG, Fox JA, Fitch RD: Treatment of adolescent Blount disease with the circular external fixation device and distraction osteogenesis. *J Pediatr Orthop* 1996;16:450–454.

In 12 treated tibias the varus deformity was reduced from an average of 18° to 2.5°. Function was improved in all patients, and there were no neurovascular complications or delayed unions.

Ferris B, Walker C, Jackson A, et al: The orthopaedic management of hypophosphatemic rickets. *J Pediatr Orthop* 1991;11:367–373.

In a review of 19 patients, three groups were identified: teenagers or young adults without knee problems, those with knee problems, and adults or elderly patients with stiff joints due to mineralization of ligaments. Diaphyseal osteotomies were performed at all ages with intramedullary nail stabilization, and metaphyseal osteotomies were most successful at or near maturity. Osteotomies were best staged.

Kanel JS, Price CT: Unilateral external fixation for corrective osteotomies in patients with rickets. *J Pediatr Orthop* 1995;15:232–235.

Corrective osteotomies with Orthofix external fixation were performed in 29 bones of 9 children with hypophosphatemic rickets. This technique allowed precise correction of the deformities without interruption of medical management.

Kasser JR: Physeal bar resections after growth arrest about the knee. *Clin Orthop* 1990;255:68–74.

Localized growth arrest about the knee can be treated with excision when less than 50% of the physis is involved and when at least 2.5 cm of growth remains. Simultaneous corrective osteotomy should be performed when the angular deformity is more than 20°.

Kline SC, Bostrum M, Griffin PP: Femoral varus: An important component in late-onset Blount's disease. *J Pediatr Orthop* 1992;12:197–206.

The significance of femoral varus should be determined preoperatively for each patient with late-onset Blount disease to avoid compensatory deformity.

Mielke CH, Stevens PM: Hemiepiphyseal stapling for knee deformities in children younger than 10 years: A preliminary report. *J Pediatr Orthop* 1996;16:423-429.

Twenty-two children with genu valgum and 3 with genu varum were treated with hemiepiphyseal stapling. The anatomic (tibiofemoral) angle and mechanical axis were improved in all patients. No physeal arrests have occurred at an average follow-up of 3 years and 3 months.

Price CT, Scott DS, Greenberg DA: Dynamic axial external fixation in the surgical treatment of tibia vara. *J Pediatr Orthop* 1995;15:236-243.

Osteotomy with dynamic external fixation was used in 31 tibiae. All osteotomies healed with no postoperative loss of correction. Advantages of this method include ease of application, adjustability, early weight-bearing, ability to lengthen the extremity, and no second operation for hardware removal.

Scheffer MM, Peterson HA: Opening-wedge osteotomy for angular deformities of long bones in children. *J Bone Joint Surg* 1994;76A:325-334.

Thirty-one osteotomies in 26 children satisfactorily corrected the deformities. Opening-wedge osteotomy with insertion of a specially prepared autogenous tricortical iliac-crest bone graft, with minimal or no internal fixation, is recommended for angular deformity of 25° or less and limb-length discrepancy that is or will be 25 mm or less at maturity.

Shoenecker PL, Johnston R, Rich MM, et al: Elevation of the medial plateau of the tibia in the treatment of Blount disease. *J Bone Joint Surg* 1992;74A:351-358.

Seven children between the ages of 10 and 13 years with severe Blount deformity were treated with elevation of the medial plateau. Results were good in five and fair in two.

Thompson GH, Carter JR: Late-onset tibia vara (Blount's disease): Current concepts. *Clin Orthop* 1990;255:24-35.

The authors present a thorough review of the topic, including classification, histopathologic analysis, etiology, and treatment.

Velazquez RJ, Bell DF, Armstrong PF, et al: Complications of the use of the Ilizarov technique in the correction of limb deformities in children. *J Bone Joint Surg* 1993;75A:1148–1156.

In 61 procedures, major complications (one that required additional surgery, caused lasting sequelae, or prolonged treatment) occurred in 38 and minor complications (one that responded to nonsurgical treatment and caused no lasting sequelae) in 50. Major complications decreased with experience, but minor complications remained relatively constant.

Zuege RC, Kempken TG, Blount WP: Epiphyseal stapling for angular deformity at the knee. *J Bone Joint Surg* 1979;61A:320–329.

This classic article describes the technique and results of hemiepiphyseal stapling to correct angular deformity.

Partial Physeal Arrest

Birch JG: Surgical technique of physeal bar resection, in Eilert RE (ed): *Instructional Course Lectures XLI.* Rosemont, IL, American Academy of Orthopaedic Surgeons, 1992, pp 445–450.

Peterson HA: Partial growth plate arrest and its treatment. *J Pediatr Orthop* 1984;4:246–258.

Both of these good review articles about partial physeal resection describe surgical technique and results.

Havranek P, Lizler J: Magnetic resonance imaging in the evaluation of partial growth arrest after physeal injuries in children. *J Bone Joint Surg* 1991;73A:1234–1241.

This article is one of several that have demonstrated the effectiveness of magnetic resonance imaging for early detection and evaluation of partial growth arrest.

Williamson RV, Staheli LT: Partial physeal growth arrest: Treatment by bridge resection and fat interposition. *J Pediatr Orthop* 1990;10:769–776.

In this series of 28 patients in whom fat was used as interposition material, results were as good as in other series. There is a good discussion.

Epiphysiolysis

Birch JG, Herring JA, Wenger DR: Surgical anatomy of selected physes. *J Pediatr Orthop* 1984;4:224–231.

This article is helpful for planning the surgical approach for partial physeal resection.

Broughton NS, Dickens DR, Cole WG, et al: Epiphyseolysis for partial growth plate arrest: Results after four years or at maturity. *J Bone Joint Surg* 1989;71B:13–16.

This article reinforces what has been learned about epiphysiolysis in a small group followed to maturity.

Carlson WO, Wenger DR: A mapping method to prepare for surgical excision of a partial physeal growth arrest. *J Pediatr Orthop* 1984;4:232–238.

This is an essential article when planning for partial physeal resection.

# Congenital Limb Deficiency and the Child Amputee

John A. Herring, MD

General

Boakes JL, Stevens PM, Moseley RF: Treatment of genu valgus deformity in congenital absence of the fibula. *J Pediatr Orthop* 1991;11:721–724.

The authors recommend that patients be followed closely until skeletal maturity. Osteotomy performed before skeletal maturity can result in recurrence of the valgus deformity.

Chenaille PJ, Horowitz ME: Purpura fulminans: A case for heparin therapy. *Clin Pediatr* 1989;28:95–98.

This brief article from the pediatric literature suggests that heparinization may reverse the coagulopathy associated with purpura fulminans. This reverse, in turn, may somewhat limit tissue destruction and improve amputation level in these patients. The article also describes full compartment fasciotomies to relieve compartment pressure associated with purpura fulminans.

Jacobsen ST, Crawford AH: Amputation following meningococcemia: A sequela to purpura fulminans. *Clin Orthop* 1984;185:214–219.

This is a review of the pathophysiology and early management of patients with purpura fulminans.

Krebs DE, Fishman S: Characteristics of the child amputee population. *J Pediatr Orthop* 1984;4:89–95.

This review of the characteristics of the patient population of 45 child amputee clinics in the United States and Canada represents a review of 4,105 patients.

Turker R, Mendelson S, Ackman J, et al: Anatomic considerations of the foot and leg in tibial hemimelia. *J Pediatr Orthop* 1996;16:445–449.

Cadaver dissections of five lower extremities revealed multiple tendon anomalies and multiple coalitions of the osseous structures of the foot. The ankle articulation was found to have a nonfunctional uniplanar motion.

Classification

Frantz CH, O'Rahilly R: Congenital skeletal limb deficiencies. *J Bone Joint Surg* 1961;43A:1202–1224.

This is a classic article with explanation of the Frantz-O'Rahilly classification of limb deficiencies. Case examples are given to clarify the classification systems.

Henkel L, Willert H-G: Dysmelia: A classification and a pattern of malformation in a group of congenital defects of the limbs. *J Bone Joint Surg* 1969;51B:399–414.

The authors provide a comprehensive classification system of congenital limb deficiencies based on a review of 287 children. Teratologic sequences are devised that demonstrate the continuous spectra of deformity from least to greatest degree of involvement.

Swanson AB, Swanson GD, Tada K: A classification for congenital limb malformation. *J Hand Surg* 1983;8:693–702.

This classification has been used especially to describe upper-extremity defects.

Congenital Constriction Band Syndrome

Askins G, Ger E: Congenital constriction band syndrome. *J Pediatr Orthop* 1988;8:461–466.

In a retrospective study of 55 patients with this syndrome, multiple extremity involvement was the most common clinical feature; 34% of the patients were premature at birth. Malformations included constriction bands, clubfoot, intrauterine amputations, syndactyly, and acrosyndactyly. The occurrence of neurologic deficits distal to the constriction bands is documented. Significant leg-length discrepancy (more than 2.5 cm) occurred in nine of 38 patients with lower extremity involvement. Surgical treatment is briefly described.

Foulkes GD, Reinker K: Congenital constriction band syndrome: A seventy-year experience. *J Pediatr Orthop* 1994;14:242–248.

Of 71 patients with congenital constriction band syndrome (CCBS), 60% had abnormal gestational histories, 50% had concurrent diagnosis, and nearly a third had clubfeet. The authors suggest the term "early amnion rupture sequence" to more accurately reflect the pathogenesis of CCBS.

Greene WB: One-stage release of congenital circumferential constriction bands. *J Bone Joint Surg* 1993;75A:650–655.

A one-stage release was performed in four extremities (three patients). No wound problems occurred, even when there had been marked swelling of the extremity distal to the band. The one-stage release made postoperative care easier and avoided additional periods of anesthesia and additional operations necessary in two- or three-stage procedures.

Upton J, Tan C: Correction of constriction rings. *J Hand Surg* 1991;16A: 947–953.

A refinement in the correction of deep and shallow constriction rings, in which subcutaneous fat and fascial flaps are advanced into the defect to prevent recurrent contour defects, is described. Of 61 constriction rings corrected with traditional serial Z-plasties, 64% had good or excellent results; of 55 treated with the newer method, 96% had good or excellent results. The authors also report fewer complications and better restoration of contour with the new technique.

Proximal Femoral Focal Deficiency

Alman BA, Krajbich JI, Hubbard S: Proximal femoral focal deficiency: Results of rotationplasty and Syme amputation. *J Bone Joint Surg* 1995;77A:1876–1882.

Comparison of rotationplasty (nine patients) and Syme amputation (seven patients) showed no difference in gross motor function or perceived physical appearance. Rotationplasty was associated with a more energy-efficient gait than was Syme amputation.

Epps CH Jr: Proximal femoral focal deficiency. *J Bone Joint Surg* 1983; 65A:867-870.

This is a concise topic review with reference to Aitken's classification and treatment recommendations.

Gillespie R, Torode IP: Classification and management of congenital abnormalities of the femur. *J Bone Joint Surg* 1983;65B:557-568.

The authors review 69 patients and divide them into two main groups. The division is made on the basis of long-term surgical and prosthetic management.

Goddard NJ, Hashemi-Nejad A, Fixsen JA: Natural history and treatment of instability of the hip in proximal femoral focal deficiency. *J Pediatr Orthop* 1995;4B:145-149.

Using the classification systems of Aitken and Fixsen and Lloyd-Roberts as applied to radiographs taken at age 12 to 15 months, the development of hip instability (formation of pseudarthrosis or complete failure of hip development) could be accurately predicted. Pseudarthrosis at the cervical level of the femur was difficult to treat surgically, but subtrochanteric pseudarthroses fused spontaneously in 30% of patients and responded well to surgical treatment when necessary.

Lange DR, Schoenecker PL, Baker CL: Proximal femoral focal deficiency: Treatment and classification in 42 cases. *Clin Orthop* 1978;135:15-25.

The authors describe the management of proximal focal femoral deficiencies in 42 patients. A new four-part classification introduced is stated to be easier to apply and more useful clinically than the Aitken classification.

Pirani S, Beauchamp RD, Li D, et al: Soft tissue anatomy of proximal femoral focal deficiency. *J Pediatr Orthop* 1991;11:563-570.

The authors examined six patients with proximal femoral deficiency using magnetic resonance imaging (MRI) to define the soft tissues. Almost all the muscles of the thigh were present and were smaller and shorter than normal, the obturator externus was longer than normal, and the sartorius was usually hypertrophied. This reference is especially useful in preparing for surgery of the hip or knee in these patients.

Steel HH, Lin PS, Betz RR, et al: Iliofemoral fusion for proximal femoral focal deficiency. *J Bone Joint Surg* 1987;69A:837–843.

This article describes a surgical procedure for fusing the femoral condyles to the pelvis, allowing the existing knee joint to act as a hip in a patient with a severe proximal femoral focal deficiency. The author reports four patients, two of whom also had Van Nes rotationplasty, and two of whom had Syme's amputations. The patients with Syme's amputations had a better result than those with the Van Nes. Two patients also required subsequent osteotomy of the femur to improve alignment.

Torode IP, Gillespie R: Rotationplasty of the lower limb for congenital defects of the femur. *J Bone Joint Surg* 1983;65B:569–573.

The operative technique for rotationplasty of the foot (Van Nes) is discussed in detail.

van der Windt D, et al: Energy expenditure during walking in subjects with tibial rotation-plasty, above-knee amputation, or hip disarticulation. *Arch Phys Med Rehabil* 1992;73:1174–1180.

This work compares tibial rotationplasty with amputation (above-knee and hip disarticulation) in patients with malignancies. Those with rotationplasty walked faster than the others, but the energy expenditure was similar for all three groups. There was no explanation for the lack of better energy consumption in the rotationplasty group.

Surgical Management

General

Benevenia J, Makley JT, Leeson MC, et al: Primary epiphyseal transplants and bone overgrowth in childhood amputations. *J Pediatr Orthop* 1992;12:746–750.

The authors compared children who had capping of the end of the residual limb with autogenous epiphyseal transplants from the amputated limb to those with standard amputations. Overgrowth was dramatically reduced (1/10) with the capping technique. They used either the distal fibula or the first metatarsal epiphysis.

Davids JR, Meyer LC, Blackhurst DW: Operative treatment of bone overgrowth in children who have an acquired or congenital amputation. *J Bone Joint Surg* 1995;77A:1490–1497.

This work describes the efficacy of iliac crest grafting to reduce overgrowth of the residual limb. Fifty-three children were reviewed after surgical treatment for bone overgrowth. They had either simple excision (31), capping with polyethylene implants (nine), or capping with iliac crest grafts (13). Eighty-four percent of all patients had recurrent overgrowth, but in those treated with iliac crest graft it did not recur as quickly. The synthetic caps failed because they loosened, fractured, or became infected. Comparison of the results of the three procedures led the authors to recommend application of a cap of autogenous bone graft from the iliac crest for treatment of established overgrowth of the bone in patients younger than 13 years of age.

O'Neal ML, Bahner R, Ganey TM, et al: Osseous overgrowth after amputation in adolescents and children. *J Pediatr Orthop* 1996;16:78–84.

The authors note that traumatic amputations overgrow more often than congenital or elective amputations. They propose a grading system from grade 1 with noncontinuous ossification to grade 4 with perforation of the skin. They suggest that the overgrowth occurs in episodes after which overgrowth may cease. Trauma was noted to initiate overgrowth in some cases.

Upper-Extremity Surgery

Gilbert A: Toe transfers for congenital hand defects. *J Hand Surg* 1982; 7:118–124.

The author describes the technique, indications, and results of microvascular transfer of the second toe to reconstruct congenital hand defects.

Swanson AB: The Krukenberg procedure in the juvenile amputee. *J Bone Joint Surg* 1964;46A:1540–1548.

This classic article describes the technique of the Krukenberg procedure. The four children described had bilateral congenital absence of the hands. The unilateral Krukenberg stump became the dominant useful extremity.

Lower-Extremity Surgery/Tibial and Fibular Hemimelia

Achterman C, Kalamchi A: Congenital deficiency of the fibula. *J Bone Joint Surg* 1979;72A:133–137.

These authors describe three types of fibular hemimelia: Ia, proximal fibula present below tibial physis and the distal fibula above talar dome; Ib, 30% to 50% of fibular length absent proximally and a distal fibula that does not support the ankle; II, complete absence. Type Ia had a final discrepancy of 13% and type II of 19%. Type Ia patients were treated with contralateral epiphysiodesis; type Ib patients had lengthenings or amputations, and type II had amputations. All had tarsal coalitions and ball and socket ankles.

Choi IH, Kumar SJ, Bowen JR: Amputation or limb-lengthening for partial or total absence of the fibula. *J Bone Joint Surg* 1990;72A:1391–1399.

This work compares limb-lengthening in the Wagner era with Syme's or Boyd's amputation in the treatment of fibular hemimelia. Many of the patients reported had congenital shortening of the femur in addition to the fibular hemimelia. Patients with no more than 15% total shortening who had stable hips and knees and a plantigrade foot did well with femoral lengthening. All those with greater degrees of shortening and those with foot deformities (ie, those with typical fibular hemimelia) had poor results after lengthening. Amputation was suggested for those with a predicted final discrepancy of 12.5 cm or more. The authors prefer the Boyd's amputation to the Syme's, but admit that it cannot be done with the typical equinus deformity of fibular hemimelia.

Davidson WH, Bohne WH: The Syme amputation in children. *J Bone Joint Surg* 1975;57A:905–909.

This review of 23 children who had Syme's amputations describes (1) the suture of extensor tendons to the heel pad, (2) the disarticulation of the ankle without disturbing the distal tibia or fibula, and (3) vascular anomalies, which can involve the posterior tibial artery.

de Bari A, Krajbich JI, Lanager F, et al: Principles of amputation surgery in children with longitudinal deficiencies of the femur. *J Bone Joint Surg* 1990;72B:1065–1069.

A modified rotationplasty (Van Ness) was performed in four children with osteosarcoma of the proximal tibia. The appearance of the leg was well acccpted by the patients and their parents and the patients were disease-free at follow-up.

Eilert RE, Jayakumar SS: Boyd and Syme ankle amputations in children. *J Bone Joint Surg* 1976;58A:1138–1141.

This is a comparison of the Boyd's and Syme's amputations in children. No distinct advantage was demonstrated for either technique. Details of heel pad management are emphasized.

Fulp T, Davids JR, Meyer LC, et al: Longitudinal deficiency of the fibula: Operative treatment. *J Bone Joint Surg* 1996;78A:674–682.

Syme amputation was performed on 15 extremities and a modified Boyd amputation on 16. Patients with Syme amputation had more problems related to reformation of the calcaneus, instability of the heel pad, prosthetic suspension, and excessive length of the residual extremity. The modified Boyd amputation improved the function of the heel pad and prosthetic suspension and provided optimum length.

Harris RI: Syme's amputation: The technical details essential for success. *J Bone Joint Surg* 1956;38B:614–632.

This classic article covers the history and technical details of the Syme's amputation.

Herring JA: Syme amputation for fibular hemimelia: A second look in the Ilizarov era, in Eilert RE (ed): *Instructional Course Lectures XLI.* Rosemont, IL, American Academy of Orthopaedic Surgeons, 1992.

The author revisits a 1986 study of fibular hemimelia patients treated with Syme's amputation in which the patients exhibited excellent athletic and social function. He points out the need for comparable functional studies of patients who have had limb lengthening and repositioning procedures. He concludes that even in this era of high technology, amputation is indicated for shortening of 35% or more, major foot deformity, or an abnormal tibiotalar articulation.

Herring JA, Barnhill B, Gaffney C: Syme amputation: An evaluation of the physical and psychological function in young patients. *J Bone Joint Surg* 1986;68A:573–578.

The authors review the functional activities of patients having Syme's amputations, most of them for fibular hemimelia. They demonstrate that these children can be expected to participate in normal sports activities, even at a competitive level. There is minimal morbidity or functional loss associated with this amputation level.

Jones D, Barnes J, Lloyd-Roberts GC: Congenital aplasia and dysplasia of the tibia with intact fibula: Classification and management. *J Bone Joint Surg* 1978;60B:31–39.

This classic article describes the currently used classification of congenital absence and dysplasia of the tibia.

Kumar A, Kruger LM: Fibular dimelia with deficiency of the tibia. *J Pediatr Orthop* 1993;13:203–209.

In their report of six patients with this condition, the authors recommend knee disarticulation in patients with an associated normal femur and femorofibular fusion in those with ipsilateral proximal focal femoral deficiency or congenital short femur. Fibulocalcaneal fusion and Boyd-type amputation provided good end-bearing stumps.

Letts M, Vinvent N: Congenital longitudinal deficiency of the fibula (fibular hemimelia): Parental refusal of amputation. *Clin Orthop* 1993;287: 160–166.

Six children whose parents had refused amputation were managed by specially designed prostheses to incorporate their foot deformity and limb-length inequality; four required subsequent corrective surgery. A more practical classification of fibular hemimelia is proposed to make treatment decisions easier for physicians and parents.

Loder RT, Herring JA: Disarticulation of the knee in children: A functional assessment. *J Bone Joint Surg* 1987;69A:1155–1160.

This study analyzes the gait and functional abilities after knee disarticulation. Mild gait deviations were documented. The functional levels of the children were shown to be satisfactory and better than those reported for above-knee amputation. Prosthetic problems were minimal. The authors conclude that this is a very satisfactory amputation level.

Loder RT, Herring JA: Fibular transfer for congenital absence of the tibia: A reassessment. *J Pediatr Orthop* 1987;7:8–13.

This review of six children who had prior Brown procedures (centralization of the fibula) for complete tibial hemimelia found no successes at follow-up. Early results were often promising, but subsequent flexion deformity and knee instability resulted in poor function. The authors recommend knee disarticulation as the primary treatment for complete fibular hemimelia.

Miller LS, Bell DF: Management of congenital fibular deficiency by Ilizarov technique. *J Pediatr Orthop* 1992;12:651–657.

The authors review 12 limbs that underwent fibular hemimelia lengthening by the Ilizarov method. A mean of 8.3 cm was gained (31% of the limb) after an average of 6 months in a frame. Laxity of the knee and ball and socket ankle abnormalities did not cause problems, but there were six major and 14 minor complications. The most significant complications included regenerate bone deformation and delayed consolidation. The technique successfully corrected the foot and ankle deformities, but functional studies were not done.

Schoenecker PL, Capelli AM, Millar EA, et al: Congenital longitudinal deficiency of the tibia. *J Bone Joint Surg* 1989;71A:278–287.

Fifty-seven tibial hemimelia patients were evaluated at an average follow-up of 9 years. For type 1 (complete tibial absence), the Brown centralization procedure was not successful, and these children were best treated with knee disarticulation. Tibiofibular synostosis procedures combined with Syme's amputation worked best for types 1b and 2. For types 3 and 4 tibial deficiencies, the Syme's amputation was the best treatment.

Simmons ED, Ginsburg GM, Hall JE: Brown's procedure for congenital absence of the tibia revisited. *J Pediatr Orthop* 1996;16:85–89.

These authors reported acceptable function after the Brown procedure for tibial hemimelia in seven knees followed up for 7 years. The key to success was the presence of at least grade III quadriceps function preoperatively, with a located patella. The difference in these patients and those reported by Loder and Herring was the presence of quadriceps function in those reported by Simmons, Ginsburg, and Hall. It is not clear why these patients had functioning quadriceps and Loder and Herring's did not when the patients were similarly classified.

Thomas IH, Williams PF: The Gruca operation for congenital absence of the fibula. *J Bone Joint Surg* 1987;69B:587–592.

This article describes a rediscovered procedure in which a tibial osteotomy attempts to create a lateral buttress for the talus. The operation is recommended for children with fibular hemimelia without a great deal of shortening or deformity at birth. The results were satisfactory in eight of nine patients.

Westin GW, Sakai DN, Wood WL: Congenital longitudinal deficiency of the fibula: Follow-up of treatment by Syme amputation. *J Bone Joint Surg* 1976;58A:492–496.

This study of 42 patients with fibular hemimelia describes the excellent functional results achieved by early Syme's amputation.

Prosthetic Management

Aitken GT: Management of severe bilateral upper limb deficiencies. *Clin Orthop* 1964;37:53–60.

This classic article details the step-by-step management, from infancy to adolescence, of children with bilateral upper-limb absence.

Aitken GT, Frantz CH: Management of the child amputee, in Reynolds FC (ed): American Academy of Orthopaedic Surgeons *Instructional Course Lectures XVII.* St. Louis, MO, CV Mosby, 1960, pp 246–295.

This classic paper covers the whole gamut of management of the child amputee. The article includes much detailed material regarding prosthetic design.

Bowker JH: Surgical techniques for conserving tissue and function in lower-limb amputation for trauma, infection, and vascular disease, in Greene WB (ed): *Instructional Course Lectures XXXIX.* Park Ridge, IL, American Academy of Orthopaedic Surgeons, 1990, pp 355–360.

Goldberg B: The orthopaedist as a prosthetic team leader: Getting the best for your patient from the team, in Greene WB (ed): *Instructional Course Lectures XXXIX.* Park Ridge, IL, American Academy of Orthopaedic Surgeons, 1990, pp 353–354.

Michael JW: Current concepts in above-knee socket design, in Greene WB (ed): *Instructional Course Lectures XXXIX.* Park Ridge, IL, American Academy of Orthopaedic Surgeons, 1990, pp 373–378.

Michael JW: Overview of prosthetic feet, in Greene WB (ed): *Instructional Course Lectures XXXIX.* Park Ridge, IL, American Academy of Orthopaedic Surgeons, 1990, pp 367–372.

Pinzur MS: New concepts in lower-limb amputation and prosthetic management, in Greene WB (ed): *Instructional Course Lectures XXXIX.* Park Ridge, IL, American Academy of Orthopaedic Surgeons, 1990, pp 361–366.

This group of chapters reviews recent advances in lower-extremity amputation and prosthetic management. Although some of the chapters emphasize the dysvascular amputee, the sections on new developments in prosthetic feet and above-knee socket design are particularly germane to the juvenile amputee.

Brown PW: Rehabilitation of bilateral lower-extremity amputees. *J Bone Joint Surg* 1970;52A:687–700.

This classic article is devoted to the complexity of overall rehabilitation of bilateral lower-extremity amputees. Four phases of adjustment are described, and the psychological aspects of rehabilitation are emphasized.

Edelstein JE, Berger N: Performance comparison among children fitted with myoelectric and body-powered hands. *Arch Phys Med Rehabil* 1993;77:376–380.

The authors found no functional advantage to the myoelectric prosthesis compared to body-powered hands in children. This finding reinforces the common opinion that myoelectric prostheses are preferred for cosmetic and comfort reasons (no straps) rather than for true functional superiority.

Lamb DW: Prosthetics in the upper extremity. *J Hand Surg* 1983;8:774–777.

This brief overview of developments in upper-extremity prosthetics covers electric and myoelectric design and improved cosmetic approaches.

Scotland TR, Galway HR: A Long-term review of children with congenital and acquired upper-limb deficiency. *J Bone Joint Surg* 1983;65B:346–349.

A review of 131 children with upper-extremity limb deficiency shows children most likely to continue using a prosthesis are those with short below-elbow absence who are fitted before they are 2 years of age. Children with above-elbow amputations and longer below-elbow amputations are unlikely to continue prosthetic use.

Waters RL, Perry J, Antonelli D, et al: Energy cost of walking of amputees: The influence of level of amputation. *J Bone Joint Surg* 1976;58A:42–46.

This study of energy expenditure during walking shows that the higher the level of amputation, the greater the energy cost. Patients usually compensate by walking more slowly. When energy demands exceed 50% of maximum aerobic capacity, rapid fatigue will occur.

Section 12

Fractures of the Spine and Spinal Cord Injuries

Richard E. McCarthy, MD

Bonadio WA: Cervical spine trauma in children: Part II. Mechanisms and manifestations of injury, therapeutic considerations. *Am J Emerg Med* 1993;11:256–278.

The author gives an in-depth discussion of cervical spinal injuries in children with clear diagrams showing the mechanisms of injuries, anatomic variations, good radiographic examples, and some tips on management. The normal anatomy and radiographic evaluation of the pediatric cervical spine are covered in a concise article in the March 1993 issue of the same journal.

Crawford AH: Operative treatment of spine fractures in children. *Orthop Clin North Am* 1990;21:325–339.

This article offers an excellent overview of treatment of pediatric spinal fractures from the cervical to the lumbar spine and gives the author's preferred method of treatment and evaluation of these injuries.

Cullen JC: Spinal lesions in battered babies. *J Bone Joint Surg* 1975; 57B:364–366.

Histories are presented of five abused patients under 2 years of age, emphasizing the need for skeletal surveys in suspected cases of maltreatment. Hyperflexion is postulated as the mechanism of injury.

Dearolf WW, Betz RR, Vogel IC, et al: Scoliosis in pediatric spinal cord-injured patients. *J Pediatr Orthop* 1990;10:214–218.

A large number of children with spinal cord injuries were evaluated over a 20-year period. Results agreed with those previously reported in that 97% of patients in the preadolescent group developed scoliosis, whereas spinal deformity occurred in the mature group at half this rate. Deformity occurred regardless of the level of the original injury. The authors found orthotics to be effective in some patients by slowing progression and delaying the need for surgery in preadolescent patients. They warned of the need to look for a posttraumatic syrinx in rapidly progressive curves, and they recommended surgery for patients older than 10 years of age with curves greater than 40°.

Dickman CA, Zabramski JM, Hadley MN, et al: Pediatric spinal cord injury without radiographic abnormalities: Report of 26 cases and review of the literature. *J Spinal Disord* 1991;4:296–305.

This is an excellent review of a large series of patients (26) with spinal cord injury without radiographic abnormalities (SCIWORA). The authors concluded that the mechanism of injury, its severity, and the prognosis of recovery were related to the patient's age. Younger children tended to have more severe injuries, and 70% of these lesions were complete. Workup should include tests to look for treatable lesions, including epidural hematomas or vertebral column instability. Immobilization in an orthosis for 3 months prevents recurrent injury and should be followed by dynamic radiographic films.

Dormans JP, Criscitiello AA, Drummond DS, et al: Complications in children managed with immobilization in a halo vest. *J Bone Joint Surg* 1995;77A:1370–1373.

The most common complications in 25 (68%) of 37 patients included pin-site infections and pin loosening. Other, less frequent complications included dural penetration, transient injury of the suborbital nerve, and objectionable pin-site scars. Younger patients who had a halo construct with more than four pins (multiple-pin constructs) had a complication rate similar to that of patients with standard four-pin halo constructs.

Grier D, Wardell S, Sarwark J, et al: Fatigue fractures of the sacrum in children: Two case reports and a review of the literature. *Skeletal Radiol* 1993;22:515–518.

This article describes a new entity in the pediatric literature: fatigue fractures of the sacrum. The patients presented had positive Faber-Patrick tests and were otherwise healthy. Awareness of this potential diagnosis will help with the differential diagnosis of low back pain in children.

Herzenberg JE, Hensinger RN, Dedrick DK, et al: Emergency transport and positioning of young children who have an injury of the cervical spine: The standard backboard may be hazardous. *J Bone Joint Surg* 1989;71A:15–22.

The cervical spines of children younger than 7 years of age are positioned in flexion when they are transported on a standard flat back board. Because of the relatively large circumference of the head in young children, the transport board must have either a recess for the occiput or some other adaptation to prevent undesirable cervical flexion during emergency transport.

McGrory BJ, Klassen RA: Arthrodesis of the cervical spine for fractures and dislocations in children and adolescents: A long-term follow-up study. *J Bone Joint Surg* 1994;76A:1606–1616.

After median 17.5-year follow-up of 41 patients, the authors concluded that spinal arthrodesis for fractures and dislocations of the cervical spine in children and adolescents can be accomplished safely, with an acceptable clinical outcome, low rate of complications, and minimum morbidity at long-term follow-up. On the basis of a new posttraumatic neck score, 76% had excellent results, 14% had good results, and 10% had fair results.

McGrory BJ, Klassen RA, Chao EY, et al: Acute fractures and dislocations of the cervical spine in children and adolescents. *J Bone Joint Surg* 1993;75A:988–995.

This is the largest review of cervical spinal injuries in children. The authors have determined that there was a clear demarcation between the characteristic of injuries in children younger than 11 years of age and those who are older, with a predominance of ligamentous injuries of the cephalic portion of the cervical spine in children younger than 11 years. They were usually due to a fall. Those older than 11 years of age were injured more often during sports and recreational activities, and the injury occurred more frequently in the caudal portion of the cervical spine.

Osenbach RK, Menezes AH: Pediatric spinal cord and vertebral column injury. *Neurosurgery* 1992;30:385–390.

The authors present an excellent review of a large series of children, birth to 16 years of age, with spinal cord or vertebral column injury, seen at one institution. They emphasize the types of injuries that occur more commonly in specific age groups, and that most injuries can be treated nonsurgically. Prognosis is correlated primarily with the severity of the initial neurologic insult. The authors recommend that children with severe spinal cord injury be closely monitored for the development of post-traumatic spinal deformity, which occurred in 12% of their patients. Children with SCIWORA constituted an interesting subset; this injury occurred primarily in a younger age group with a high incidence of complete neurologic injury.

Rathbone D, Johnson G, Letts M: Spinal cord concussion in pediatric athletes. *J Pediatr Orthop* 1992;12:616–620.

This topic has been controversial, especially in regard to the pediatric athlete. These authors found that although 12 children had been treated for transient sensory or motor loss after a spinal injury, only seven met the criteria for spinal stenosis as defined by Hinck or Torg who had previously discussed this topic. In children, other factors, such as hyperflexibility of the pediatric spine, may be as important in the pathomechanics of cord compression as the bony criteria of other authors. The authors recommend that athletes not be allowed to return to contact sports after having sustained cord concussion.

Rumball K, Jarvis J: Seat-belt injuries of the spine in young children. *J Bone Joint Surg* 1992;74B:571–574.

Numerous articles have been published recently on identification of problems associated with lap belt injuries in young children and the complex of associated abdominal injury associated with the seat belt sign. This article proposes a classification system that may help in the early evaluation of the injury and potentially reduce the delay in diagnosis.

Shacked I, Ram Z, Hadani M: The anterior cervical approach for traumatic injuries to the cervical spine in children. *Clin Orthop* 1993;292:144–150.

These authors discuss their experience with six patients. According to their description, a technique that is not often used in children offered distinct advantages in patients with neurologic loss and vertebral deformity after traumatic injury. The authors have a good follow-up with improvement in the neurologic status of their patients.

Sturm PF, Glass RB, Sivit CJ, et al: Lumbar compression fractures secondary to lap-belt use in children. *J Pediatr Orthop* 1995;15:521–523.

Of seven children (average age 7 years) with lumbar spine compression fractures due to lap-belt use, four had associated abdominal injuries and one died of an associated head injury. The authors hypothesize that the mechanism of injury was similar to that in flexion-distraction injuries, but the increased elasticity in the posterior ligamentous complex in children may result in compression fracture rather than the expected flexion-distraction injury. More than 50% of the authors' patients had abdominal injuries, and the fracture treatment was nonsurgical.

Yngve DA, Harris WP, Herndon WA, et al: Spinal cord injury without osseous spine fracture. *J Pediatr Orthop* 1988;8:153–159.

Patients (18) with spinal cord injury without osseous spine fracture were younger (mean age 6 years) than those (55) with osseous spine fracture (mean age 16 years). Patients without osseous fractures should be followed for the development of late spinal deformity that may require orthotic support or surgical stabilization.

Section 13

Trauma: Upper Extremity

William C. Warner, Jr., MD

Sternoclavicular Joint

Rockwood CA Jr: Dislocations of the sternoclavicular joint, in Evans EB (ed): American Academy of Orthopaedic Surgeons *Instructional Course Lectures XXIV.* St. Louis, MO, CV Mosby, 1975, pp 144–159.

This is a review of the anatomy, mechanism of injury, diagnosis, and treatment of sternoclavicular fractures and dislocations. Results indicate that these fractures and dislocations will remodel in patients up to 25 years of age and only conservative care is necessary.

Anterior Dislocations

Cope R, Riddervold HO, Shore JL, et al: Dislocations of the sternoclavicular joint: Anatomic basis, etiologies, and radiologic diagnosis. *J Orthop Trauma* 1991;5:379–384.

The authors describe the use of plain radiographic views and computed tomography (CT) scan stress maneuver to diagnose sternoclavicular fracture-separations.

de Jong KP, Sukul DM: Anterior sternoclavicular dislocation: A long-term follow-up study. *J Orthop Trauma* 1990;4:420–423.

Good results at long-term follow-up were obtained in 13 patients treated nonsurgically.

Posterior Dislocations

Lewonowski K, Bassett GS: Complete posterior sternoclavicular epiphyseal separation: A case report and review of the literature. *Clin Orthop* 1992;281:84–88.

The anatomy, diagnosis, treatment, and complications of posterior sternoclavicular fracture-separations were described and one case is reported.

Fractures of the Clavicle

Eidman DK, Siff SJ, Tullos HS: Acromioclavicular lesions in children. *Am J Sports Med* 1981;9:150–154.

This is a review of acromioclavicular joint lesions in 25 children and adolescents, one of whom had failure through the physis of the coracoid process. Conservative treatment is advocated for patients younger than 13 years of age.

Havranek P: Injuries of the distal clavicular physis in children. *J Pediatr Orthop* 1989;9:213–215.

Of 10 distal clavicular fractures in children and adolescents, nine were treated nonsurgically. All fractures healed without functional sequelae, but open reduction is recommended for significantly displaced fractures to prevent residual deformity about the shoulder.

Lewonowski K, Bassett GS: Complete posterior sternoclavicular epiphyseal separation: A case report and review of the literature. *Clin Orthop* 1992;281:84–88.

The anatomy, diagnosis, treatment, and complications of posterior sternoclavicular fracture-separations are described and one case is reported.

Oppenheim WL, Davis A, Growdon WA, et al: Clavicle fractures in the newborn. *Clin Orthop* 1990;250:176–180.

In this large retrospective review of live births, 2.7 per 1,000 had fractures of the clavicle. The fractures were associated with heavy neonates and shoulder dystocia. Brachial plexus palsy occurred in one of the 19 patients with clavicular fractures.

Rockwood CA: Abstract: Fracture of the outer clavicle in children and adults. *J Bone Joint Surg* 1982;64B:642.

This brief report describes the attachment of the intact periosteum to the intact coracoclavicular ligaments in fracture-dislocations of the distal clavicle. Conservative treatment is recommended for patients up to 16 years of age.

Fractures of the Proximal Humerus

Baxter MP, Wiley JJ: Fractures of the proximal humeral epiphysis: Their influence on humeral growth. *J Bone Joint Surg* 1986;68B:570–573.

In this review of 57 patients with proximal humeral fractures (2- to 8-year follow-up), shortening of the humerus and residual varus angulation were not significant regardless of treatment. Favorable results were obtained with nonsurgical treatment.

Beaty JH: Fractures of the proximal humerus and shaft in children, in Eilert RE (ed): *Instructional Course Lectures XLI*. Park Ridge, IL, American Academy of Orthopaedic Surgeons, 1992, pp 369–372.

This is a good review of treatment of fractures of the proximal humerus and shaft in pediatric patients.

Broker FH, Burbach T: Ultrasonic diagnosis of separation of the proximal humeral epiphysis in the newborn. *J Bone Joint Surg* 1990;72A:187–191.

The authors report ultrasonic diagnosis of proximal humeral epiphyseal separations in four newborns.

Larsen CF, Kiær T, Lindequist S: Fractures of the proximal humerus in children: Nine-year follow-up of 64 unoperated on cases. *Acta Orthop Scand* 1990;61:255–257.

In this report of 64 children with humeral fractures treated nonsurgically, only seven had minor residual complaints.

Shoulder Dislocations

Marans HJ, Angel KR, Schemitsch EH, et al: The fate of traumatic anterior dislocation of the shoulder in children. *J Bone Joint Surg* 1992;74A:1242–1244.

This is a review of 21 children treated for anterior traumatic dislocations of the shoulder, all of whom had one or more recurrent dislocations. Immobilization of 6 weeks had no effect on the rate of recurrent dislocation.

Elbow: General

Beaty JH, Kasser JR: Fractures about the elbow, in Jackson DW (ed): *Instructional Course Lectures 44.* Rosemont, IL, American Academy of Orthopaedic Surgeons, 1995, pp 199–215.

This is an overview of elbow injuries, treatment, and complications.

Haraldsson S: On osteochondrosis deformans juvenilis capituli humeri, including investigation of intra-osseous vasculature in the distal humerus. *Acta Orthop Scand* 1959;38(suppl):1–232.

This monograph reviews in detail the ossification process and vascular supply (gross and microscopic) of the elbow.

Morrissy RT, Wilkins KE: Deformity following distal humerus fracture in children. *J Bone Joint Surg* 1984;66A:557–562.

The authors report five children who had a rare complication of distal humeral fractures. The so-called "fishtail" deformity of the distal humerus may be caused by compromise of the vascular supply to the trochlea.

Silberstein JJ, Brodeur AE, Graviss ER: Some vagaries of the capitellum. *J Bone Joint Surg* 1979;61A:244–247.
Silberstein MJ, Brodeur AE, Graviss ER, et al: Some vagaries of the medial epicondyle. *J Bone Joint Surg* 1981;63A:524–528.
Silberstein MJ, Brodeur AE, Graviss ER, et al: Some vagaries of the olecranon. *J Bone Joint Surg* 1981;63A:722–725.
Silberstein MJ, Brodeur AE, Graviss ER: Some vagaries of the lateral epicondyle. *J Bone Joint Surg* 1981;64A:444–448.
Silberstein MJ, Brodeur AI, Graviss ER: Some vagaries of the radial head and neck. *J Bone Joint Surg* 1982;64A:1153–1157.

This series of five articles describes in detail normal ossification, variations in development, and fracture patterns that may be confused with normal ossification.

Yates C, Sullivan JA: Arthrographic diagnosis of elbow injuries in children. *J Pediatr Orthop* 1987;7:54–60.

In this prospective study of arthrograms made after elbow injuries in 36 patients, arthrography altered the initial diagnosis and treatment in 19%.

Yoo CI, Suh JT, Suh KT, et al: Avascular necrosis after fracture-separation of the distal end of the humerus in children. *Orthopedics* 1992;15:959–963.

Avascular necrosis of the trochlea occurred in 80 patients with fracture-separations of the distal humerus.

Supracondylar Humeral Fractures

Biyani A, Gupta SP, Sharma JC: Determination of medial epicondylar epiphyseal angle for supracondylar humerus fractures in children. *J Pediatr Orthop* 1993;13:94–97.

The authors describe a radiographic angle, the medial epicondylar epiphyseal (MEE) angle, used to evaluate of the accuracy of reduction of 20 supracondylar fractures. The angle was determined by measurement of 100 radiographs of normal children.

Celiker O, Pestilci FI, Tuzuner M: Supracondylar fracture of the humerus in children: Analysis of the results in 142 patients. *J Orthop Trauma* 1990;4:265–269.

Results were compared of closed reduction and casting (76% good or excellent results), overhead skeletal traction (100% good or excellent results), and open reduction and internal fixation (60% good or excellent results). Elbow stiffness was more frequent after open reduction, but varus or valgus angular deformities were less frequent.

France J, Strong M: Deformity and function in supracondylar fractures of the humerus in children variously treated by closed reduction and splinting, traction, and percutaneous pinning. *J Pediatr Orthop* 1992;12: 494–498.

Methods used to treat 84 patients were compared. Closed reduction and percutaneous pinning resulted in better humerocapitellar angles, better maintenance of reduction, and better clinical results.

Williamson DM, Coates CJ, Miller RK, et al: Normal characteristics of the Baumann (humerocapitellar) angle: An aid in assessment of supracondylar fractures. *J Pediatr Orthop* 1992;12:636–639.

The Baumann angle was evaluated in 114 normal children. The mean Baumann angle was 72° (standard deviation = 4°), and 95% of normal elbows had Baumann angles between 64° and 81°.

Nonsurgical Treatment

Alburger PD, Weidner PL, Betz RR: Supracondylar fractures of the humerus in children. *J Pediatr Orthop* 1992;12:16–19.

Of 39 children treated with delayed closed reduction after 3 to 5 days of side-arm traction, good or excellent results were obtained in 92%, with no vascular problems or Volkmann contractures.

Dunlop J: Transcondylar fractures of the humerus in childhood. *J Bone Joint Surg* 1939;21:59–73.

Hey-Groves EW: Direct skeletal traction in the treatment of fractures. *Br J Surg* 1928;16:149–157.

Palmer EE, Niemann KMW, Vesely D, et al: Supracondylar fracture of the humerus in children. *J Bone Joint Surg* 1978;60A:653–656.

Smith FM: Kirschner wire traction in elbow and upper arm injuries. *Am J Surg* 1947;74:770–787.

These articles describe traction treatment of supracondylar humeral fractures in children.

Closed Reduction and Percutaneous Pinning

Boyd DW, Aronson DD: Supracondylar fractures of the humerus: A prospective study of percutaneous pinning. *J Pediatr Orthop* 1992;12:789–794.

Good results were obtained when Baumann's angle was used as criterion for acceptable reduction. Use of two lateral pins for fixation is recommended.

Jones KG: Percutaneous pin fixation of fractures of the lower end of the humerus. *Clin Orthop* 1967;50:53–59.

This early description of the use of percutaneous pin fixation for supracondylar humeral fractures includes descriptions of surgical techniques and pitfalls.

Kallio PE, Foster BK, Paterson DC: Difficult supracondylar fractures in children: Analysis of percutaneous pinning technique. *J Pediatr Orthop* 1992;12:11–15.

Results were acceptable after fixation of 55 supracondylar humeral fractures with lateral divergent pins.

Mehserle WL, Meehan PL: Treatment of the displaced supracondylar fracture of the humerus (type III) with closed reduction and perctuaneous cross-pin fixation. *J Pediatr Orthop* 1991;11:705–711.

Good results were achieved with crossed K-wire fixation of type III fractures. Baumann's angle and the lateral humeral capitellar angle were useful guides for evaluating maintenance of fracture reduction.

Paradis G, Lavallee P, Gagnon N, et al: Supracondylar fractures of the humerus in children: Technique and results of crossed percutaneous K-wire fixation. *Clin Orthop* 1993;297:231–237.

The authors report good results after closed reduction and crossed K-wire percutaneous pinning of 26 supracondylar fractures.

Pirone AM, Graham HK, Krajbich JI: Management of displaced extension-type supracondylar fractures of the humerus in children. *J Bone Joint Surg* 1988;70A:641–650.

In this retrospective study of 230 patients with type III supracondylar humeral fractures, closed reduction and casting resulted in significantly fewer good results and more complications. Percutaneous pinning provided the most good results and is recommended as the treatment of choice for most fractures. Skeletal traction, however, provided acceptable results in some patients who had significant soft-tissue swelling.

Thometz JG: Techniques for direct radiographic visualization during closed pinning of supracondylar humerus fractures in children. *J Pediatr Orthop* 1990;10:555–558.

This is a description of techniques in which a modification of Dunlop's extension traction was used to allow direct fluoroscopic evaluation of Baumann's angle, the contour of the distal humerus, the pin insertion site, and the angle of pin insertion.

Topping RE, Blanco JS, Davis TJ: Clinical evaluation of crossed-pin versus lateral-pin fixation in displaced supracondylar humerus fractures. *J Pediatr Orthop* 1995;15:435–439.

After comparison of the results of crossed-pin fixation in 27 fractures to those of lateral-pin fixation in 20 fractures, the authors conclude that crossed-pin fixation offers no clinically significant advantage over two laterally placed pins.

Zionts LE, McKellop HA, Hathaway R: Torsional strength of pin configurations used to fix supracondylar fractures of the humerus in children. *J Bone Joint Surg* 1994;76A:253–256.

Results of this study show that crossed medial and lateral Kirschner-wire (K-wire) fixation provided better rotational stability than lateral pins.

Open Reduction

Ramsey RH, Griz J: Immediate open reduction and internal fixation of severely displaced supracondylar fractures of the humerus in children. *Clin Orthop* 1973;90:131–132.

Shifrin PG, Gehring HW, Iglesais LJ: Open reduction and internal fixation of displaced supracondylar fractures of the humerus in children. *Orthop Clin North Am* 1976;7:573–581.

Weiland AJ, Meyer S, Tolo VT, et al: Surgical treatment of displaced supracondylar fractures of the humerus in children: Analysis of fifty-two cases followed for five to fifteen years. *J Bone Joint Surg* 1978;60A: 657–661.

These three articles describe the indications, techniques, and pitfalls of open reduction and internal fixation of supracondylar humeral fractures.

Complications (Neurovascular)

Campbell CC, Waters PM, Emans JB, et al: Neurovascular injury and displacement in type III supracondylar humerus fractures. *J Pediatr Orthop* 1995;15:47–52.

This is a report of neurovascular injuries in 29 (49%) of 59 children with type III fractures. Posterolateral displacement was associated with median nerve injuries and posteromedial displacement with radial nerve injuries; brachial artery injuries occurred with both types of displacement.

Clement DA: Assessment of a treatment plan for managing acute vascular complications associated with supracondylar fractures of the humerus in children. *J Pediatr Orthop* 1990;10:97–100.

This is a description of anatomic findings in nine children with ischemia of the forearm associated with supracondylar fractures. Surgical procedures are discussed, and clinical results are reviewed.

Cramer KE, Green NE, Devito DP: Incidence of anterior interosseous nerve palsy in supracondylar humerus fractures in children. *J Pediatr Orthop* 1993;13:502–505.

This is a retrospective review of 101 supracondylar humeral fractures in children, 15% of whom had neural lesions. Reported incidence of anterior interosseous nerve lesion is higher than in previous reports.

Culp RW, Osterman L, Davidson RS, et al: Neural injuries associated with supracondylar fractures of the humerus in children. *J Bone Joint Surg* 1990;72A:1211–1215.

This is a report of 18 neural injuries in 13 children with supracondylar fractures. Nine neural lesions resolved spontaneously, neurolysis was performed on eight nerves, and nerve grafting was required for one. Recommended initial treatment consists of observation and supportive therapy; exploration and neurolysis are indicated if no evidence of neural function is present 5 months after injury.

Royce RO, Dutkowsky JP, Kasser JR, et al: Neurologic complications after K-wire fixation of supracondylar humerus fractures in children. *J Pediatr Orthop* 1991;11:191–194.

Of 143 supracondylar fractures treated with K-wire fixation, four (3%) had neurologic complications: two late ulnar neuropraxias, one ulnar nerve injury, and one radial nerve injury. All patients regained full neurologic function.

Shaw BA, Kasser JR, Emans JB, et al: Management of vascular injuries in displaced supracondylar humerus fractures without arteriography. *J Orthop Trauma* 1990;4:25–29.

The authors provide guidelines for when arterial exploration is indicated in a child with a displaced supracondylar fracture and vascular insufficiency.

Complications (Deformity)

DeRosa GP, Graziano GP: A new osteotomy for cutibus varus. *Clin Orthop* 1988;236:160–165.

The authors describe a step-cut technique of distal humeral valgus osteotomy fixed with one cortical screw. Excellent or good results were obtained in ten of 11 patients in whom the procedure was performed.

LaBelle H, Bunnel WP, Duhaime M, et al: Cubitus varus deformity following supracondylar fractures of the humerus in children. *J Pediatr Orthop* 1982;2:539–546.

This is a review of 63 patients with cubitus varus deformities, in whom no growth inhibition was apparent. The primary cause of deformity was inadequate reduction with medial tilt. All patients had normal function, and osteotomy was performed to correct cosmetic defects. Results were unsatisfactory in 33%.

Oppenheim WL, Clader TJ, Smith C, et al: Supracondylar humeral osteotomy for traumatic childhood cubitus varus deformity. *Clin Orthop* 1984;188:34–39.

This is a review of a large series of osteotomies for cubitus varus, in which 24% of patients had complications. The authors delineate important technical points to decrease the complication rate.

Uchida Y, Ogata K, Sugioka Y: A new three-dimensional osteotomy for cubitus varus deformity after supracondylar fracture of the humerus in children. *J Pediatr Orthop* 1991;11:327–331.

The authors describe a technique for correction of cubitus varus deformity in 12 patients. Eleven patients had excellent results and one had a good result.

Fractures of the Lateral Humeral Condyle

Badelon O, Bensahel H, Mazda K, et al: Lateral humeral condylar fractures in children: A report of 47 cases. *J Pediatr Orthop* 1988;8:31–34.

This article describes a radiographic classification that can be used to decide whether surgical or nonsurgical treatment is needed.

Davids JR, Maguire MF, Mubarak SJ, et al: Lateral condylar fracture of the humerus following posttraumatic cubitus varus. *J Pediatr Orthop* 1994;14:466–470.

Five of six lateral condylar fractures in children with cubitus varus deformities occurred after malunited extension-type supracondylar fractures and one after a lateral condylar fracture complicated by lateral overgrowth. Biomechanical analysis suggests that torsional moment and shear force generated across the capitellar physis by a routine fall are increased by varus malalignment. Posttraumatic cubitus varus deformity may predispose a child to subsequent lateral condylar fracture and should be viewed as more than a cosmetic deformity.

Finnbogason T, Karlsson G, Lindberg L, et al: Nondisplaced and minimally displaced fractures of the lateral humeral condyle in children: A prospective radiographic investigation of fracture stability. *J Pediatr Orthop* 1995;15:422–425.

Radiographic evaluation of 112 children identified criteria that allowed separation of fractures into "stable," "uncertain," and "unstable or high-risk" fractures. Displacement occurred in none of 65 stable fractures, in 17% of 35 uncertain fractures, and in 42% of 12 unstable fractures.

Flynn JC: Nonunion of slightly displaced fractures of the lateral humeral condyle in children: An update. *J Pediatr Orthop* 1989;9:691–696.

This is an update of the author's 1975 series of 31 fractures, in which he reiterates his treatment recommendation of early stabilization and bone grafting, provided that the fragment is in acceptable position and that the patient has open physes.

Foster DE, Sullivan JA, Gross RH: Lateral humeral condylar fractures in children. *J Pediatr Orthop* 1985;5:16–22.

This review of 53 patients with 56 lateral humeral condylar fractures indicates that closed treatment produced satisfactory results if the initial displacement was not more than 2 mm.

Hardacre JA, Nahigan SH, Froimson AI, et al: Fractures of the lateral condyle of the humerus in children. *J Bone Joint Surg* 1971;53A:1083–1095.

This report of 52 lateral condylar fractures details treatment, results, and complications.

Jakob R, Fowles JV, Rang M, et al: Observations concerning fractures of the lateral humeral condyle in children. *J Bone Joint Surg* 1975;57B:430–436.

Wadsworth TG: Injuries of the capitular (lateral humeral condylar) epiphysis. *Clin Orthop* 1972;85:127–142.

These classic articles are reviews of types of displacement, treatment, and complications of lateral condylar fractures.

Masada K, Kawai H, Kawabata H, et al: Osteosynthesis for old, established non-union of the lateral condyle of the humerus. *J Bone Joint Surg* 1990;72A:32–40.

Seventeen patients were treated with osteosynthesis of the nonunion combined with neurolysis and anterior transposition of the ulnar nerve, with or without corrective osteotomy of the humerus. Pain and apprehension were relieved, but range of motion decreased in most patients. Osteosynthesis is recommended for treatment of lateral humeral condylar nonunions only if the patient has serious pain or apprehension due to lateral instability.

Mintzer CM, Waters PM, Brown DJ, et al: Percutaneous pinning in the treatment of displaced lateral condyle fractures. *J Pediatr Orthop* 1994;14:462–465.

This is a report of percutaneous pinning of 12 lateral humeral condylar fractures with more than 2 mm of displacement and arthrographic documentation of no articular incongruity.

Roye DP Jr, Bini SA, Infosino A: Late surgical treatment of lateral condylar fractures in children. *J Pediatr Orthop* 1991;11:195–199.

The authors describe the technique of functional reduction in four children with symptomatic nonunions of lateral condylar fractures 8 weeks and 2, 5, and 14 years after injury.

Fractures of the Medial Humeral Condyle

Fowles JV, Kassab MT: Displaced fractures of the medial humeral condyle in children. *J Bone Joint Surg* 1980;62A:1159–1163.

This report of seven medial humeral condylar fractures emphasizes frequency of misdiagnosis or delayed diagnosis, which can cause a poor result.

Papavasiliou V, Nenopoulos S, Venturis T: Fractures of the medial condyle of the humerus in childhood. *J Pediatr Orthop* 1987;7:421–423.

In this report of 15 medial humeral condylar fractures for which treatment was based on amount of displacement, open reduction and internal fixation of displaced fractures obtained good clinical results.

Fractures of the Medial Humeral Epicondyle

Dias JJ, Johnson GV, Hoskinson J, et al: Management of severely displaced medial epicondyle fractures. *J Orthop Trauma* 1987;1:59–62.

The authors report good results after nonsurgical treatment of 20 medial epicondylar fractures associated with elbow dislocation. One patient had slight impairment of elbow function, and none had late onset of ulnar neuritis.

Fowles JV, Kassab MT, Moula T: Untreated intra-articular entrapment of the medial humeral epicondyle. *J Bone Joint Surg* 1984;66B:562–565.

This is a report of six patients with untreated intra-articular entrapment of the medial epicondyle after elbow dislocation. After treatment, initiated at an average of 14 weeks after injury, all patients had improved function.

Fowles JV, Slimane N, Kassab MT: Elbow dislocation with avulsion of the medial humeral epicondyle. *J Bone Joint Surg* 1990;72B:102–104.

This is a comparison of results after closed and open reduction; more motion was lost in those treated with open reduction.

Hines RF, Herndon WA, Evans JP: Operative treatment of medial epicondyle fractures in children. *Clin Orthop* 1987;223:170–174.

This is a report of 31 medial epicondylar fractures. Good results were obtained with surgical treatment in fractures displaced more than 2 mm if arthrotomy was not required. Elbow motion was decreased if arthrotomy was required for removal of an entrapped fragment.

Woods GM, Tullos HG: Elbow instability and medial epicondyle fracture. *Am J Sports Med* 1977;5:23–30.

The authors describe use of the gravity stress radiograph to determine elbow instability after medial epicondylar fracture. Surgery is recommended for unstable fractures and for throwing athletes.

T-condylar Fractures of the Distal Humerus

Jarvis JG, D'Astous JL: The pediatric T-supracondylar fracture. *J Pediatr Orthop* 1984;4:697–699.

This report of 16 T-condylar fractures contains recommendation for open reduction, internal fixation, and early mobilization. Little functional disability occurred despite some loss of elbow motion.

Distal Humeral Epiphyseal Separation

Abe M, Ishizu T, Nagaoka T, et al: Epiphyseal separation of the distal end of the humeral epiphysis: A follow-up note. *J Pediatr Orthop* 1995; 15:426–434.

Of 21 children with fracture-separations of the distal humerus, 15 developed cubitus varus deformities, 9 of whom regained nearly normal carrying angles after closing-wedge osteotomy.

Davidson RS, Markowitz RI, Dormans J, et al: Ultrasonographic evaluation of the elbow in infants and young children after suspected trauma. *J Bone Joint Surg* 1994;76A:1804–1813.

The authors report the use of ultrasonography in seven infants and one child with suspected elbow trauma. Three had physeal separations, two had supracondylar fractures, two had no skeletal injury, and one had an avulsion fracture of the lateral epicondyle.

de Jager LT, Hoffman EB: Fracture-separation of the distal humeral epiphysis. *J Bone Joint Surg* 1991;73B:143–146.

This report of 12 injuries contains a recommendation for closed reduction and pinning in children younger than 2 years of age because of increased incidence of cubitus varus deformity (30%). Arthrography may be needed for diagnosis and evaluation of reduction.

DeLee JC, Wilkins KE, Rogers LF, et al: Fracture-separation of the distal humeral epiphysis. *J Bone Joint Surg* 1980;62A:46–51.

In this report of 16 fracture-separations of the distal humeral epiphysis, patients are grouped according to age and radiographic appearance to define treatment principles. The frequency of child abuse in infants with this injury is noted.

Holda ME, Manoli A II, LaMont RI: Epiphyseal separation of the distal end of the humerus with medial displacement. *J Bone Joint Surg* 1980;62A:51–57.

Mizuno K, Hirohata K, Kashiwagi D: Fracture-separation of the distal humeral epiphysis in young children. *J Bone Joint Surg* 1979;61A: 570–573.

These articles describe risks of complications after this injury; Holda and associates report a high incidence of cubitus varus.

Elbow Dislocation

Beaty JH, Donati NL: Recurrent dislocation of the elbow in a child: Case report and review of the literature. *J Pediatr Orthop* 1991;11:392–396.

This is a report of an 8-year-old boy with six recurrent elbow dislocations in 2 years. Transfer of the biceps and central slip of the triceps stabilized the elbow.

Borris LC, Lassen MR, Christensen CS: Elbow dislocation in children and adults: A long-term follow-up of conservatively treated patients. *Acta Orthop Scand* 1987;58:649–651.

In this report of 63 elbow dislocations, 23 were in children. All had satisfactory results with closed reduction.

Carlioz H, Abols Y: Posterior dislocation of the elbow in children. *J Pediatr Orthop* 1984;4:8–12.

This is a report of 58 elbow dislocations in children, 64% of whom had associated fractures. Closed reduction failed in 10% of patients; in two of these failures, inverted osteochondral fragments detached from the articular surface of the ulna prevented reduction. Neurovascular complications were transient.

DeLee JC: Transverse divergent dislocation of the elbow in a child: Case report. *J Bone Joint Surg* 1981;63A:322–323.

Sovio OM, Tredwell SJ: Divergent dislocation of the elbow in a child. *J Pediatr Orthop* 1986;6:96–97.

These case reports of divergent dislocations describe the reduction maneuver.

Monteggia Fracture-Dislocation

Bado JL: The Monteggia lesion. *Clin Orthop* 1967;50:71–86.

This is a summary of the original 1962 text that gives the classic description of Monteggia injuries and classifies them into four types. This is the standard classification system for these injuries.

Bell-Tawse AJS: The treatment of malunited anterior Monteggia fractures in children. *J Bone Joint Surg* 1965;47B:718–723.

The author describes the use of a strip of the triceps aponeurosis for reconstructing the orbicular ligament in radial head dislocations that are recognized late.

Best TN: Management of old unreduced Monteggia fracture dislocations of the elbow in children. *J Pediatr Orthop* 1994;14:193–199.

The natural history of unreduced Monteggia fracture-dislocations may not be benign, and surgical treatment 6 years or less after the initial injury is described, as is the surgical technique used in six patients. Complete correction of the ulnar deformity is the essential feature of a stable result.

Letts M, Locht R, Weins J: Monteggia fracture-dislocations in children. *J Bone Joint Surg* 1985;67B:724–727.

The authors report 28 Monteggia fracture-dislocations and describe a classification system.

Olney BW, Menelaus MB: Monteggia and equivalent lesions in childhood. *J Pediatr Orthop* 1989;9:219–223.

In this report of 102 Monteggia fracture-dislocations in children, ten of 14 type I equivalent lesions required open reduction. Varus angulation was common at follow-up, although angulation of up to 25° was acceptable with little functional loss.

Stoll TM, Willis RB, Paterson DC: Treatment of the missed Monteggia fracture in the child. *J Bone Joint Surg* 1992;74B:436–440.

This is a report of eight children with missed Monteggia fracture-dislocations. Of six patients with open reduction, five required ulnar osteotomy for reduction. Open reduction is recommended only for children 10 years of age or younger and can be attempted up to 4 years after injury.

Fractures of the Radial Neck

Bernstein SM, McKeever P, Bernstein L: Percutaneous reduction of displaced radial neck fractures in children. *J Pediatr Orthop* 1993;13:85–88.

The authors describe their technique of percutaneous reduction and report good results.

D'souza S, Vaishya R, Klenerman L: Management of radial neck fractures in children: A retrospective analysis of one hundred patients. *J Pediatr Orthop* 1993;13:232–238.

The authors of this report of 100 radial neck fractures provide criteria for translation and angulation that can be treated nonsurgically.

Fowles JV, Kassab MT: Observations concerning radial neck fractures in children. *J Pediatr Orthop* 1986;6:51–57.

The authors report 23 radial neck fractures. Fractures with more than 60° of angulation were treated with open reduction and internal fixation. Oblique K-wire fixation is recommended.

Rodriguez-Merchan EC: Percutaneous reduction of displaced radial neck fractures in children. *J Trauma* 1994;37:812–814.

In this report of 23 displaced radial neck fractures, the degree of initial displacement is correlated with functional outcome.

Steinberg EL, Golomb D, Salama R, et al: Radial head and neck fractures in children. *J Pediatr Orthop* 1988;8:35–40.

This is a review of the long-term results of fractures of the radial head and neck in 42 children. Primary angulation was the most important factor affecting results.

Fractures of the Olecranon

Graves SC, Canale ST: Fractures of the olecranon in children: Long-term followup. *J Pediatr Orthop* 1993;13:239–241.

The authors report 41 olecranon fractures in children. Satisfactory results were obtained with nonsurgical treatment in 93% of fractures with less than 5 mm of displacement; 78% of displaced fractures that required surgery had satisfactory results.

Papavasiliou VA, Beslikas TA, Nenopoulos S: Isolated fractures of the olecranon in children. *Injury* 1987;18:100–102.

In this report of 15 isolated olecranon fractures in children, two major groups are described (intra-articular and extra-articular). Subclassifications are based on the amount of displacement.

Nursemaid Elbow

Salter RB, Zaltz C: Anatomic investigations of the mechanism of injury and pathologic anatomy of "pulled elbow" in young children. *Clin Orthop* 1971;77:134–143.

This is a review of the pathology, anatomy, and treatment of nursemaid elbow.

Snellman O: Subluxation of the head of the radius in children. *Acta Orthop Scand* 1959;28:311–315.

This report of 474 children with nursemaid elbow includes description of the pathologic mechanism of injury and results of treatment.

Fractures of the Forearm

Amit Y, Salai M, Chechik A, et al: Closed intramedullary nailing for the treatment of diaphyseal forearm fractures in adolescence: A preliminary report. *J Pediatr Orthop* 1985;5:143–146.

The authors report satisfactory results in 20 adolescents with diaphyseal forearm fractures treated with closed intramedullary nailing. The surgical technique is described.

Bailey DA, Wedge JH, McCulloch RG, et al: Epidemiology of fractures of the distal end of the radius in children as associated with growth. *J Bone Joint Surg* 1989;71A:1225–1231.

Results of this study of 7,315 fractures show that peak incidence coincides with peak velocity of growth in boys and girls. Because the peak incidence of fracture could not be explained solely by an incease in physical activity, the authors hypothesize that it may be related to a temporary increase in bone porosity.

Daruwalla JS: A study of radioulnar movements following fractures of the forearm in children. *Clin Orthop* 1979;139:114–120.

Friberg KS: Remodeling after distal forearm fractures in children. (I. The effect of residual angulation on the spatial orientation of the epiphyseal plates; II. The final orientation of the distal and proximal epiphyseal plates of the radius; and III. Correction of residual angulation in fractures of the radius.) *Acta Orthop Scand* 1979;50:537–546, 731–739, 741–749.

Högström H, Nilsson BE, Willner S: Correction with growth following diaphyseal forearm fracture. *Acta Orthop Scand* 1976;47:299–303.

Nilsson BE, Obrant K: The range of motion following fracture of the shaft of the forearm in children. *Acta Orthop Scand* 1977;48:600–602.

These analyses of forearm fractures provide guidelines for determining which fractures remodel and which have residual angulation or loss of motion. Common prognostic factors can be determined for evaluating the adequacy of reduction.

Fuller DJ, McCullough CJ: Malunited fractures of the forearm in children. *J Bone Joint Surg* 1982;64B:364–367.

This is a report of 49 children with malunited forearm fractures. Fractures of the distal third of the radius and ulna had satisfactory remodeling in children younger than 14 years of age, but diaphyseal fractures satisfactorily remodeled only in children younger than 8 years of age.

Kasser JR: Forearm fractures, in Eilert RE (ed): *Instructional Course Lectures XLI.* Park Ridge, IL, American Academy of Orthopaedic Surgeons, 1992, pp 391–396.

The author reviews the different types of forearm fractures in children and the treatment options for these fractures.

Kay S, Smith C, Oppenheim WL: Both-bone midshaft forearm fractures in children. *J Pediatr Orthop* 1986;6:306–310.

This is a report of 26 children with both-bone forearm fractures. Closed treatment gave excellent results in children younger than 10 years of age. In children between 10 and 16 years of age, results were less predictable with closed treatment, and many required open reduction and internal fixation.

Lascombes P, Prevot J, Ligier JN, et al: Elastic stable intramedullary nailing in forearm shaft fractures in children: 85 cases. *J Pediatr Orthop* 1990;10:167–171.

At 3.5-year follow-up, 92% had excellent results with full range of motion; there were no nonunions or infections. This method is recommended for displaced forearm fractures in children older than 10 years of age and in younger children when conservative treatment fails.

Matthews LS, Kaufer H, Garver DF, et al: The effect on supination-pronation of angular malalignment of fractures of both bones of the forearm: An experimental study. *J Bone Joint Surg* 1982;64A:14–17.

In this study 10° of angulation resulted in no significant loss of motion, but 20° of angulation resulted in loss of 30% of supination and pronation.

Nimityongskul P, Anderson LD, Sri P: Plastic deformation of the forearm: A review and case reports. *J Trauma* 1991;31:1678–1685.

This is a literature review and report of four children with plastic deformation of the forearm. Manipulation and correction of deformities of 15° or more is recommended in children older than 10 years of age and of 20° or more in children between 6 and 10 years of age. No treatment is required in children younger than 5 years of age because of potential for remodeling.

Price CT, Scott DS, Kurzner ME, et al: Malunited forearm fractures in children. *J Pediatr Orthop* 1990;10:705–712.

Of 47 patients with radiographic malunions after closed reduction, 39 returned for clinical follow-up. All patients were satisfied with the clinical result, and 92% had good or excellent motion. Distal fractures had a better prognosis than proximal fractures. Closed treatment is recommended for forearm fractures in children, and good results are obtained in most patients despite radiographic malunion.

Sanders WE, Heckman JD: Traumatic plastic deformation of the radius and ulna: A closed method of correction of deformity. *Clin Orthop* 1984;188:58–67.

The authors describe deformities that occur with plastic deformation of the radius and ulna, emphasizing that this injury may not be recognized. The method of reduction is described.

Tarr RR, Garfinkel AJ, Sarmiento A: The effects of angular and rotational deformities of both bones of the forearm. *J Bone Joint Surg* 1984;66A:65–70.

The results of this study demonstrate that 10° of angulation of the forearm has little effect on pronation and supination.

Tredwell SJ, Van Peteghem K, Clough M: Pattern of forearm fractures in children. *J Pediatr Orthop* 1984;4:604–608.

This article is an analysis of 500 forearm fractures in children; it provides a good overview of fracture patterns, incidences, and percentages.

Verstreken L, Delronge G, Lamoureux J: Shaft forearm fractures in children: Intramedullary nailing with immediate motion. A preliminary report. *J Pediatr Orthop* 1988;8:450–453.

The authors describe the technique and report six forearm fractures for which intramedullary nailing was used to maintain alignment after closed treatment failed.

Vittas D, Larsen E, Torp-Pedersen S: Angular remodeling of midshaft forearm fractures in children. *Clin Orthop* 1991;265:261–264.

The authors report 36 children with angulated midshaft forearm fractures. In children younger than 11 years of age, 13° of correction was obtained, but in children older than 11 years of age, the amount of remodeling was unpredictable.

Voto SJ, Weiner DS, Leighley B: Redisplacement after closed reduction of forearm fractures in children. *J Pediatr Orthop* 1990;10:79–84.

The authors report 90 forearm fractures, of which 7% redisplaced or angulated after closed reduction. Nonphyseal fractures were safely remanipulated up to 24 days after injury.

Walker JL, Rang M: Forearm fractures in children: Cast treatment with the elbow extended. *J Bone Joint Surg* 1991;73B:299–301.

Of 15 fractures treated with cast immobilization with the elbow extended, only one had more than 15° of angulation at the time of union. All patients obtained normal elbow motion at 2 weeks and full forearm rotation at follow-up. Although the extended-elbow cast is awkward, it provides an alternative to internal fixation for some unstable fractures.

Galeazzi Fracture-Dislocation

Landfried MJ, Stenclik M, Susi JG: Variant of Galeazzi fracture-dislocation in children. *J Pediatr Orthop* 1991;11:332–335.

This is a report of a type of Galeazzi fracture-dislocation with soft-tissue interposition blocking closed reduction.

Letts M, Rowhani N: Galeazzi-equivalent injuries of the wrist in children. *J Pediatr Orthop* 1993;13:561–566.

In this report of 10 Galeazzi fractures in children, the six who had Galeazzi-equivalent fractures had less favorable results than those with classic Galeazzi fractures. A classification system is described.

Mikic ZD: Galeazzi fracture-dislocations. *J Bone Joint Surg* 1975;57A:1071–1080.

This is the report of large series of Galeazzi fracture-dislocations in adults and children. Nonsurgical management was successful only in children (14 patients); adults required surgical treatment.

Walsh HP, McLaren CA, Owen R: Galeazzi fractures in children. *J Bone Joint Surg* 1987;69B:730–733.

In this report of 41 Galeazzi fractures in children, joint disruption was not identified on initial examination in 41% of patients. Acceptable results were obtained with nonsurgical management. Placing the forearm in supination during cast immobilization is recommended.

Wrist Injuries

Christodoulou AG, Colton CL: Scaphoid fractures in children. *J Pediatr Orthop* 1986;6:37–39.

This is a report of 77 children with scaphoid fractures. In most patients, union was obtained with cast immobilization.

Golz RJ, Grogan DP, Greene TL, et al: Distal ulnar physeal injury. *J Pediatr Orthop* 1991;11:318–326.

The authors describe injury to the distal ulnar physis, which results in premature physeal closure and ulnar shortening.

Letts M, Esser D: Fractures of the triquetrum in children. *J Pediatr Orthop* 1993;13:228–231.

This is a report of 15 children with triquetral fractures, most of which were flake fractures. Three fractures were missed on initial evaluation. Missed diagnosis or incorrect diagnosis as wrist "sprain" is frequent in children with these injuries.

Mussbichler H: Injuries of the carpal scaphoid in children. *Acta Radiol* 1961;56:361–368.

The author reviewed 100 scaphoid fractures in patients younger than 15 years of age. Dorsal radial avulsions were seen in 52%, and fewer than

15% had waist fractures. All healed within 6 weeks. The need for radiographic views in extreme pronation is emphasized.

Southcott R, Rosman MA: Non-union of carpal scaphoid fractures in children. *J Bone Joint Surg* 1977;59B:20-23.

Eight nonunions were treated successfully with bone grafting.

Vahvanen V, Westerlund M: Fracture of the carpal scaphoid in children: A clinical and roentgenological study of 108 cases. *Acta Orthop Scand* 1980;51:909-913.

This is a report of 108 scaphoid fractures, most of which were distal. All healed with conservative treatment. Classification of various fracture types had no clinical signficance.

Fractures of the Hand

Barton NJ: Fractures of the phalanges of the hand in children. *Hand* 1979;2:134-143.

This article is a description of patterns of finger fractures in a large series. Although fingertip injuries were common in children, few were joint injuries. Physeal fractures were most often Salter-Harris type II injuries.

Bogumill GP: A morphologic study of the relationship of collateral ligaments to growth plates in the digits. *J Hand Surg* 1983;8:74-79.

Hankin FM, Janda DH: Tendon and ligament attachments in relationship to growth plates in a child's hand. *J Hand Surg* 1989;14B:315-318.

These are anatomic studies. The authors describe soft-tissue attachments from the physes of the fingers in an attempt to explain physeal injuries of the hand.

Dixon GL Jr, Moon NF: Rotational supracondylar fractures of the proximal phalanx in children. *Clin Orthop* 1972;83:151-156.

This is a description of rotational deformity after phalangeal neck fractures. This deformity usually requires surgical intervention.

Fischer MD, McElfresh EC: Physeal and periphyseal injuries of the hand: Patterns of injury and results of treatment. *Hand Clin* 1994;10:287–301.

Injury patterns and results of treatment of hand fractures in children are reviewed.

Leonard MH, Dubravcik P: Management of fractured fingers in the child. *Clin Orthop* 1970;73:160–168.

The authors report 263 phalangeal fractures in children; 75% were treated with simple splintage, 15% required manipulation, and only 10% required surgery (a third of these were phalangeal neck fractures). Slightly fewer than half of the fractures were physeal injuries.

Seymour N: Juxta-epiphyseal fracture of the terminal phalanx of the finger. *J Bone Joint Surg* 1966;48B:347–349.

Mallet finger deformity in children is described as a physeal separation rather than an avulsion of the tendon. Conservative management and preservation of the nail are emphasized.

Miscellaneous

Abraham E: Remodeling potential of long bones following angular osteotomies. *J Pediatr Orthop* 1989;9:37–43.

This study of immature monkeys was undertaken to demonstrate the potential for remodeling in valgus, varus, and flexion deformities. The periosteum and the physis contributed equally to correction of angular deformities.

Mabrey JD, Fitch RD: Plastic deformation in pediatric fractures: Mechanism and treatment *J Pediatr Orthop* 1989;9:310–314.

This review of the mechanism and treatment of plastic deformation of the radius and ulna includes discussion of molecular, histologic, and biomechanical properties of pediatric bones that lead to plastic deformation.

Moseley CF: General features of fractures in children, in Eilert RE (ed): *Instructional Course Lectures XLI.* Park Ridge, IL, American Academy of Orthopaedic Surgeons, 1992, pp 337–346.

This review of unique features of children's fractures includes discussions of growth arrest, bony bars, growth stimulation, remodeling, and mechanical properties of children's bones.

Injuries to the Physis

Poland J: *Traumatic Separation of the Epiphyses.* London, England, Smith, Elder & Co, 1898.

This is one of the most complete works written on physeal injuries; it still is considered a classic.

Pritchett JW: Growth plate activity in the upper extremity. *Clin Orthop* 1991;268:235–242.

Growth predictions are given for the proximal and distal humerus, radius, and ulna; these predictions can be used in predicting shortening and the need for epiphysiodesis.

Salter RB, Harris WR: Injuries involving the epiphyseal plate. *J Bone Joint Surg* 1963;45A:587–622.

This classic article provides original classification of physeal injuries into five different types; this is still the most widely accepted classification.

Child-Abuse Syndrome

Kempe CH, Helfer RE: *The Battered Child,* ed 3. Chicago, IL, University of Chicago Press, 1980.

Kempe CH, Silverman FN, Steele BF, et al: The battered-child syndrome. *JAMA* 1962;181:17–24.

These are discussions of the total picture of the child-abuse syndrome, with clear delineation of radiologic manifestations.

King J, Diefendorf D, Apthorp J, et al: Analysis of 429 fractures in 189 battered children. *J Pediatr Orthop* 1988;8:585–589.

This is a report of 429 fractures, half of which were single transverse fractures of long bones. The authors emphasize that single diaphyseal fractures are more common in battered children than the so-called pathognomonic multiple fractures.

Loder RT, Bookout C: Fracture patterns in battered children. *J Orthop Trauma* 1991;5:428–433.

This is a report of 75 battered children, most of whom did not have classic child-abuse fracture patterns. An isolated fracture without signs of other trauma was most common: 41% of long bone fractures were transverse and only 28% were "corner" fractures.

Nimityongskul P, Anderson LD: The likelihood of injuries when children fall out of bed. *J Pediatr Orthop* 1987;7:184–186.

This is a report of 76 children from newborns to 16 years of age who were reported to have fallen out of bed while in the hospital. Severe head, neck, spine, and extremity injuries were extremely rare in these children, and child abuse should be suspected if a child is said to have fallen out of bed at home.

Overuse Syndromes

Albanese SA, Palmer AK, Kerr DR, et al: Wrist pain and distal growth plate closure of the radius in gymnasts. *J Pediatr Orthop* 1989;9:23–28.

This report of wrist pain in three competitive gymnasts indicates that all had radiographic evidence of premature physeal closure that resulted in shortening of the radius and alterations in the normal distal radioulnar joint.

Barnett LS: Little League shoulder syndrome: Proximal humeral epiphysiolysis in adolescent baseball pitchers. A case report. *J Bone Joint Surg* 1985;67A:495–496.

This article is a case report, review of the literature, and discussion of the diagnosis and treatment of this condition.

Cahill BR, Tullos HS, Fain RH: Little League shoulder. *Am J Sports Med* 1974;2:150–153.

A chronic stress fracture of the proximal humeral physis in a young pitcher is described.

Caine D, Roy S, Singer KM, et al: Stress changes of the distal radial growth plate: A radiographic survey and review of the literature. *Am J Sports Med* 1992;20:290–298.

The authors review clinical and radiographic findings in "gymnast's wrist."

Gugenheim JJ Jr, Stanley RF, Woods GW, et al: Little League survey: The Houston study. *Am J Sports Med* 1976;4:189–200.

Larson RL, Singer KM, Bergstrom R, et al: Little League survey: The Eugene study. *Am J Sports Med* 1976;4:201–209.

These articles describe the long-term effects of throwing in young individuals. Long-term effects were minimal when moderation in games was practiced.

Maffulli N, Chan D, Alridge MJ: Overuse injuries of the olecranon in young gymnasts. *J Bone Joint Surg* 1992;74B:305–308.

This is a report of overuse injuries in ten patients, all but one of whom responded to conservative treatment.

Yong-Hing K, Wedge JH, Bowen CV: Chronic injury to the distal ulnar and radial growth plates in an adolescent gymnast: A case report. *J Bone Joint Surg* 1988;70A:1087–1089.

This is a case report of chronic injury to the distal radius in a young gymnast.

Section 14

Fractures of the Pelvis and Lower Extremities

Stephen D. Heinrich, MD

Ablin DS, Greenspan A, Reinhart MA: Pelvic injuries in child abuse. *Pediatr Radiol* 1992;22:454–457.

Pelvic injuries associated with child abuse are reviewed through three case reports.

Bond SJ, Gotschall CS, Eichelberger MR: Predictors of abdominal injury in children with pelvic fracture. *J Trauma* 1991;31:1169–1173.

Fifty-four of 2,248 children admitted to a regional pediatric trauma center with blunt trauma had a boney injury to the pelvis. The probability of abdominal injury was less than 1% in children with an isolated pubic fracture, 15% for iliac or sacral fractures, and 60% for multiple fractures of the pelvic ring.

Garvin KL, McCarthy RE, Barnes CL, et al: Pediatric pelvic ring fractures. *J Pediatr Orthop* 1990;10:577–582.

Of 29 patients with pelvic fractures, 67% had associated injuries and 30% had long-term morbidity or mortality. The high probability of associated injuries must be appreciated in these patients, because even minimal bony injury may be associated with life-threatening visceral injuries.

Magid D, Fishman EK, Ney DR, et al: Acetabular and pelvic fractures in the pediatric patient: Value of two- and three-dimensional imaging. *J Pediatr Orthop* 1992;12:621–625.

This article highlights the use of two- and three-dimensional computerized tomography in the evaluation of the child with a complex pelvic fracture.

McIntyre RC Jr, Bensard DD, Moore EE, et al: Pelvic fracture geometry predicts risk of life-threatening hemorrhage in children. *J Trauma* 1993; 35:423–429.

Other authors have concluded that pelvic fractures in children are rarely a source of life-threatening hemorrhage. This study determined that children with bilateral, anterior, and posterior pelvic fractures were at significantly increased risk of life-threatening hemorrhage when compared with children who have unilateral anterior and/or posterior pelvic fractures. The authors urge a prompt multispecialty approach to children with a high risk of life-threatening hemorrhage as determined by pelvic fracture geometry.

Metzmaker JN, Pappas AM: Avulsion fractures of the pelvis. *Am J Sports Med* 1985;13:349–358.

All 27 patients with avulsion fractures treated nonsurgically had excellent results except for one of six ischial tuberosity avulsions. The authors recommend nonsurgical treatment.

Sundar M, Carty H: Avulsion fractures of the pelvis in children: A report of 32 fractures and their outcome. *Skeletal Radiol* 1994;23:85–90.

This is an excellent review of the experiences of the Royal Liverpool Children's Hospital with avulsion fractures of the pediatric pelvis. Eight of 12 patients with ischial avulsions reported significant reduction in their sporting ability.

Wootton JR, Cross MJ, Holt KW: Avulsion of the ischial apophysis: The case for open reduction and internal fixation. *J Bone Joint Surg* 1990; 72B:625–627.

This is a report of three patients with chronic disability after nonunion of ischial tuberosity avulsion.

Hip Dislocations

Barquet A: Natural history of avascular necrosis following traumatic hip dislocation in childhood: A review of 145 cases. *Acta Orthop Scand* 1982;53:815–820.

This article reviews the outcome of 145 patients followed to maturity and defines two groups. Osteonecrosis in younger children behaved like Legg-Calvé-Perthes disease. In children older than 12, the course was similar to osteonecrosis in adults. The incidence of deformities was high.

Barquet A: Traumatic anterior dislocation of the hip in childhood. *Injury* 1982;13:435–440.

This article reviews combined data reported in the world literature of 111 anterior hip dislocations in children. The ratio of anterior to posterior dislocation is the same in children as in adults. The Allis method is the most successful method of reduction. Anterior dislocations are associated with a high prevalence of concomitant injuries.

Gartland JJ, Benner JH: Traumatic dislocations in the lower extremity in children. *Orthop Clin North Am* 1976;7:687–700.

This is a review of the literature and a summary of 248 hip dislocations in children.

Fractures of the Femoral Neck and Peritrochanteric Region

Davison BL, Weinstein SL: Hip fractures in children: A long-term follow-up study. *J Pediatr Orthop* 1992;12:355–358.

The authors report the long-term follow-up (average 16 years) of 19 children with hip fractures. Nine of the 19 fractures were complicated by osteonecrosis of the capital femoral epiphysis. Of the patients who developed osteonecrosis, 78% required additional surgery. A delayed or nonunion occurred in approximately 31% of the patients. Coxa vara was identified in five of the 15 patients with follow-up radiographs.

Hughes LO, Beaty JH: Fractures of the head and neck of the femur in children. *J Bone Joint Surg* 1994;76A:283–291.

This article is an excellent review of the anatomy, classification, treatment guidelines, and complications associated with fractures of the proximal femur in children.

Ratliff AHC: Fractures of the neck of the femur in children, in Salvati EA (ed): *The Hip: Proceedings of the Ninth Open Scientific Meeting of the Hip Society, 1981.* St. Louis, MO, CV Mosby, 1981, pp 188–218.

This extensive review of 168 patients discusses incidences, types, complication rates, and treatment principles. This supersedes an earlier review of 71 patients (*J Bone Joint Surg* 1962;44B:522-542) and elaborates on the classification of osteonecrosis.

Wolfgang GL: Stress fracture of the femoral neck in a patient with open capital femoral epiphyses. *J Bone Joint Surg* 1977;59A:680–681.

This article reviews the world literature on stress fractures of the femoral neck. Most are in young male adults. It describes a stress fracture in a 10-year-old female.

Femoral Shaft Fractures

Aronson DD, Singer RM, Higgins RF: Skeletal traction for fractures of the femoral shaft in children: A long-term study. *J Bone Joint Surg* 1987; 69A:1435–1439.

Traction pins placed obliquely are more often associated with fracture angulation than pins placed horizontally. Fractures in children more than 11 years old should be reduced without overriding.

Aronson J, Tursky EA: External fixation of femur fractures in children. *J Pediatr Orthop* 1992;12:157–163.

Forty-four diaphyseal femoral fractures were treated with external fixation. All healed in satisfactory position. There were no refractures.

Beaty JH, Austin SM, Warner WC, et al: Interlocking intramedullary nailing of femoral-shaft fractures in adolescents: Preliminary results and complications. *J Pediatr Orthop* 1994;14:178–183.

The authors report the Campbell Clinic experience of stabilizing 31 femoral shaft fractures with interlocking intramedullary nails in 30 children. No angular or rotational malunions occurred. Two patients had overgrowth of more than 2.5 cm. One adolescent developed a segmental osteonecrosis of the capital femoral epiphysis.

Bohn WW, Durbin RA: Ipsilateral fractures of the femur and tibia in children and adolescents. *J Bone Joint Surg* 1991;73A:429–439.

This is an excellent review of 44 patients. Complications were greatest in children older than 10 years and for juxta-articular fractures.

Brouwer KJ, Molenaar JC, van Linge B: Rotational deformities after femoral shaft fractures in childhood: A retrospective study 27-32 years after the accident. *Acta Orthop Scand* 1981;52:81–89.

Clinical examination and anteversion radiographs found only one patient with rotational asymmetry. The authors conclude that some patients probably had rotational malalignment at time of union but that it spontaneously resolved in all but one.

Buehler KC, Thompson JD, Sponseller PD, et al: A prospective study of early spica casting outcomes in the treatment of femoral shaft fractures in children. *J Pediatr Orthop* 1995;15:30–35.

The authors propose the "telescope test" for early spica casting. When gentle longitudinal compression of the thigh under anesthesia produces less than 25 mm of overlap, then the fracture can be safely treated with a spica cast.

Canale ST, Tolo VT: Fractures of the femur in children. *J Bone Joint Surg* 1995;77A:294–315.

This is an excellent, concise review of pediatric femoral fractures from hip to knee.

Heinrich SD, Drvaric DM, Darr K, et al: The operative stabilization of pediatric diaphyseal femur fractures with flexible intramedullary nails: A prospective analysis. *J Pediatr Orthop* 1994;14:501–507.

The surgical technique is described. Indications for pediatric femoral fracture stabilization with flexible nails are reviewed.

Hennrikus WL, Kasser JR, Rand F, et al: The function of the quadriceps muscle after a fracture of the femur in patients who are less than seventeen years old. *J Bone Joint Surg* 1993;75A:508–513.

Of 33 patients with closed femoral shaft fractures, 13 (39%) had a persistent deficit in the strength of the quadriceps an average of 33 months after injury. Fourteen (42%) had an average loss of 10 mm in thigh circumference, and 16 (48%) had an average loss of 10° of knee flexion. Despite persistent weakness of the quadriceps, none had a clinical problem at latest follow-up.

Herndon WA, Mahnken RF, Yngve DA, et al: Management of femoral shaft fractures in the adolescent. *J Pediatr Orthop* 1989;9:29–32.

Reeves RB, Ballard RI, Hughes JL: Internal fixation versus traction and casting of adolescent femoral shaft fractures. *J Pediatr Orthop* 1990; 10:592–595.

These two reports compare nonsurgical to surgical results and support surgical management of femoral fractures in adolescents.

Hresko MT, Kasser JR: Physeal arrest about the knee associated with nonphyseal fractures in the lower extremity. *J Bone Joint Surg* 1989;71A: 698–703.

The authors describe seven patients who developed physeal arrest of the distal femur or proximal tibia associated with fractures elsewhere in the lower extremity not involving the physis. Recognition of growth disturbance was delayed an average of 0.8 years. This article provides another reason why children with long bone fractures should be followed beyond the time of initial bone healing.

Hughes BF, Sponseller PD, Thompson JD: Pediatric femur fractures: Effects of spica cast treatment on family and community. *J Pediatr Orthop* 1994;15:457–460.

In 23 children treated with spica casting, mobility was identified by families as the major problem. Other adaptations necessary with this treatment method are highlighted to aid in advance planning.

Kregor PJ, Song KM, Routt MIC Jr, et al: Plate fixation of femoral shaft fractures in multiply injured children. *J Bone Joint Surg* 1993;75A: 1774–1780.

Fifteen fractures in 12 patients (average age 8 years) with polytrauma were treated with compression plating. All fractures healed, and anatomic alignment was obtained in 14; one healed with 13° of anterior angulation. Overgrowth of the injured femur averaged 0.9 cm in seven patients who had an uninjured contralateral femur.

Martin-Ferrero MA, Sanchez-Martin MM: Prediction of overgrowth in femoral shaft fractures in children. *Int Orthop* 1986;10:89–93.

Seventy-one patients were followed with radiographs. Femoral overgrowth was greatest in children between 3 and 9 years of age, in those with severe initial displacement, and in those who healed without overriding.

Martinez AG, Carroll NC, Sarwark JF, et al: Femoral shaft fractures in children treated with early spica cast. *J Pediatr Orthop* 1991;11:712–716.

In 51 patients (age 3 to 11 years) with femoral shaft fractures treated with early spica casting, shortening of more than 20 mm was the most common complication, occurring in 22 (43%). Factors associated with unacceptable shortening were shortening of more than 10 mm at the time of cast application, shortening of more than 20 mm at initial examination, and increasing age. One criticism of this report is that patients were only followed to union of the fracture.

McCartney D, Hinton A, Heinrich SD: Operative stabilization of pediatric femur fractures. *Orthop Clin North Am* 1994;25:635–650.

This is an excellent review of the indications, techniques, and results of surgical stabilization of proximal, diaphyseal, and distal pediatric femoral fractures.

Newton PO, Mubarak SJ: Financial aspects of femoral shaft fracture treatment in children and adolescents. *J Pediatr Orthop* 1994;14:508–512.

Total charges were lowest for those treated with early spica casting ($5,494) and highest for those treated with skeletal traction and intramedullary nailing ($21,093 and $21,359, respectively). Skin traction and home Neufeld traction were associated with significant savings over in-hospital skeletal traction and intramedullary nailing.

O'Malley DE, Mazur JM, Cummings RJ: Femoral head avascular necrosis associated with intramedullary nailing in an adolescent. *J Pediatr Orthop* 1995;15:21–23.

The authors describe the pediatric vascular anatomy and emphasize the risk of this complication in skeletally immature patients.

Raney EM, Ogden JA, Grogan DP: Premature greater trochanteric epiphysiodesis secondary to intramedullary femoral rodding. *J Pediatr Orthop* 1993;13:516–520.

This article discusses the change in growth, the resulting deformities, and how this technique predisposes the proximal femur to a subsequent growth disturbance.

Reeves RB, Ballard RI, Hughes JL: Internal fixation versus traction and casting of adolescent femoral shaft fractures. *J Pediatr Orthop* 1990;10:592–595.

Of 90 patients with 96 femoral shaft fractures, 49 (52 fractures) were treated with rigid internal fixation and 41 (44 fractures) were treated with traction and casting. Those treated with traction and casting had an average hospital stay of 26 days, while the surgical group had an average of 9 days and had fewer complications than the nonsurgical group.

Shapiro F: Fractures of the femoral shaft in children: The overgrowth phenomenon. *Acta Orthop Scand* 1981;52:649–655.

This is a report of 74 patients followed with orthoroentgenograms from time of fracture healing until skeletal maturity. Most overgrowth is completed by 18 months but may continue for 3.5 years and occasionally longer. Average overgrowth was 0.92 cm.

Stannard JP, Christensen KP, Wilkins KE: Femur fractures in infants: A new therapeutic approach. *J Pediatr Orthop* 1995;15:461–466.

The authors describe the use of the Pavlik harness for 16 children from birth to age 18 months.

Viljanto J, Kiviluoto H, Paananen M: Remodelling after femoral shaft fracture in children. *Acta Chir Scand* 1975;141:360–365.

This is one of the few articles that follows and quantitates angular malalignment. The greater the angle, the greater the remodeling. Varus remodels 40%, valgus remodels 60%, and anterior or posterior angulation, 70%. Remodeling continued for up to 5 years.

Ward WT, Levy J, Kaye A: Compression plating for child and adolescent femur fractures. *J Pediatr Orthop* 1992;12:626–632.

Twenty-five femoral fractures were stabilized with AO compression plate fixation. Most of the patients had an associated severe head injury or polytrauma. Twenty-three (92%) fractures healed in an average of 11 weeks, leg-length discrepancy was not a clinical problem, and nursing care and rehabilitation were simplified in all children.

Weiss AP, Schenck RC Jr, Sponseller PD, et al: Peroneal nerve palsy after early cast application for femoral fractures in children. *J Pediatr Orthop* 1992;12:25–28.

Children who have an early hip spica cast applied for a femoral fracture and have the hip and knee in 90° of flexion are at significant risk for developing a peroneal nerve palsy if the cast is wedged to correct malalignment.

Patellar Fractures

Houghton GR, Ackroyd CE: Sleeve fractures of the patella in children: A report of three cases. *J Bone Joint Surg* 1979;61B:165–168.

Wu CD, Huang SC, Liu TK: Sleeve fracture of the patella in children: A report of five cases. *Am J Sports Med* 1991;19:525–528.

These two articles describe the mechanism of injury and difficulties of diagnosis for this unique pediatric fracture.

Maguire JK, Canale ST: Fractures of the patella in children and adolescents. *J Pediatr Orthop* 1993;13:567–571.

Ray JM, Hendrix J: Incidence, mechanism of injury, and treatment of fractures of the patella in children. *J Trauma* 1992;32:464–467.

Two series of patellar fractures in children are reported.

Fractures of the Distal Femoral Epiphysis

Lombardo SJ, Harvey JP Jr: Fractures of the distal femoral epiphyses: Factors influencing prognosis. A review of thirty-four cases. *J Bone Joint Surg* 1977;59A:742–751.

Riseborough EJ, Barrett IR, Shapiro F: Growth disturbances following distal femoral physeal fracture-separations. *J Bone Joint Surg* 1983;65A:885–893.

These two papers report a high incidence of physeal arrest and angular deformity after distal femoral physeal fracture. Growth disturbance correlated with severity of initial trauma and displacement. The Salter-Harris classification was unreliable for predicting growth disturbance.

Thomson JD, Stricker SJ, Williams MM: Fractures of the distal femoral epiphyseal plate. *J Pediatr Orthop* 1995;15:474–478.

Retrospective analysis of 30 consecutive fractures of the distal femoral physis showed the best results occurred when fractures were anatomically reduced and fixed with pins. No fractures with internal fixation displaced, while 43% of those without fixation displaced during cast treatment.

Fractures of the Intercondylar Eminence of the Tibia

Janarv PM, Westblad P, Johansson C, et al: Long-term follow-up of anterior tibial spine fractures in children. *J Pediatr Orthop* 1995;15:63–68.

Sixty-one tibial eminence fractures were evaluated at an average follow-up of 16 years. Most type III injuries had an open reduction and internal fixation. Results were excellent or good in 87%. Pathologic sagittal plane laxity occurred in 38% but was not related to poor subjecive function. Arthroscopic evaluation of type II and III lesions is recommended to rule out associated meniscal and/or articular damage. Recommendations for treatment are type I; closed reduction and casting; type II, arthroscopically controlled reduction and casting; and type III, arthroscopic reduction and fixation.

McLennan JG: Lessons learned after second-look arthroscopy in type III fractures of the tibial spine. *J Pediatr Orthop* 1995;15:59–62.

Ten patients with type III fractures had arthroscopy for other conditions 6 years after treatment at an average age of 17 years. Four patients had closed reduction (group I), three had arthroscopic reduction and casting (group 2) and three had arthroscopic reduction and fixation (group 3). All were measured and graded using objective and functional tests. The patients' primary complaints were anterior knee pain and not instability. Patellar malacic changes were seen primarily in group I. Offset of > 3 mm was seen in groups I and II, suggesting loss of reduction and malunion. Sagittal laxity was greatest in group I and least in group 3; functional tests were best in group 3.

Medler RG, Jansson KA: Arthroscopic treatment of fractures of the tibial spine. *Arthroscopy* 1994;10:292–295.

Mah JY, Otsuka NY, McLean J: An arthroscopic technique for the reduction and fixation of tibial-eminence fractures. *J Pediatr Orthop* 1996;16:119–121.

These papers report an arthroscopic technique to evaluate and stabilize tibial eminence fractures in children.

Meyers MH, McKeever FM: Fracture of the intercondylar eminence of the tibia. *J Bone Joint Surg* 1970;52A:1677–1684.

This classic article describes a classification based on the degree of displacement. It recommends open reduction and internal fixation of fractures with wide displacement.

Wiley JJ, Baxter MP: Tibial spine fractures in children. *Clin Orthop* 1990; 255:54–60.

This is an excellent evaluation (with a discussion of the pertinent anatomy) of tibial spine fractures in children. Anterior cruciate laxity appears in many children with tibial spine fractures that have been reduced anatomically. This laxity does not appear to lead to clinical symptoms.

Willis RB, Blokker C, Stoll TM, et al: Long-term follow-up of anterior tibial eminence fractures. *J Pediatr Orthop* 1993;13:361–364.

Fifty patients were evaluated at an average of 4 years after fracture. Sagittal anterior increase in translation was clinically evident in 64% and by arthrometer testing in 74%. Twenty-nine of the 50 had type III injuries, 16 treated by open reduction and fixation. Patients treated by closed techniques had equal results to those managed surgically. Twenty percent of all patients had a positive pivot shift. No patient complained of instability.

Fractures Involving the Proximal Tibial Physis and Tuberosity

Burkhart SS, Peterson HA: Fractures of the proximal tibial epiphyses. *J Bone Joint Surg* 1979;61A:996–1002.

This paper reports 28 fractures. Type IV Salter Harris fractures most often result from lawn mower injuries. Most type I and III injuries occur in adolescents. The article recommends stress films if diagnosis is in doubt. Type III injuries often are associated with avulsion of the tibial tubercle.

Chow SP, Lam JJ, Leong JC: Fracture of the tibial tubercle in the adolescent. *J Bone Joint Surg* 1990;72B:231–234.

Patients with type I or II tibial tubercle avulsions can be treated without surgical intervention with good results. Type II fractures involving the knee joint should be fixed internally.

Shelton WR, Canale ST: Fractures of the tibia through the proximal tibial epiphyseal cartilage. *J Bone Joint Surg* 1979;61A:167–173.

This paper reports 39 fractures, including two with popliteal artery disruption. Other complications include compartment syndrome, peroneal nerve palsy, and associated ligamentous injuries. Age range and fracture patterns were similar to those in Burkhart and Peterson's series.

Fractures of the Proximal Tibial Metaphyses

Balthazar DA, Pappas AM: Acquired valgus deformity of the tibia in children. *J Pediatr Orthop* 1984;4:538–541.

This article offers a complete review of the development of this deformity, which can be secondary to overgrowth, incomplete reduction, or both. It warns against osteotomy because of recurring deformity.

Ogden JA, Ogden DA, Pugh L, et al: Tibia valga after proximal metaphyseal fractures in childhood: A normal biologic response. *J Pediatr Orthop* 1995;15:489–494.

Detailed measurements in 19 patients indicate that asymmetric overgrowth is the most likely cause of this phenomenon.

Zionts LE, MacEwen GD: Spontaneous improvement of post-traumatic tibia valga. *J Bone Joint Surg* 1986;68A:680–687.

The authors of this classic article recommend a conservative approach to valgus deformity after tibial metaphyseal fracture.

Fractures of the Tibial Shaft

Briggs TW, Orr MM, Lightowler CD: Isolated tibial fractures in children. *Injury* 1992;23:308–310.

Isolated tibial fractures account for at least one third of all injuries to the tibia. These fractures can displace into varus during the first 2 weeks after injury and, therefore, must be followed closely.

Buckley SL, Smith G, Sponseller PD, et al: Open fractures of the tibia in children. *J Bone Joint Surg* 1990;72A:1462–1469.

Kreder HJ, Armstrong P: A review of open tibia fractures in children. *J Pediatr Orthop* 1995;15:482–488.

Hope PG, Cole WG: Open fractures of the tibia in children. *J Bone Joint Surg* 1992;74B:546–553.

These three large series indicate that open tibial fractures in children have complications similar to those in adults.

Dreder HJ, Armstrong P: A review of open tibia fractures in children. *J Pediatr Orthop* 1995;15:482–488.

In a retrospective study of 56 open tibial fractures in 55 children, the mortality rate was 7%, and the prevalence of infection was 14%. The most important variables affecting infection were the presence of neurovascular injury and delay in surgical treatment: delay of more than 6 hours was correlated with a 25% infection rate, compared to 12% for those treated within 6 hours of injury. Patient age was the most significant factor affecting time to union.

Hansen BA, Greiff J, Bergmann F: Fractures of the tibia in children. *Acta Orthop Scand* 1976;47:448–453.

Longitudinal studies in 102 children are reported. This is a good source for statistics regarding incidence, age group, and time of healing. Angulation was corrected only by 10%, ceased at 18 months postinjury, and was independent of age at the time of fractures.

Hope PG, Cole WG: Open fractures of the tibia in children. *J Bone Joint Surg* 1992;74B:546–553.

Open tibial fractures in children are associated with frequent early and late complications. In 92 children, short-term complications were similar to those in adults, but long-term follow-up (1.5 to 9.8 years) showed a high prevalence of continuing morbidity, including pain (50%), restriction of athletic activity (23%), joint stiffness (23%), cosmetic defects (23%), and minor leg-length discrepancies (64%).

Shannak AO: Tibial fractures in children: Follow-up study. *J Pediatr Orthop* 1988;8:306–310.

The author reports 117 tibial shaft fractures treated by above-the-knee casting with or without traction. The average growth acceleration was 4 mm. A residual angular deformity was least likely to correct if it had been in a posterior direction. Valgus malunion was the next least likely to correct spontaneously. Valgus and posterior angulation persisted and, therefore, should be avoided. Shortening of more than 10 mm could not be accepted because of the small fracture-induced growth acceleration.

Fractures of the Distal Tibial Metaphysis and Physis

Dias LS, Tachdjian MO: Physeal injuries of the ankle in children: Classification. *Clin Orthop* 1978;136:230–233.

The authors describe a classification modifying the Lauge-Hansen "mechanism of injury" system and apply it to patients with open physes. The article describes four major groups: supination-inversion, supination-plantarflexion, supination-external rotation, and pronation-eversion-external rotation.

Ertl JP, Barrack RL, Alexander AH, et al: Triplane fracture of the distal tibial epiphysis: Long-term follow-up. *J Bone Joint Surg* 1988;70A:967–976.

This is a report of the long-term follow-up (3 to 13 years) of intra-articular fractures of the distal tibia/fibula in children and adolescents. Although symptoms were absent at early follow-up, about half of the patients were symptomatic at long-term evaluation. Residual displacement of 2 mm or more at the weightbearing surface was associated with suboptimal results.

Kleiger B, Mankin HJ: Fracture of the lateral portion of the distal tibial epiphysis. *J Bone Joint Surg* 1964;46A:25–32.

This is the original description of the juvenile Tillaux fracture. It describes the early closure of the medial aspect of the physis, leaving the lateral portion open in adolescence.

Kling TF Jr: Operative treatment of ankle fractures in children. *Orthop Clin North Am* 1990;21:381–392.

This is a description of pediatric physeal ankle injuries.

Spiegel PG, Cooperman DR, Laros GS: Epiphyseal fractures of the distal ends of the tibia and fibula: A retrospective study of two hundred and thirty-seven cases in children. *J Bone Joint Surg* 1978;60A:1046–1050.

A report of 184 fractures notes a high risk for growth arrest after Salter-Harris type III and IV fractures with displacement of more than 2 mm.

Fractures of the Foot

Berndt AL, Harty M: Transchondral fractures (osteochondritis dissecans) of the talus. *J Bone Joint Surg* 1959;41A:988–1020.

This is the most complete review of the types, mechanisms of injury, and treatment of this injury in the orthopaedic literature.

Canale ST, Belding RH: Osteochondral lesions of the talus. *J Bone Joint Surg* 1980;62A:97–102.

A review of 29 patients showed that lateral lesions associated with trauma were more likely to be symptomatic. The paper gives treatment recommendations using Berndt and Harty classifications.

Cole RJ, Brown HP, Stein RE, et al: Avulsion fracture of the tuberosity of the calcaneus in children: A report of four cases and review of the literature. *J Bone Joint Surg* 1995;77A:1568–1571.

Of four children with this injury, three required open reduction and internal fixation because satisfactory closed reduction could not be obtained. All four had good results with no functional loss.

Dvaric DM, Schmitt EW: Irreducible fracture of the calcaneus in a child. *J Orthop Trauma* 1988;2:154–157.

A 4-year 8-month-old boy sustained a fracture of the anterior process of the calcaneus that required open reduction. The authors review treatment guidelines for calcaneal fractures in children.

Izant RJ Jr, Rothmann BF, Frankel VH: Bicycle spoke injuries of the foot and ankle in children: An underestimated "minor" injury. *J Pediatr Surg* 1969;4:654–656.

This classic paper describes the pathology of this injury and emphasizes that soft-tissue injury is the major component. The extent of the injury may not be apparent initially, and an associated fracture may exist. Pathology is similar to that seen in a wringer injury in the upper extremity.

Jensen I, Wester JU, Rasmussen F, et al: Prognosis of fracture of the talus in children: 21 (7-34)-year follow-up of 14 cases. *Acta Orthop Scand* 1994;65:398–400.

The talar neck was fractured in ten children and the talar body in four. Three displaced fractures were reduced and immobilized; nondisplaced fractures were treated conservatively. All fractures healed, but patients with displaced fractures had exercise-induced pain at follow-up.

Laliotis N, Pennie BH, Carty H, et al: Toddler's fracture of the calcaneum. *Injury* 1993;24:169–170.

Seven calcaneal fractures in children younger than 3 years of age occurred without history of significant injury. In five, the fracture was not visible on plain radiographs and the diagnosis was made by scintigraphy.

Mulfinger GL, Trueta J: The blood supply of the talus. *J Bone Joint Surg* 1970;52B:160–167.

This article describes the blood supply of the talus as coming from three sources. It points out the vulnerability of the neck to developing osteonecrosis in fractures.

Owen RJ, Hickey FG, Finlay DB: A study of metatarsal fractures in children. *Injury* 1995;26:537–538.

A review of radiographs of 388 children with foot injuries identified 62 metatarsal and seven tarsal fractures in 60 children. The most common fracture was of the fifth metatarsal (42%); 90% of these children were older than 10 years. In children younger than 5 years, first metatarsal fractures occurred in 73%. Overall, 6.5% of all fractures and 20% of first metatarsal fractures were unreccognized on initial examination.

Pinckney LE, Currarino G, Kennedy LA: The stubbed great toe: A cause of occult compound fracture and infection. *Radiology* 1981;138:375–377.

Salter I physeal separation of the distal phalanx may be associated with nail bed injury while the nail obscures the diagnosis as an open fracture.

Schanz K, Rasmussen F: Calcaneus fracture in the child. *Acta Orthop Scand* 1987;58:507–509.

Of 80 fractures in 78 children, fewer than half were intra-articular fractures, in contrast to the same fractures in adults, probably because fewer children sustained the fracture in a fall. Associated injuries were more common in children who were traffic accident victims.

Schindler A, Mason DE, Allington MJ: Occult fracture of the calcaneus in toddlers. *J Pediatr Orthop* 1996;16:201–205.

In five children aged 14 to 33 months, initial radiographs were negative and physical examination did not localize a fracture. Radiographs after 2 weeks revealed an arc of sclerosis across the tuberosity of the calcaneus. Bone scan was not instrumental in making the diagnosis in any patient.

Schmidt TL, Weiner DS: Calcaneal fractures in children: An evaluation of the nature of the injury in 56 children. *Clin Orthop* 1982;171:150–155.

This article reviews patterns of calcaneal injuries in children. Compared with adults, children have a higher incidence of injury by lawn mower or direct blows, a higher incidence of other associated fractures, and fewer intra-articular fractures.

Polytrauma/Multiple Fractures

Cramer KE: The pediatric polytrauma patient. *Clin Orthop* 1995;318: 125–135.

This is an excellent review with 109 references.

Dormans JP, Azzoni M, Davidson RS, Drummond DS: Major lower extremity lawn mower injuries in children. *J Pediatr Orthop* 1995; 15:78–82.

Of 16 children with 18 lower-extremity mower-related injuries, 11 were not operators of the mower. Fourteen of the 18 injured limbs required eventual amputation. A classification of lawn mower injuries is proposed to help predict outcome of limb salvage procedures.

Section 15

Bone and Joint Infections

Laurie O. Hughes, MD

Green NE, Edwards K: Bone and joint infections in children. *Orthop Clin North Am* 1987;18:555–576.

This thorough and still-current review article is extensively referenced and includes discussions of the major forms of orthopaedic infection affecting children. Special patient populations, such as neonates and sickle cell patients, are also discussed.

Norden C, Gillespie WJ, Nade S (eds): *Infections in Bones and Joints*. Boston, MA, Blackwell Scientific, 1994.

This is a current general reference text covering all forms of musculoskeletal sepsis in children and adults.

Etiology

Alderson M, Speers D, Emslie K, et al: Acute haematogenous osteomyelitis and septic arthritis: A single disease. An hypothesis based upon the presence of transphyseal blood vessels. *J Bone Joint Surg* 1986;68B:268–274.

This is an elegant histologic study in which the authors demonstrated in the avian model the spread of hematogenous bacterial infection across the physis via transphyseal blood vessels. The pathogenesis of concurrent septic arthritis and osteomyelitis is described. Similarity between this model and the pathogenesis of this disease in infants is proposed.

Morrissy RT, Haynes DW: Acute hematogenous osteomyelitis: A model with trauma as an etiology. *J Pediatr Orthop* 1989;9:447–456.

The authors of this classic article used a rabbit model to investigate the role of trauma in the development of acute hematogenous osteomyelitis. Almost all the animals with coexistent fracture of the proximal tibial metaphysis and bacteremia developed osteomyelitis. Osteomyelitis did not develop in bacteremic animals without fracture. The authors suggest that trauma in combination with bacteremia is a major etiologic factor in the development of acute hematogenous osteomyelitis.

Evaluation

Canale ST, Harkness RM, Thomas PA, et al: Does aspiration of bones and joints affect results of later bone scanning? *J Pediatr Orthop* 1985;5:23–26.

Canine studies indicated that, when osteomyelitis or pyarthrosis is clinically suspected, joint aspiration can be performed without fear of producing a false-positive bone scan.

Herndon WA, Alexieva BT, Schwindt ML, et al: Nuclear imaging for musculoskeletal infections in children. *J Pediatr Orthop* 1985;5:343–347.

This retrospective review of bone scans of 63 children documents the limitations of nuclear imaging in certain clinical situations. The bone scan was found to be unreliable in detecting musculoskeletal infections in neonates, and less accurate in the foot than in the rest of the skeleton.

Howard CB, Einhorn M, Dagan R, et al: Fine-needle bone biopsy to diagnose osteomyelitis. *J Bone Joint Surg* 1994;76B:311–314.

In 30 patients with suspected osteomyelitis, fine needle bone biopsy was found to have a sensitivity of 87% and a specificity of 93%. The authors recommend fine needle bone biopsy under intravenous sedation and ultrasonic radiographic control in cases of suspected osteomyelitis. Their technique is described.

Mah ET, LeQuesne GW, Gent RJ, et al: Ultrasonic features of acute osteomyelitis in children. *J Bone Joint Surg* 1994;76B:969–974.

Deep soft-tissue swelling was the earliest sign of osteomyelitis; in the next stage periosteal evaluation and a thin layer of subperiosteal fluid were present and in some patients this progressed to form a subperiosteal abscess. The later stages were characterized by cortical erosion, common in those with symptoms of more than a week's duration.

Mazur JM, Ross G, Cummings J, et al: Usefulness of magnetic resonance imaging for the diagnosis of acute musculoskeletal infections in children. *J Pediatr Orthop* 1995;15:144–147.

Magnetic resonance imaging (MRI) was found to be extremely sensitive (0.97) and specific (0.92) in diagnosing the infection, with only one false positive and one false negative in 43 children. Bone scans are more likely to yield false positive and negative examinations. MRI is especially useful with conflicting clinical data and infections of the spine or pelvis.

Tuson CE, Hoffman EB, Mann MD: Isotope bone scanning for acute osteomyelitis and septic arthritis in children. *J Bone Joint Surg* 1994;76B:306–310.

In a prospective study of 86 children with suspected hematogenous osteomyelitis or septic arthritis, the technetium scan was found to have an overall accuracy of 81%. A cold scan was found to have a predictive value of 100%, while the predictive value of a hot scan was 82%. Characteristic scan appearances of septic arthritis and osteomyelitis are described.

Unkila-Kallio L, Kallio MJ, Peltola H: The usefulness of C-reactive protein levels in the identification of concurrent septic arthritis in children who have acute hematogenous osteomyelitis: A comparison with the usefulness of the erythrocyte sedimentation rate and the white blood-cell count. *J Bone Joint Surg* 1994;76A:848–853.

When the C-reactive protein on the third day was more than 1.5 times the level at the time of admission, the likelihood ratio that septic arthritis was also present was 6.5. Changes in the erythrocyte sedimentation rate gave the same information, but later.

Miscellaneous

Aprin H, Turen C: Pyogenic sacroiliitis in children. *Clin Orthop* 1993;287:98–106.

Pyogenic sacroiliitis is an often-missed diagnosis for which a high degree of clinical suspicion is essential. Workup and treatment recommendations are emphasized in this review of seven children with the disease.

Selected Bibliography of Pediatric Orthopaedics

Carr AJ, Cole WG, Roberton DM, et al: Chronic multifocal osteomyelitis. *J Bone Joint Surg* 1993;75B:582–591.

This paper outlines in detail the guidelines for the diagnosis, treatment, and prognosis of chronic multifocal osteomyelitis. It is based on a review of 22 patients with an average 6-year follow-up for this rare disorder.

Craigen MA, Watters J, Hackett JS: The changing epidemiology of osteomyelitis in children. *J Bone Joint Surg* 1992;74B:541–545.

In a 20-year period (1970 to 1990), there was a 50% reduction in the occurrence of osteomyelitis, mainly in long-bone infections and those due to *Staphylococcus aureus*. The number of complications also was reduced.

Epps CH Jr, Bryant DD III, Coles MJ, et al: Osteomyelitis in patients who have sickle-cell disease: Diagnosis and management. *J Bone Joint Surg* 1991;73A:1281–1294.

Osteomyelitis resolved in 29 (97%) of 30 affected bones after surgical decompression followed by a minimum of 6 weeks of parenteral antibiotic therapy. Complications included adhesive pericapsulitis of the shoulder, osteonecrosis of the humeral head, and pathological fracture of the femur. *Staphylococcus aureus* was isolated in cultures from eight of 15 patients, *Salmonella* from six, and *Proteus mirabilis* from one.

Green NE: Musculoskeletal infections in children: Part VI. Disseminated gonococcal infections and gonococcal arthritis, in Evarts MC (ed): American Academy of Orthopaedic Surgeons *Instructional Course Lectures XXXII*. St. Louis, MO, CV Mosby, 1983, pp 48–50.

This is a thorough review of the most common cause of septic arthritis in the adolescent population.

Gregg-Smith SJ, Pattison RM, Dodd CA, et al: Septic arthritis in haemophilia. *J Bone Joint Surg* 1993;75B:368–370.

The authors report septic arthritis in six patients with hemophilia. This previously rare complication is now increasingly common. The authors suggest that the increased incidence is due to the prevalence of HIV infection among hemophiliacs and to the intravenous self-administration of factor concentrate. They recommend aspiration of the joint and antibiotic therapy rather than arthrotomy.

Hamdy RC, Lawton L, Carey T, et al: Subacute hematogenous osteomyelitis: Are biopsy and surgery always indicated? *J Pediatr Orthop* 1996;16:220–223.

Of 44 patients with subacute hematogenous osteomyelitis, the group treated with antibiotics alone responded equally as well to treatment as did the group treated with surgical debridement and antibiotics. The authors recommend nonsurgical treatment in most patients and discuss the indications for surgery.

Jacobs RF, McCarthy RE, Elser JM: *Pseudomonas* osteochondritis complicating puncture wounds of the foot in children: A 10-year evaluation. *J Infect Dis* 1989;160:657–661.

This is to date the largest series and longest follow-up of patients with *Pseudomonas* osteochondritis and septic arthritis following nail puncture wound to the foot. In the absence of undetected septic arthritis, clinical cure was achieved with surgical debridement followed by 7 days of intravenous antibiotics. This article establishes the standard of care for this disease.

McNeill TW: Spinal infections, in Greene WB (ed): *Instructional Course Lectures XXXIX*. Park Ridge, IL, American Academy of Orthopaedic Surgeons, 1990, pp 515–524.

The author reviews the etiology, diagnosis, and treatment of diskitis, pyogenic osteomyelitis, and tubercular and fungal disease of the spine in children and adults. The extensive reference section includes several important papers on pediatric spinal infection.

Watts HG, Lifeso RM: Tuberculosis of bone and joints. *J Bone Joint Surg* 1996;78A:288–298.

This up-to-date review of skeletal tuberculosis in children and adults covers epidemiology, diagnosis, and treatment of the disease and cites numerous classic studies.

Treatment

Choi IH, Pizzutillo PD, Bowen JR, et al: Sequelae and reconstruction after septic arthritis of the hip in infants. *J Bone Joint Surg* 1990;72A:1150–1165.

Thirty-four hips in 31 children who had septic arthritis of the hip before the age of 1 year were reviewed radiographically and functionally. Poor functional results correlated with higher degrees of residual deformity. The most significant prognostic factor was delay in diagnosis and treatment. The authors propose a classification system based on the radiographic results and make treatment recommendations for each class.

Daoud A, Saighi-Bouaouina A: Treatment of sequestra, pseudarthroses, and defects in the long bones of children who have chronic hematogenous osteomyelitis. *J Bone Joint Surg* 1989;71A:1448–1468.

In this study of 34 patients with hematogenous osteomyelitis of the long bones, the status of the periosteum was found to be of primary importance in determining the prognosis and treatment. Patients with periosteal new bone (involucrum) may be treated with sequestrectomy and immobilization alone. In the absence of an involucrum, staged bone grafting and surgical fixation are recommended. Early sequestrectomy is emphasized.

Lauschke FH, Frey CT: Hematogenous osteomyelitis in infants and children in the northwestern region of Namibia: Management and two-year results. *J Bone Joint Surg* 1994;76A:502–510.

Seventy-five children were divided into three groups: those with early acute (seven), those with late acute (18), and those with chronic (30) osteomyelitis. The bones most affected were the tibia (22) and femur (19). The most frequent infecting organism was penicillin-resistant *Staphylococcus aureus* (76%). The seven patients with early acute osteomyelitis and four of the 18 with late acute responded to antibiotic treatment only; antibiotic treatment and surgical treatment were required in 14 of the 18 with late acute osteomyelitis and in all 30 with chronic osteomyelitis.

Prober CG: Current antibiotic therapy of community-acquired bacterial infections in hospitalized children: Bone and joint infections. *Pediatr Infect Dis J* 1992;11:156–159.

This article outlines current standards in antibiotic treatment of pediatric bone and joint infections. The pathophysiology and diagnostic criteria for pediatric musculoskeletal sepsis are also well covered.

Ring D, Johnston CE II, Wenger DR: Pyogenic infectious spondylitis in children: The convergence of discitis and vertebral osteomyelitis. *J Pediatr Orthop* 1995;15:652–660.

Results of a study of 47 patients support the contention that so-called diskitis is pyogenic infectious spondylitis in children and suggest that specific treatment and intravenous antibiotics are more likely to lead to rapid relief of symptoms and signs without recurrence.

Shaw BA, Kasser JR: Acute septic arthritis in infancy and childhood. *Clin Orthop* 1990;257:212–225.

The authors thoroughly review the diagnosis, pathophysiology, and treatment of septic arthritis in the pediatric population. Treatment recommendations are discussed in detail.

Outcome Studies

Betz RR, Cooperman DR, Wopperer JM, et al: Late sequelae of septic arthritis of the hip in infancy and childhood. *J Pediatr Orthop* 1990; 10:365–372.

This is a multicenter retrospective analysis of 28 patients (32 hips), each with a minimum 20-year follow-up for septic arthritis of the hip. Leg length discrepancy averaged 3 to 3.5 cm. Preservation of hip motion, however slight, gave better results. Surgery resulted in stiffness in the group with onset before the age of 3 months. The authors include treatment recommendations based on these results.

Fink CW, Nelson JD: Septic arthritis and osteomyelitis in children. *Clin Rheum Dis* 1986;12:423–435.

Five hundred ninety-one patients with septic arthritis and 340 with osteomyelitis were followed up for 25 to 30 years. Patterns of joint involvement, infecting organism, presenting symptoms, and diagnostic criteria are noted for both osteomyelitis and septic arthritis. Comparison is made between this series and previous reports.

Peters W, Irving J, Letts M: Long-term effects of neonatal bone and joint infection on adjacent growth plates. *J Pediatr Orthop* 1992;12:806–810.

Six patients were noted at long-term follow-up to have residual growth plate deformity following septic arthritis and osteomyelitis in the neonatal period. In five of the six, the deformity was not appreciated until a mean age of 9 years. Follow-up of such children until skeletal maturity is recommended.

Scott RJ, Christofersen MR, Robertson WW Jr, et al: Acute osteomyelitis in children: A review of 116 cases. *J Pediatr Orthop* 1990;10:649–652.

Most patients present early in the course of their disease and may have no findings other than local tenderness and an elevated sedimentation rate. Sixty-four (55%) of the 116 patients were successfully treated nonsurgically.

Section 16

Neuromuscular Diseases

John G. Birch, MD

General

Dormans JP, Templeton JJ, Edmonds C, et al: Intraoperative anaphylaxis due to exposure to latex (natural rubber) in children. *J Bone Joint Surg* 1994;76A:1688–1691.

Of 21 patients with intraoperative anaphylactic reactions to latex, 12 had spina bifida, six had cerebral palsy, one had exstrophy of the bladder, one had VATER syndrome, and one had Duchenne muscular dystrophy. Manifestations of the allergic reaction included a rash (15), hypotension (15), tachycardia (11), bronchospasm (ten), bradycardia (two), and cardiac arrest (two). All patients responded to management; there were no deaths.

Dubowitz V: *Color Atlas of Muscle Disorders in Childhood.* Chicago, IL, Year Book Medical, 1989.

This book contains clinical photographs, histologic examples, and brief outlines of the clinical features and natural history of the muscular dystrophies, spinal muscular atrophy, and hereditary motor and sensory neuropathies. This is an excellent quick pictorial reference to many neuromuscular disorders.

Shapiro F, Specht L: The diagnosis and orthopaedic treatment of childhood spinal muscular atrophy, peripheral neuropathy, Friedreich ataxia, and arthrogryposis. *J Bone Joint Surg* 1993;75A:699–714.

This review article summarizes a diagnostic approach to the disorders in the title as well as an overview of the genetic aspects, natural history, and results of orthopaedic treatment of these conditions. This is an excellent up-to-date review of these disorders with an extensive bibliography of 92 references.

Shapiro F, Specht L: The diagnosis and orthopedic treatment of inherited muscular diseases of childhood. *J Bone Joint Surg* 1993;75A:439–454.

This review article presents a diagnostic approach, which includes a description of proper muscle biopsy technique, to children with suspected muscular disease. Current genetic knowledge, clinical features, natural history, and results of orthopaedic treatment are summarized for Duchenne, Becker, Emery-Dreifuss, facioscapulohumeral, and limb-girdle muscular dystrophies, as well as for the myotonias. An extensive bibliography is included. This review article and its companion by the same authors provide the reader with an excellent source of up-to-date information on neuromuscular diseases in children.

Duchenne Muscular Dystrophy

Bonnet I, Burgot D, Bonnard C, et al: Surgery of the lower limbs in Duchenne muscular dystrophy. *Fr J Orthop Surg* 1991;5:160–168.

Seventy-one patients with Duchenne muscular dystrophy (DMD) underwent lower extremity surgery to prolong walking ability (28 patients), restore walking ability (23 patients), or remove deformity for sitting purposes (20 patients). The mean age at which walking ability was lost was 9 years, 7 months; ability to walk was prolonged to a mean age of 12 years in the first two groups. Results were considered good or excellent in 85% of patients overall.

Galaski CSB, Delaney C, Morris P: Spinal stabilization in Duchenne muscular dystrophy. *J Bone Joint Surg* 1992;74B:210–214.

This report compares two groups of patients with DMD: 32 treated by spinal fusion and 23 who refused surgery. Forced vital capacity, which diminished an average 8% per year in the patients who refused surgery, remained stable for 3 years in the patients who underwent surgery. Scoliosis remained stable in the surgically treated patients but increased from an average 37° to 89° at 5-year follow-up. There were no deaths, deep infections, pseudarthroses, or instrumentation failures in the surgically treated patients. The authors recommend posterior spinal fusion and segmental instrumentation when scoliosis measures 20° in these patients.

Kurz LT, Mubarak SJ, Schultz P, et al: Correlation of scoliosis and pulmonary function in Duchenne muscular dystrophy. *J Pediatr Orthop* 1983;3:347–353.

Pulmonary function peaks at the age when standing ceases. It decreased by 4% each year and with each 10° increase in curvature. Early spinal instrumentation is indicated in order to slow rate of decline of pulmonary function.

Miller F, Moseley CF, Koreska J, et al: Pulmonary function and scoliosis in Duchenne dystrophy. *J Pediatr Orthop* 1988;8:133–137.

Pulmonary function (% FVC) declines most rapidly during the adolescent growth spurt. Surgery does not influence the rate of pulmonary function deterioration.

Miller F, Moseley CF, Koreska J: Spinal fusion in Duchenne muscular dystrophy. *Dev Med Child Neurol* 1992;34:775–786.

The authors describe the results of spinal fusion in 86 patients with progressive spinal deformity. The patients with surgically stabilized spines were more comfortable over time than those with DMD who were not fused; however, deteriorating pulmonary function was not affected by the fusion. Factors noted to improve quality of life included segmental instrumentation, fusion from T2 to the pelvis, correcting or balancing scoliosis, creating normal sagittal plane alignment, and correcting pelvic obliquity.

Miller RG, Chalmers AC, Dao H, et al: The effect of spine fusion on respiratory function in Duchenne muscular dystrophy. *Neurology* 1991;41:38–40.

No differences in declining respiratory function were noted between a group of surgically and nonsurgically treated patients. The authors note, however, that all surgically treated patients reported either improved sitting comfort, appearance, or both.

Mubarak SJ, Morin WD, Leach J: Spinal fusion in Duchenne muscular dystrophy: Fixation and fusion to the sacropelvis? *J Pediatr Orthop* 1993;13:752–757.

Wheelchair-bound patients with DMD underwent Luque segmental instrumentation and fusion. Twelve patients were instrumented to the sacropelvis, and ten were instrumented to L5. The authors recommend surgery for curves of more than 20° and if forced vital capacity is more than 40%; they indicate that if treatment is initiated early, Luque instrumentation and fusion from T2-3 to L5 should be sufficient.

Oda T, Shimizu N, Yonenobu K, et al: Longitudinal study of spinal deformity in Duchenne muscular dystrophy. *J Pediatr Orthop* 1993; 13:478–488.

This is a longitudinal review of radiographic and clinical data in 46 patients with DMD in whom the natural course and its clinical relevance are examined.

Smith AD, Koreska J, Moseley CF: Progression of scoliosis in Duchenne muscular dystrophy. *J Bone Joint Surg* 1989;71A:1066–1074.

A retrospective review of 51 boys with DMD who were not treated by spinal fusion. Scoliosis progressed beyond 90° in 25 before they died. Most ultimately had trouble sitting because of deformity or pain. Vital capacity was less than 40% of normal by the time the curve had progressed beyond 35°. The authors recommend consideration of spinal fusion before the curve exceeds 35° in all patients with DMD who are unable to walk.

Smith SE, Green NE, Cole RJ, et al: Prolongation of ambulation in children with Duchenne muscular dystrophy by subcutaneous lower limb tenotomy. *J Pediatr Orthop* 1993;13:336–340.

Twenty-nine patients who had hip, knee, and ankle tenotomies were compared to 25 children who declined surgery. Patients with tenotomies continued ambulation with braces to a mean age of 12 years and 8 months, while those without surgery ceased ambulating at a mean age of 10 years. The authors suggest that tenotomy is effective in allowed braced ambulation well beyond what the natural history would allow.

Other Muscular Dystrophies

Bunch WH, Siegel IM: Scapulothoracic arthrodesis in facioscapulohumeral muscular dystrophy. *J Bone Joint Surg* 1993;74A:372–376.

The authors present results of arthrodesis of the scapula to the thorax in 12 patients followed up for 3 to 21 years. The indications, surgical technique, and aftercare are well described. Abduction arc improved an average of 60°. One patient had a transient brachial plexus palsy, another a stiff shoulder. Patient satisfaction was high (11 of 12 patients) because carrying, lifting, and other arm-lifting activities were improved postoperatively and maintained for a long time because of the slow progression of the underlying muscular weakness.

LeTournel E, Fardeau M, Lytle JO, et al: Scapulothoracic arthrodesis for patients who have facioscapulohumeral muscular dystrophy. *J Bone Joint Surg* 1990;72A:78–84.

The authors present results of an average 69-month follow-up of nine patients who underwent 16 scapulothoracic fusions. Results remained stable in follow-up. Complications of surgery included pneumothorax, fracture of the scapula, and pseudarthrosis. A detailed description of the surgery is included. No bone grafting or spica immobilization was used in the later patients in the study.

Shapiro F, Specht L: Orthopedic deformities in Emery-Dreifuss muscular dystrophy. *J Pediatr Orthop* 1991;11:336–340.

Patients with Emery-Dreifuss muscular dystrophy present in the first few years of life with muscle weakness, awkward gait, and toe-walking. Ankle equinus, elbow flexion, and neck extension contractures all develop subsequently. This paper documents four patients with this rare X-linked recessive form of muscular dystrophy. The authors emphasize the importance of recognizing the disorder because the patients develop initially asymptomatic heart block, which leads to sudden death unless it is recognized and prevented by pacemaker insertion.

Spinal Muscular Atrophy

Brown JC, Zeller JL, Swank SM, et al: Surgical and functional results of spine fusion in spinal muscular atrophy. *Spine* 1989;14:763–770.

The authors compare two groups of patients treated by spinal fusion for scoliosis and spinal muscular atrophy: one (34 patients) treated with Harrington instrumentation, and the other (six patients) with Luque segmental wire fixation. The only surgical complication was wire breakage in one patient. Postoperative gains were modest. Sitting endurance was improved in only 10% of patients, while mobile arm supports, lapboards, and reachers were required postoperatively because of the change in sitting posture. The authors conclude that patients and families must be informed of the changes that occur in functional activity after surgery.

Granata C, Merlini L, Magni E, et al: Spinal muscular atrophy: Natural history and orthopaedic treatment of scoliosis. *Spine* 1989;14:760–762.

The authors describe the natural history of scoliosis in 32 patients with mild spinal muscular atrophy and 31 with intermediate spinal muscular atrophy. Spinal deformity usually occurs by age 6, and progression is certain without treatment. Bracing may slow curve progression. Early surgical stabilization is recommended to prevent pulmonary compromise and functional loss.

Merlini L, Granata C, Bonfiglioli S, et al: Scoliosis in spinal muscular atrophy: Natural history and management. *Dev Med Child Neurol* 1989;31:501–508.

This is a review of the literature on scoliosis in spinal muscular atrophy as well as a report on the natural history of 109 patients over a 12-year period. All 18 children with the severe form died at an average age of under 6 months. The maximal functional ability of the 52 with the intermediate form was unaided sitting. Five of these patients died between the ages of 5 and 13 years. Sixteen of the 39 with mild involvement lost the ability to walk between the ages of 4 and 15 years; the others continued to walk during the period of study (age range 3 to 36 years). Scoliosis was documented in 24 with intermediate and 16 with mild forms. The predominant curve type was a single thoracolumbar curve. A total contact underarm orthosis was prescribed for all nonambulatory patients, but curves in this group progressed an average 8° per year in the brace. The authors were unable to determine whether braces slowed the rate of progression of scoliosis. Seven patients had spinal fusion at an average curve magnitude of 94°. Satisfactory cosmetic results and no impairment of function were reported with stable fusion.

Phillips DP, Roye DP Jr, Farcy JP, et al: Surgical treatment of scoliosis in a spinal muscular atrophy population. *Spine* 1990;15:942–945.

Thirty-one patients with spinal muscular atrophy with an average follow-up of 11.5 years were analyzed with respect to treatment of scoliosis. The average age at which scoliosis was documented was 8.8 years. Nine patients were operated on. Surgery improved sitting balance and endurance. The authors recommend aggressive management of scoliosis in these patients because of their prolonged survival.

Thompson CE, Larsen LJ: Recurrent hip dislocation in intermediate spinal atrophy. *J Pediatr Orthop* 1990;10:638–641.

Hip deformity and progressive dislocation can occur in patients with spinal muscular atrophy. Four patients treated for unilateral hip dislocation suffered redislocation, and no functional benefit was achieved. Because neither pain nor functional deficits resulted from the dislocations, the authors conclude that hip surgery appears unwarranted.

Charcot-Marie-Tooth Disease

Mann DC, Hsu JD: Triple arthrodesis in treatment of fixed cavovarus deformity in adolescent patients with Charcot-Marie-Tooth disease. *Foot Ankle* 1992;13:1–6.

Twelve feet in ten patients with Charcot-Marie-Tooth disease were evaluated an average of 7.5 years after triple arthrodesis for cavovarus foot deformity. Nine patients had undergone posterior tibial tendon transfer at some point during the course of treatment. Nine feet, including one undergoing revision of the triple arthrodesis, were plantigrade and asymptomatic, with or without radiographic evidence of a pseudarthrosis. Three feet were nonplantigrade and symptomatic in spite of radiographic union. The authors were not able to determine from the retrospective study whether nonplantigrade feet represented progression of the disease or inadequate correction.

Pailthorpe CA, Benson MK: Hip dysplasia in hereditary motor and sensory neuropathies. *J Bone Joint Surg* 1992;74:538–540.

This is a report of four patients with hip dysplasia who ultimately proved to have peripheral neuropathies of the hereditary motor and sensory neuropathy, type I and II (Charcot-Marie-Tooth disease). The authors point out that patients with these neuropathies may be at risk for progressive dysplasia, and that unexplained progressive dysplasia may be due to the presence of the neuropathy.

Roper BA, Tibrewal SB: Soft tissue surgery in Charcot-Marie-Tooth disease. *J Bone Joint Surg* 1989;71B:17–20.

Eighteen feet in 10 patients with Charcot-Marie-Tooth disease were evaluated an average of 14 years after soft-tissue reconstruction of cavovarus feet. All feet were graded satisfactory at follow-up, with no feet requiring triple arthrodesis. However, two patients had recurrence of deformity, which required a second soft-tissue procedure.

Walker JL, Nelson KR, Heavilon JA, et al: Hip abnormalities in children with Charcot-Marie-Tooth disease. *J Pediatr Orthop* 1994;14:54–59.

Retrospective radiographic review of 74 children with Charcot-Marie-Tooth (CMT) disease revealed hip dysplasia in six (8%) and minor hip abnormalities, most commonly increased neck-shaft angles, in 21 other patients. Most patients with hip dysplasia were asymptomatic.

Westmore RS, Drennan JC: Long-term results of triple arthrodesis in Charcot-Marie-Tooth disease. *J Bone Joint Surg* 1989;71A:417–422.

Thirty triple arthrodeses performed in 16 patients with Charcot-Marie-Tooth disease were evaluated an average of 21 years after surgery. Fourteen feet were rated poor, nine fair, five good, and only two feet were rated excellent. Six patients subsequently had ankle arthrodesis for degenerative changes. The authors conclude that triple arthrodesis should be reserved for only the most severe foot deformities in Charcot-Marie-Tooth disease.

Friedreich's Ataxia

Aronsson DD, Stokes IA, Ronchetti PJ, et al: Comparison of curve shape between children with cerebral palsy, Friedreich's ataxia, and adolescent idiopathic scoliosis. *Dev Med Child Neurol* 1994;36:412–418.

The authors compare curve shape in these three conditions.

Beauchamp M, Labelle H, Duhaime M, et al: Natural history of muscle weakness in Friedreich's ataxia and its relation to loss of ambulation. *Clin Orthop* 1995;311:270–275.

Thirty-three patients with Friedreich's ataxia were followed prospectively with careful muscular strength assessment for an average of 6 years. Weakness usually was manifest in hip extension first, followed by variable further lower extremity weakness. Patients began to use a wheelchair at an average age of 18 years, and became completely unable to walk by age 20.5 years. Because muscle strength was still 70% of normal at initiation of wheelchair use, the authors conclude that muscle weakness is not the primary cause of loss of walking ability.

Cady RB, Bobechko WP: Incidence, natural history and treatment of scoliosis in Friedreich's ataxia. *J Pediatr Orthop* 1984;4:673–676.

This is a study of 42 patients with Freidreich's ataxia. The incidence of scoliosis is high. Curves tend to progress with disease severity. Bracing has no role in treatment. Early surgical stabilization is indicated in progressive curves.

Labelle H, Tohme S, Duhaime M, et al: Natural history of scoliosis in Friedreich's ataxia. *J Bone Joint Surg* 1986;68A:564–572.

In this retrospective review of 56 patients with Friedreich's ataxia, all had scoliosis measuring at least 10°. Thirty-six of these patients followed up for more than 10 years were noted to fall into one of two groups: those whose curves progressed, measuring more than 60° (20 patients) and those whose curves stabilized at under 40° (16 patients). The authors recommend that curves under 40° be observed, those greater than 60° be fused, and those between 40° and 60° observed or fused, depending on individual circumstances.

Arthrogryposis Multiplex Congenita

Bayne LG: Hand assessment and management of arthrogryposis multiplex congenita. *Clin Orthop* 1985;194:68–73.

This is a general article on the potential solutions to hand and wrist deformities in arthrogryposis, particularly pronation contracture of the forearm, proximal interphalangeal joint flexion contractures, and ulnar deviation of the fingers.

Carlson WO, Speck GJ, Vicari V, et al: Arthrogryposis multiplex congenita. *Clin Orthop* 1985;194:115–123.

The authors present a follow-up study of 34 patients at an average age of 27 years. The nature and frequency of deformities of the upper and lower extremities and spine are documented. Thirteen of 22 potentially employable patients were actually employed, and 11 were married. Half of the patients were independently ambulatory, while eight were nonambulatory. The authors recommend properly sequenced orthopaedic procedures as well as early efforts to promote independence in activities of daily living, mobility, and education.

Daher YH, Lonstein JE, Winter RB, et al: Spinal deformities in patients with arthrogryposis: A review of 16 patients. *Spine* 1985;10:609–613.

This is a literature review and results of management of a small group of patients with arthrogryposis.

DelBello DA, Watts HG: Distal femoral extension osteotomy for knee flexion contracture in patients with arthrogryposis. *J Pediatr Orthop* 1996;16:122–126.

Thirty-two severe knee flexion contractures were treated by distal femoral extension osteotomy. The average contracture correction was 43°, but during the 32-month follow-up an average of 22° of correction was lost at a rate of almost 1° per month. The ambulatory levels of all patients increased at least one level.

Goldberg M: *The Dysmorphic Child: An Orthopedic Perspective.* New York, NY, Raven Press, 1987.

Chapter one of this excellent text reviews classic arthrogryposis multiplex congenita as well as the more common recognizable disorders that often are confused with the classic variety.

Sarwarak JF, MacEwen GD, Scott CI: Amyoplasia: A common form of arthrogryposis. *J Bone Joint Surg* 1990;72A:465–469.

The most common, clinically recognizable form of arthrogryposis is termed amyoplasia and also is known as arthrogryposis multiplex congenita. This article reviews current understanding of the pathogenesis and orthopaedic management of these patients.

Sodergard J, Ryoppy S: Foot deformities in arthrogryposis multiplex congenita. *J Pediatr Orthop* 1994;14:768–772.

Foot deformities are common in patients with arthrogryposis. This article is a review of 52 patients with arthrogryposis, 43 of whom had foot deformities. Congenital clubfoot was the most common (72 feet, 52 of which required surgery). Forty-three feet suffered recurrent deformity. Talectomy and decancellations (removal of cancellous bone from the cuboid and talus) were effective in treating recurrences. Calcaneovalgus feet and true vertical tali were treated nonsurgically in this series. The authors recommend extensive soft-tissue procedures for nonplantigrade feet prior to walking, and bony procedures to manage recurrent deformities in the older patients. Recurrence and unsatisfactory long-term results were common.

Sodergard J, Ryoppy S: Knee in arthrogryposis multiplex congenita. *J Pediatr Orthop* 1990;10:177–182.

This paper summarizes the treatment and function of 58 knees in 30 patients with arthrogryposis who were treated for knee deformity. They were part of a total patient population of 50 who were followed up for 1 to 36 years. There were slightly more extension contractures than flexion contractures. Two thirds of patients with extension contractures were successfully managed nonsurgically. Flexion contractures were more disabling, required surgery more often (usually soft-tissue release and femoral shortening, extension osteotomy), and were prone to recurrence. The authors recommended treatment, however, because all patients so treated became functional walkers. Patients followed into adulthood seemed to be at an above-average risk for developing osteoarthritis.

Solund K, Sonne-Holm S, Kjolbye, JE: Talectomy for equinovarus deformity in arthrogryposis: A 13 (2-20) year review of 17 feet. *Acta Orthop Scand* 1991;62:372–374.

This is a 13-year follow-up of 17 feet in ten children treated by talectomy for severe, rigid clubfoot deformity. Most of the feet had undergone multiple previous procedures with recurrence. Fourteen of the feet were satisfactory in follow-up, although five of them had required at least one further procedure. Three were unsatisfactory because of recurrent deformity and required specialized footwear. The authors recommend talectomy with pinning of the calcaneus to the tibia either for recurrent deformity or as the primary procedure for clubfeet in arthrogryposis.

Staheli LT, Chew DE, Elliott JS, et al: Management of hip dislocations in children with arthrogryposis. *J Pediatr Orthop* 1987;7:681–685.

Eighteen patients from a total population of 131 children with arthrogryposis had a total of 24 dislocations (12 unilateral and six bilateral). Six hips were treated with closed reduction, five by anterior open reduction, and 13 by medial open reduction. At follow-up, range of motion was best in patients treated by medial open reduction, and hip function was rated good in 12 of 13; the other was fair after developing osteonecrosis. The authors recommend medial open reduction between 3 and 6 months of age with 5 to 6 weeks of casting postoperatively.

Szöke G, Staheli LT, Jaffe K, et al: Medial-approach open reduction of hip dislocation in amyoplasia-type arthrogryposis. *J Pediatr Orthop* 1996;16:127–130.

Open reduction through a medial approach obtained good results in 80% of 25 hip dislocations in 16 patients (average age 8.9 months) with amyoplasia-type arthrogryposis. Stiffness or asymmetry did not occur in any of the nine patients with bilateral reductions.

Thomas B, Schopler S, Wood W, et al: The knee in arthrogryposis. *Clin Orthop* 1985;194:87–92.

Seventy-four of 104 patients with arthrogryposis had flexion contracture, extension contracture, or instability. Nonsurgical therapy without prolonged casting or bracing rarely improved the arc of knee motion. Surgical treatment tended to change the location of the arc of motion without substantially changing the total arc. Osteotomies to extend the knee were prone to recurrence of the deformity in the skeletally immature child. Overall, 26% of patients treated for knee deformity had either unsuccessful efforts of correction or recurrence.

Williams PF: Management of upper limb problems in arthrogryposis. *Clin Orthop* 1985;194:60–67.

This is a general article on the problems and potential solutions, with respect to activities of daily living. No specific patient results are presented.

Miscellaneous

Bell DF, Moseley CF, Koreska J: Unit rod segmental spinal instrumentation in the management of patients with progressive neuromuscular spinal deformity. *Spine* 1989;14:1301–1307.

The authors report the use of a 1/4" U-shaped rod (unit rod) with sublaminar wires for posterior spine fusion to the pelvis in 34 nonambulatory patients with neuromuscular scoliosis. Major complications were two implant failures that required revision and two patients with intraoperative blood loss, which necessitated completion of the procedure in a second stage. The authors recommended this instrumentation for treatment of patients with progressive neuromuscular scoliosis.

Broom MJ, Banta JV, Renshaw TS: Spinal fusion augmented by Luque-rod segmental instrumentation for neuromuscular scoliosis. *J Bone Joint Surg* 1989;71A:32–44.

This article reviews the results of posterior spinal fusion and Luque-rod segmental instrumentation in 74 patients with a variety of neuromuscular disorders, including nine with muscular dystrophy and four with spinal muscular atrophy. Curves averaged 73° preoperatively, 38° postoperatively with an average loss of correction of 4° at 42-month average follow-up. Complications included one death, one late neurologic complication, three repeated surgeries for pseudarthrosis, and eight superficial and three deep wound infections. Seven patients required proximal extension of their fusions for progression, and the authors recommend that fusion extend to T3 or above. This study provides a good summary of the treatment and attendant complications of neuromuscular scoliosis.

Section 17

Cerebral Palsy

Peter A. DeLuca, MD

General

Albright AL, Barron WB, Fasick MP, et al: Continuous intrathecal baclofen infusion for spasticity of cerebral origin. *JAMA* 1993;270: 2475–2477.

Severe spasticity in 37 patients was significantly reduced at 24-month follow-up. This neurosurgical treatment provides a hopeful treatment for severely involved spastic patients.

Bleck EE: Management of the lower extremities in children who have cerebral palsy. *J Bone Joint Surg* 1990;72A:140–144.

Bleck EE (ed): Orthopaedic management in cerebral palsy, in *Clinics in Developmental Medicine.* London, England, MacKeith Press, vol 99/100, 1987, pp 1–485.

Gage JR (ed): Gait analysis in cerebral palsy, in *Clinics in Developmental Medicine.* London, England, MacKeith Press, 1991, vol 121.

Renshaw TS, Green NE, Griffin PP, et al: Cerebral palsy: Orthopaedic management. *J Bone Joint Surg* 1995;77A:1590–1606.

These resources provide in-depth reviews of orthopaedic management schemes for cerebral palsy (CP). Although each is heavily based in its authors' biases, they provide excellent summations of the available literature.

Campos da Paz A, Burnett SM, Braga LW: Walking prognosis in cerebral palsy: A 22-year retrospective analysis. *Dev Med Child Neurol* 1994; 36:130–134.

The prognosis for ambulation is favorable if children develop head control by 9 months of age, sitting at 24 months, and crawling by 30 months. Attaining these milestones by 20, 36, and 61 months, respectively, held poor prognosis for walking.

Koman LA, Mooney JF III, Smith B, et al: Management of cerebral palsy with botulinum-A toxin: Preliminary investigation. *J Pediatr Orthop* 1993;13:489–495.

After intramuscular injection of Botox in 27 patients, reduction in spasticity was apparent in 12 to 72 hours, the effect of Botox after target threshold was reached lasted 3 to 6 months, and no major side effects occurred. This method may allow delay of surgical intervention until the child is older and at less risk for complications.

Sussman MD (ed): *The Diplegic Child: Evaluation and Management.* Rosemont, IL, American Academy of Orthopaedic Surgeons, 1992.

This symposium is a multiauthored review of state-of-the-art opinions concerning spastic diplegic CP.

Upper Extremity

Beach WR, Strecker WB, Coe J, et al: Use of the Green transfer in treatment of patients with spastic cerebral palsy: 17-year experience. *J Pediatr Orthop* 1991;11:731–736.

A 17-year review of Green procedures and transfer of the flexor carpi ulnaris (FCU) in treatment of spastic forearm pronation, wrist volarflexion, and ulnar deviation deformities reveals a cosmetic (88%) and functional (79%) improvement. Supination improved markedly when a pronator procedure was also performed. Patients older than 12 years of age had less functional improvement.

Goldner JL: Surgical reconstruction of the upper extremity in cerebral palsy. *Hand Clin* 1988;4:223–265.

This article reviews treatment principles for the management of hand deformities in patients with CP. Such treatment should provide a balanced grasp and release, a reasonable range of pronation and supination of the forearm, and should maintain sufficient strength for hand function.

Goldner JL, Koman LA, Gelberman R, et al: Arthrodesis of the metacarpophalangeal joint of the thumb in children and adults: Adjunctive treatment of thumb-in-palm deformity in cerebral palsy. *Clin Orthop* 1990;253: 75–89.

A hypermobile hyperextension or hyperflexion deformity of the metacarpophalangeal (MCP) joint associated with thumb-in-palm deformity was treated by MCP arthrodesis with or without intrinsic muscle lengthening and/or extrinsic tendon transfer in 22 adults and 68 children. Forty-four of the 50 children followed to maturity had improved function. There was no significant disturbance in growth of those thumbs that had MCP joint fusion when the physes were open.

Hoffer MM: The use of the pathokinesiology laboratory to select muscles for tendon transfers in the cerebral palsy hand. *Clin Orthop* 1993;288: 135–138.

Fine wire electromyography was used in 119 CP patients to determine appropriateness of the flexor carpi radialis or brachioradialis as transfers to augment release. Only one half of the muscles were found to be suitable.

Hoffer MM, Lehman M, Mitani M: Long-term follow-up on tendon transfers to the extensors of the wrist and fingers in patients with cerebral palsy. *J Hand Surg* 1986;11A:836–840.

Tendon transfers to improve wrist and finger extension were successful in patients with good hand placement, sensibility, and motor control. Transfers to the finger extensors improved finger extension and release, and preserved grasp; however, 40% of patients with transfers to the wrist extensors had extension contractures with difficulty in release.

Hoffer MM, Zeitzew S: Wrist fusion in cerebral palsy. *J Hand Surg* 1988;13A:667–670.

Wrist fusion was a very effective procedure for 19 patients with severe wrist and finger flexion deformities, and allowed for improved hygiene and cosmesis.

Manske PR: Cerebral palsy of the upper extremity. *Hand Clin* 1990;6: 697–709.

The author reviews the surgical concepts of releasing spastic muscles and transferring tendons that contribute to deformities so that they may serve to correct the deformity. The patient's voluntary use of the extremity is essential.

Strecker WB, Emanuel JP, Dailey L, et al: Comparison of pronator tenotomy and pronator rerouting in children with spastic cerebral palsy. *J Hand Surg* 1988;13A:540–543.

In patients with pronation contracture of the forearm, pronator teres rerouting (41) produced greater active forearm supination than did pronator teres tenotomy (16) (78° versus 54°).

Thometz JG, Tachdjian M: Long-term follow-up of the flexor carpi ulnaris transfer in spastic hemiplegic children. *J Pediatr Orthop* 1988;8:407–412.

Twenty-five patients had transfer of the flexor carpi ulnaris to the radial wrist extensors at an average age of 8 years and were followed up for 8 years. Results were excellent or good in 60%. Although wrist dorsiflexion improved, active palmarflexion frequently was lost. The authors recommend that a patient have good digital extension (with the wrist extended passively above neutral) to be considered for the transfer.

Selective Posterior Dorsal Rhizotomy

Arens LJ, Peacock WJ, Peter J: Selective posterior rhizotomy: A long-term follow-up study. *Childs Nerv Syst* 1989;5:148–152.

Fifty-one spastic children maintained tone reduction between 5 and 8 years after selective posterior lumbar rhizotomy. The best results were in patients younger than 8 years of age at surgery. There were no spinal abnormalities or significant sensory problems. Postrhizotomy orthopaedic surgery for fixed-joint contractures generally brought further improvement.

Boscarino LF, Ounpuu S, Davis RB III, et al: Effects of selective dorsal rhizotomy on gait in children with cerebral palsy. *J Pediatr Orthop* 1993;13:174–179.

One year postoperative gait analysis in 19 patients noted improved sagittal plane hip, knee, and ankle motion with no change in the coronal plane motion of the pelvis and hip. The only major negative change observed was an increase in anterior pelvic tilt for independent ambulators.

Peter JC, Arens LJ: Selective posterior lumbosacral rhizotomy in teenagers and young adults with spastic cerebral palsy. *Br J Neurosurg* 1994;8:135–139.

Thirty teenagers and young adults with CP who had selective posterior lumbosacral rhizotomy for spasticity had satisfactory long-term tone reduction. Sitting and standing were improved in 21 and 17, respectively, and walking patterns of the 25 of 26 spastic diplegic patients were improved. There was no incontinence; however, five patients had leg dysaesthetic sensations and seven had patchy inconsistent areas of pinprick loss. Touch was preserved in all. Twenty-three patients were unequivocally positive about the benefits of this procedure.

Vaughan CL, Berman B, Peacock WJ: Cerebral palsy and rhizotomy: A three-year follow-up evaluation with gait analysis. *J Neurosurg* 1991; 74:178–184.

Gait analysis of 14 patients was performed at 1 and 3 years after selective rhizotomy. Knee motion improved by 1 year and normalized by 3 years. Stride length and walking speed improved, while cadence remained unchanged.

Foot Deformities

Varus Foot

Asirvatham R, Watts HG, Rooney RJ: Tendo achilles tenodesis to the fibula: A retrospective study. *J Pediatr Orthop* 1991;11:652–656.

Gait was improved in a third of 48 postpolio patients. When the hindfoot was stabilized, gait improved in 40%; when it was not stabilized, only 22% had improved gait. Excessive equinus developed in 18 patients, all of whom were younger than 12 years of age at the time of surgery.

Barnes MJ, Herring JA: Combined split anterior tibial-tendon transfer and intramuscular lengthening of the posterior tibial tendon: Results in patients who have a varus deformity of the foot due to spastic cerebral palsy. *J Bone Joint Surg* 1991;73A:734–738.

Combined split anterior tibial-tendon transfer and intramuscular lengthening of the posterior tibial tendon, with and without concomitant lengthening of the Achilles tendon, corrected flexible varus in 20 spastic CP patients followed up for 6 years. Fixed varus or weakness in the anterior tibialis led to the four poor results.

Hoffer MM, Barakat G, Koffman M: 10-year follow-up of split anterior tibial tendon transfer in cerebral palsied patients with spastic equinovarus deformity. *J Pediatr Orthop* 1985;5:432–434.

Split anterior tibial tendon transfer was successful in 20 of 21 patients. This procedure was performed when there was dynamic hindfoot varus and continuous anterior tibial muscle activity. Achilles and posterior tibial lengthening were added when there was fixed equinovarus.

Johnson WL, Lester EL: Transposition of the posterior tibial tendon. *Clin Orthop* 1989;245:223–227.

The posterior tibial tendon was rerouted by the technique described by Baker and Hill in 35 feet in children with dynamic varus deformities due to spastic CP. At 11.4-year follow-up, there was no overcorrection in the ten having an isolated transfer, but three of 25 having other procedures developed cavus due to excessive weakening of the triceps surae.

McCall RE, Frederick HA, McCluskey GM, et al: The Bridle procedure: A new treatment for equinus and equinovarus deformities in children. *J Pediatr Orthop* 1991;11:83–89.

This procedure combines tritendon anastomosis between the posterior tibialis, anterior tibialis, and peroneus longus with Achilles tendon lengthening. Of 107 procedures performed on patients with cerebral palsy, 74% obtained excellent or good results.

Medina PA, Karpman RR, Young AT: Split posterior tibial tendon transfer for spastic equinovarus foot deformity. *Foot Ankle* 1989;10:65–67.

A variation of split posterior tibial tendon transfer in the treatment of spastic equinovarus deformity of the foot is to transfer to the peroneus brevis. Eleven of 13 patients had good results at a mean follow-up of 21 months.

Root L, Miller SR, Kirz P: Posterior tibial-tendon transfer in patients with cerebral palsy. *J Bone Joint Surg* 1987;69A:1133–1139.

Fifty-seven posterior tibial-tendon transfers through the interosseous membrane to the dorsum of the foot were performed in 51 patients with CP, who were followed up for a mean of 9.3 years (range, 5 to 26 years).

Good or excellent results were obtained in 39 patients. For success, the foot had to be passively correctable to at least a neutral position and the tendon had to be passed superficial to the extensor retinaculum and inserted into the lateral cuneiform bone. The heel cord should be lengthened before the tendon transfer.

Saji MJ, Upadhyay SS, Hsu LC, et al: Split tibialis posterior transfer for equinovarus deformity in cerebral palsy: Long-term results of a new surgical procedure. *J Bone Joint Surg* 1993;75B:498–501.

Transfers of the anterior half of the split tibialis posterior to the dorsum of the foot through the interosseous membrane are reported good or excellent at 8 years in 23 feet in 18 children.

Sutherland DH: Varus foot in cerebral palsy: An overview, in Heckman JD (ed): *Instructional Course Lectures 42*. Rosemont, IL, American Academy of Orthopaedic Surgeons, 1993, pp 539–543.

This is a good review of the varus foot. Gait analysis and EMG help define muscle abnormalities but fail to fully define the pathology. Biomechanical studies of foot and ankle function are explored.

Valgus Foot

Alman BA, Craig CL, Zimbler S: Subtalar arthrodesis for stabilization of valgus hindfoot in patients with cerebral palsy. *J Pediatr Orthop* 1993; 13:634–641.

Twenty-nine patients (53 feet) were followed up an average of 8.9 years after Grice extra-articular subtalar arthrodesis. Talar head uncovering is a useful and reproducible method for evaluation of hindfoot valgus in these patients. Five spastic quadriplegic patients had progressive hindfoot or ankle deformity at latest follow-up. The 17 less severely involved patients had no recurrence.

Drvaric DM, Schmitt EW, Nakano JM: The Grice extra-articular subtalar arthrodesis in the treatment of spastic hindfoot valgus deformity. *Dev Med Child Neurol* 1989;31:665–669.

The Grice extra-articular subtalar arthrodesis was evaluated in 102 feet of 60 ambulatory patients with spasticity at an average of 5 years postoperatively. Results were satisfactory in 96 feet (94%).

Gallien R, Morin F, Marquis F: Subtalar arthrodesis in children. *J Pediatr Orthop* 1989;9:59–63.

The authors present a clinical and radiologic retrospective study of 51 feet in 30 patients with CP, myelomeningocele, and agenesis of the corpus callosum with valgus deformity of the feet treated with three different types of subtalar extra-articular and intra-articular arthrodesis. The combined Grice-Green-Batchelor procedure gave the best results, with 84% excellent and satisfactory results, with bony union in 96% of the feet at 4 years. They emphasize the importance of weightbearing anteroposterior films of the ankles to analyze the true location of the deformity.

Guttmann GG: Subtalar arthrodesis in children with cerebral palsy: Results using iliac bone plug. *Foot Ankle* 1990;10:206–210.

Twenty-six extra-articular subtalar arthrodeses using an iliac crest bone plug and muscle balancing were performed on 15 patients with flexible planovalgus feet due to CP. At average 6.8-year follow-up, satisfactory results were achieved in 88.4% of the patients.

Koman LA, Mooney JF III, Goodman A: Management of valgus hindfoot deformity in pediatric cerebral palsy patients by medial displacement osteotomy. *J Pediatr Orthop* 1993;13:180–183.

Medial displacement osteotomy of the calcaneus gave excellent correction of valgus in 17 of 18 feet that were followed up for an average of 42 months. The distal fragment was displaced 50% or more and transfixed with two parallel pins.

Tenuta J, Shelton YA, Miller F: Long-term follow-up of triple arthrodesis in patients with cerebral palsy. *J Pediatr Orthop* 1993;13:713–716.

Triple arthrodesis is reviewed at mean follow-up of 17.8 years in 24 patients (35 feet). Twenty-three feet had planovalgus deformities and 12 had equinovarus deformities. Forty-three percent of the feet had degenerative changes at the ankle joint; however, they were not correlated with pain, distance limitations, residual deformity, or patient satisfaction. Patient satisfaction was correlated to persistent pain and residual deformity, which were themselves strongly correlated with residual planovalgus deformity.

Hip

Aronson DD, Zak PJ, Lee CL, et al: Posterior transfer of the adductors in children who have cerebral palsy: A long-term study. *J Bone Joint Surg* 1991;73A:59–65.

Seventy-eight posterior transfers of the adductors of the hip in 42 spastic children reviewed at an average of 5.7 years were successful in improving or maintaining abduction, extension, functional walking, and stability of the hip in 88%.

Bagg MR, Farber J, Miller F: Long-term follow-up of hip subluxation in cerebral palsy patients. *J Pediatr Orthop* 1993;13:32–36.

At 19-year follow-up, varus osteotomy prevented dislocation of 64 subluxated hips in 45 spastic quadriplegic patients when combined with muscle releases. Nine dislocated hips had the most degenerative arthritis, pain, and the least movement. Subluxated hips also had more degenerative arthritis but approximately the same level of pain as reduced hips.

Baxter MP, D'Astous JL: Proximal femoral resection-interposition arthroplasty: Salvage hip surgery for the severely disabled child with cerebral palsy. *J Pediatr Orthop* 1986;6:681–685.

Proximal femoral resection-interposition arthroplasty was successful for five painful, spastic hip dislocations in four CP patients. Limited follow-up of 6 months to 5 years shows comfortable seating with no significant loss of motion, bony ankylosis or impingement, myositis ossificans, or recurrence of pain.

Brunner R, Baumann JU: Clinical benefit of reconstruction of dislocated or subluxated hip joints in patients with spastic cerebral palsy. *J Pediatr Orthop* 1994;14:290–294.

Femoral and pelvic osteotomy, an anterior iliopsoas transfer, and soft-tissue surgery were used on 64 dislocated hips in 47 spastic patients. Pain relief and improved sitting were maintained at 6.8 years' follow-up, but radiographs showed three redislocations and 23 poorly covered.

Buly RL, Huo M, Root L, et al: Total hip arthroplasty in cerebral palsy: Long-term follow-up results. *Clin Orthop* 1993;296:148–153.

Nineteen cemented total hip arthroplasties (THA) were performed in 18 patients with cerebral palsy at an average age of 30 years. Four hips required bone graft augmentation of the deficient acetabulum, and spica casts were used in 16 of 18 patients to minimize the incidence of dislocation and trochanteric nonunion. Seventeen of 18 patients (94%) had pain relief and improved function after arthroplasty, and survivorship analysis was 95% at 10 years for loosening.

Erken EH, Bischof FM: Iliopsoas transfer in cerebral palsy: The long-term outcome. *J Pediatr Orthop* 1994;14:295–298.

Eight subluxated and 39 dislocated hips in 33 total-body involvement, nonambulatory patients with spastic CP underwent iliopsoas transfers as part of the surgery for hip instability. Forty-five of the 47 hips were located at mean 8-year follow-up, but sitting ability did not improve in any patient and had in fact deteriorated in 50%.

Herndon WA, Bolano L, Sullivan JA: Hip stabilization in severely involved cerebral palsy patients. *J Pediatr Orthop* 1992;12:68–73.

Thirty-two patients (48 hips) with total body involved CP underwent adductor and psoas release, anterior branch obturator neurectomy, and proximal femoral shortening osteotomy for hip subluxation or dislocation. Twenty-eight hips were rated good, 15 were rated fair, and five were rated poor at 43-month follow-up. Best results were found when there was less dysplasia and when surgery achieved good reduction. Early surgery correlates best with good outcome.

Hoffer MM, Stein GA, Koffman M, et al: Femoral varus-derotation osteotomy in spastic cerebral palsy. *J Bone Joint Surg* 1985;67A:1229–1235.

At minimum 7-year follow-up, 20 of 25 hips treated by varus-derotation osteotomy and muscle releases remained well centered with improved center edge and neck shaft angles. Four hips remained subluxated but less subluxated than before the osteotomy. One hip remained dislocated. The authors emphasize the importance of combining muscle balancing with correction of bony deformity.

McHale KA, Bagg M, Nason SS: Treatment of the chronically dislocated hip in adolescents with cerebral palsy with femoral head resection and subtrochanteric valgus osteotomy. *J Pediatr Orthop* 1990;10:504–509.

Femoral head resection with valgus subtrochanteric osteotomy was successful for six chronically dislocated and painful hips in five nonambulatory adolescent CP patients. This procedure was successful because pain, perineal care, and seating were improved. Complications, such as proximal migration of the remaining femur, recurrence of adduction deformity, hip stiffness, and excessive heterotopic bone formation, common to other procedures used for this condition, did not occur.

Mubarak SJ, Valencia FG, Wenger DR: One-stage correction of the spastic dislocated hip: Use of pericapsular acetabuloplasty to improve coverage. *J Bone Joint Surg* 1992;74A:1347–1357.

Eighteen subluxated or dislocated hips with severe acetabular dysplasia in 11 children between 5 and 13 years of age who had spastic CP were treated with release of the adductors, psoas, and proximal hamstrings; a femoral-shortening varus derotation osteotomy; and a pericapsular pelvic osteotomy. Seventeen hips remained anatomically reduced at average 6 years, 10 months of follow-up. The pelvic osteotomy was designed to increase superolateral coverage of the femoral head in the elongated acetabulum, which had erosion of the superior and lateral aspects.

Payne LZ, DeLuca PA: Heterotopic ossification after rhizotomy and femoral osteotomy. *J Pediatr Orthop* 1993;13:733–738.

Fifteen patients with CP underwent selective posterior rhizotomy (SPR) and subsequent proximal femoral varus derotation osteotomy (VDO). Heterotopic ossification (HO) around the hip after VDO was noted in four of the eight patients with spastic quadriplegia (seven of 26 hips, 27%), but not noted in the seven patients with spastic diplegia. A radiographic review of 118 hips with a femoral VDO in the 69 patients with CP who did not undergo SPR during the same period showed no HO.

Pope DF, Bueff HU, DeLuca PA: Pelvic osteotomies for subluxation of the hip in cerebral palsy. *J Pediatr Orthop* 1994;14:724–730.

Stability was maintained in 19 of 23 hips in 21 patients treated with pelvic osteotomies (ten Salter, seven Chiari, six Steel) followed up for an average of 6 years. Redirectional osteotomy did not produce posterior instability.

Root L, Goss JR, Mendes J: The treatment of the painful hip in cerebral palsy by total hip replacement or hip arthrodesis. *J Bone Joint Surg* 1986;68A:590–598.

Six of eight hip arthrodeses and 13 of 15 replacements improved pain and function in painful degenerative spastic hip disease.

Szalay EA, Roach JW, Houkom JA, et al: Extension-abduction contracture of the spastic hip. *J Pediatr Orthop* 1986;6:1–6.

Patients with athetosis or rigidity are those most likely to develop extension-abduction contractures either spontaneously or following adductor releases. Treatment in 27 patients was directed at improving sitting by either physical therapy (11), wheelchair modification (six), or femoral shortening, rotation osteotomy with muscle release (12).

Ankle Equinus Deformity

Graham HK, Fixsen JA: Lengthening of the calcaneal tendon in spastic hemiplegia by the White slide technique: A long-term review. *J Bone Joint Surg* 1988;70A:472–475.

The White slide technique produced excellent correction of equinus in 35 spastic hemiplegic patients at 14 to 20 years' follow-up. The complications and recurrence rates were low.

Rose SA, DeLuca PA, Davis RB III, et al: Kinematic and kinetic evaluation of the ankle after lengthening of the gastrocnemius fascia in children with cerebral palsy. *J Pediatr Orthop* 1993;13:727–732.

Joint kinematic and kinetic evaluation 1 year following lengthening of the gastrocnemius fascia (Baker) in 21 independent ambulators (24 sides) showed improved ankle range of motion during gait, a decrease in the abnormal energy generated around the ankle in midstance, and a statistically significant increase in the energy generated in late stance for push-off.

Segal LS, Thomas SE, Mazur JM, et al: Calcaneal gait in spastic diplegia after heel cord lengthening: A study with gait analysis. *J Pediatr Orthop* 1989;9:697-701.

Through gait analysis, 30% (six of 20 spastic diplegics) prevalence of calcaneal gait at more than 5 years following surgery suggests that an increased incidence of calcaneal gait may be present after heel-cord lengthening.

Strecker WB, Via MW, Oliver SK, et al: Heel cord advancement for treatment of equinus deformity in cerebral palsy. *J Pediatr Orthop* 1990;10:105-108.

One hundred patients with at least 30 months' follow-up after anterior transpositions of the Achilles tendon had good correction of equinus without the complications of calcaneal gait or recurrence of equinus.

Knee Dysfunction

Damron TA, Breed AL, Cook T: Diminished knee flexion after hamstring surgery in cerebral palsy patients: Prevalence and severity. *J Pediatr Orthop* 1993;13:188-191.

Isolated hamstring tenotomy in 52 patients with CP resulted in reduced prone knee flexion in 71% at 3 years, 4 months. Thirteen percent of ambulators eventually required a rectus femoris transfer to correct the resultant stiff-legged gait.

Hadley N, Chambers C, Scarborough N, et al: Knee motion following multiple soft-tissue releases in ambulatory patients with cerebral palsy. *J Pediatr Orthop* 1992;12:324-328.

In 45 extremities, rectus femoris transfer with hamstring lengthening significantly improved total knee range of motion, minimum knee flexion in stance, timing of maximum knee flexion, and slope of the knee flexion curve at toe off as documented by gait analysis.

Hsu LC, Li HS: Distal hamstring elongation in the management of spastic cerebral palsy. *J Pediatr Orthop* 1990;10:378–381.

Forty of 49 patients with spastic CP evaluated 4.4 years following distal hamstring lengthening had improvements in gait patterns and 18 increased a functional grade. Complications included transient stiff-legged gait and exaggerated lumbar lordosis, which responded to physical therapy.

Ounpuu S, Muik E, Davis RB III, et al: Rectus femoris surgery in children with cerebral palsy: Part I. The effect of rectus femoris transfer location on knee motion. *J Pediatr Orthop* 1993;13:325–330.

Rectus femoris transfer to either the sartorius (62 sides), semitendinosus (19 sides), or the gracilis (14 sides) muscles, or laterally to the iliotibial band (10 sides) was performed in 78 children (105 sides) with CP. Gait analysis demonstrated increased knee range of motion with increased extension at initial contact and in midstance and maintained knee flexion in swing. There were no statistically significant differences between the four transfer sites, nor were there transverse plane (rotational) effects.

Ounpuu S, Muik E, Davis RB III, et al: Rectus femoris surgery in children with cerebral palsy: Part II. A comparison between the effect of transfer and release of the distal rectus femoris on knee motion. *J Pediatr Orthop* 1993;13:331–335.

Gait analysis was performed one year following rectus femoris transfer in 105 lower limbs, and distal rectus femoris release in 31. Results suggest that the rectus femoris should be transferred and not released when knee range of motion is more than 80%. There were no significant changes in knee motion after either rectus femoris transfer or distal release when preoperative knee range of motion was more than 80% of normal.

Sutherland DH, Davids JR: Common gait abnormalities of the knee in cerebral palsy. *Clin Orthop* 1993;288:139–147.

From gait analysis of more than 588 patients with CP, four primary gait abnormalities of the knee were identified: jump knee, crouch knee, stiff knee, and recurvatum knee. The most common etiologies and the consequences for gait of each disorder are considered.

Sutherland DH, Santi M, Abel MF: Treatment of stiff-knee gait in cerebral palsy: A comparison by gait analysis of distal rectus femoris transfer versus proximal rectus release. *J Pediatr Orthop* 1990;10:433–441.

Gait analysis was reviewed after proximal release (12 patients) or distal transfer (ten patients) of the rectus femoris for treatment of knee stiffness in swing phase. Peak knee flexion was increased 9.1° in swing phase by proximal rectus release and 16.2° by distal rectus transfer, whereas hip motion was not affected.

Thometz J, Simon S, Rosenthal R: The effect on gait of lengthening of the medial hamstrings in cerebral palsy. *J Bone Joint Surg* 1989;71A:345–353.

Gait analysis following lengthening of the medial hamstrings in 31 patients with spastic CP showed that the contours of the postoperative motion graphs of the knees changed very little. Although extension of the knee in stance phase improved postoperatively, the improvement was accompanied by decreased flexion of the knee during swing phase. When spasticity of both the hamstrings and the quadriceps was noted on the preoperative EMG, motion of the knee in the sagittal plane was markedly restricted.

Gait Analysis

Gage JR, DeLuca PA, Renshaw TS: Gait analysis: Principles and applications. Emphasis on its use in cerebral palsy. *J Bone Joint Surg* 1995; 77A:1607–1623.

This is a good overview of gait analysis presented in a concise, understandable manner.

Lee EH, Goh JC, Bose K: Value of gait analysis in the assessment of surgery in cerebral palsy. *Arch Phys Med Rehabil* 1992;73:642–646.

The results of surgery that was performed based on the recommendations of three-dimensional gait analysis were superior to those surgeries that were different than recommended.

Nene AV, Evans GA, Patrick JH: Simultaneous multiple operations for spastic diplegia: Outcome and functional assessment of walking in 18 patients. *J Bone Joint Surg* 1993;75B:488–494.

After simultaneous multiple operations in 18 children with spastic diplegia, 14 had reduction in the physiologic cost index. The more involved patients took up to 2 years to reach an improvement plateau. Distal transfer of the rectus femoris, when it was shown to be contracting inappropriately, improved the knee flexion arc during walking from a mean of 28.3° to 45.2°. Intrapelvic intramuscular psoas tenotomy produced an improvement of hip flexion deformity in 15 of 17 patients without the loss of muscle power to initiate the swing phase.

Norlin R, Tkaczuk H: One session surgery on the lower limb in children with cerebral palsy: A five-year follow-up. *Int Orthop* 1992;16:291–293.

Twenty-three children with CP were reviewed after 5 years by footswitch measurements and assessment of video recordings. Gait improvements continued with normal growth-related development, and there were no recurrences.

Miscellaneous

Dennis SC, Green NE: Hereditary spastic paraplegia. *J Pediatr Orthop* 1988;8:413–417.

Twenty-six patients with autosomally dominant hereditary spastic paraplegia are reviewed. Although a slow progression of spastic paraparesis, it is frequently misdiagnosed as CP. Each child was treated when necessary with appropriate tendon lengthenings.

Koman LA, Mooney JF III, Smith BP, et al: Management of spasticity in cerebral palsy with botulinum-A toxin: Report of a preliminary, randomized, double-blind trial. *J Pediatr Orthop* 1994;14:299–303.

A randomized, double-blind, placebo-controlled study of the efficacy of local intramuscular injections of botulinum-A toxin in the management of dynamic equinus deformity associated with CP showed improvement in five of six patients (using the authors' Physician Rating Scale).

Section 18

Myelomeningocele

John M. Mazur, MD
John A. Churchill, MD

General Overview

Beaty JH, Canale ST: Orthopaedic aspects of myelomeningocele. *J Bone Joint Surg* 1990;72A:626–630.

This is a comprehensive review article summarizing the orthopaedic management of patients who have myelomeningocele. The authors prepared this review based on an open forum attended by recognized leaders in this field. It includes an overview, orthotic management, and treatment of spinal, hip, and foot deformities.

Centers for Disease Control and Prevention: Recommendations for use of folic acid to reduce number of spina bifida cases and other neural tube defects. *JAMA* 1993;269:1233–1238.

Available evidence indicates that 0.4 mg (400 mg) per day of folic acid will reduce the number of neural tube defects, including spina bifida and anencephaly. The United States Public Health Service recommends that all women of childbearing age who are capable of becoming pregnant should consume 0.4 mg of folic acid per day to reduce their risk of having a child with spina bifida. Women who have had a child with a neural tube defect are at a high risk of having a subsequent affected child and should seek genetic counseling.

Chatkupt S, Skurnick JH, Jaggi M, et al: Study of genetics, epidemiology, and vitamin usage in familial spina bifida in the United States in the 1990s. *Neurology* 1994;44:65–70.

Although folic acid may decrease the incidence of spina bifida, it is not the only factor; other genetic susceptibilities and environmental factors may be involved. Of 70 families with multiple occurrences of spina bifida, 50% reported some German ancestry and 49% reported some Irish ancestry; only one family reported African-American ancestry. The number of collateral cases on the maternal side analyzed by category of kinship were significantly higher than those on the paternal side. Prenatal diagnosis with alpha-fetoprotein screening may be appropriate in genetically susceptible individuals.

Elias ER, Sadeghi-Nejad AB: Precocious puberty in girls with myelodysplasia. *Pediatrics* 1994;93:521–522.

This article is important for the orthopaedist dealing with children affected with myelodysplasia who are likely to be skeletally mature earlier than the general population. This early maturity is an important issue in timing operations such as epiphysiodesis in which bone age is critical. The precocious puberty is believed to be secondary to hydrocephalus, whether treated, mild, or nonprogressive.

Harris MB, Banta JV: Cost of skin care in the myelomeningocele population. *J Pediatr Orthop* 1990;10:355–361.

Skin care preventing skin breakdown is often neglected by patients. Because of this, 75% of spina bifida patients experience pressure sores needlessly, increasing the hospital days and cost of treatment in this patient population.

Hori A: A review of the morphology of spinal cord malformations and their relation to neuro-embryology. *Neurosurg Rev* 1993;16:259–266.

This is the most up-to-date study of the morphologic characteristics of spinal dysraphic disorders. The major focus is on the anomalies of the ascending and descending pathways of the spinal tracts. These neuroembryologic considerations do much to clarify the pathogenesis and pathophysiology of spina bifida.

Luthy DA, Wardinsky T, Shurtleff DB, et al: Cesarean section before the onset of labor and subsequent motor function in infants with meningomyelocele diagnosed antenatally. *N Engl J Med* 1991;324:662–666.

Authors of this landmark article showed that for the fetus with uncomplicated meningomyelocele, delivery by cesarean section before the onset of labor may result in better subsequent motor function than vaginal delivery or delivery by cesarean section after a period of labor.

Mazur JM, Menelaus MB: Neurologic status of spina bifida patients and the orthopedic surgeon. *Clin Orthop* 1991;264:54–64.

The authors emphasize the importance of the neurologic examination in planning the orthopaedic treatment of children with spina bifida. The status of the neurologic deficit remains the most important factor in determining the myelomeningocele patient's ultimate functional abilities. Determination of the neurosegmental level of the lesion, recognition of spasticity and progressive paralysis, the potential for deformity, and functional expectations are described.

McDonald CM, Jaffe KM, Shurtleff DB, et al: Modifications to the traditional description of neurosegmental innervation in myelomeningocele. *Dev Med Child Neurol* 1991;33:473–481.

This important article alters the classic description of the neurosegmental innervation in myelomeningocele. The authors emphasize the need to classify children with myelomeningocele according to specific muscle strength rather than by neurosegmental level.

Oakley GP Jr, Erickson JD, James LM, et al: Prevention of folic acid-preventable spina bifida and anencephaly. *Ciba Found Symp* 1994;181:212–231.

One of the most exciting medical findings of the last part of the 20th century is that folic acid, a simple, widely available, water-soluble vitamin, can prevent spina bifida and anencephaly in 400,000 infants each year worldwide. The results of the British Medical Research Council's randomized controlled trial proved that folic acid can prevent spin bifida and anencephaly. Current policy discussions concern whether to permit manufacturers of vitamins or food products to claim that folic acid will prevent spina bifida and anencephaly and whether to allow a food staple to be fortified with folic acid.

Omtzigt JGC, Los FJ, Hagenaars AM, et al: Prenatal diagnosis of spina bifida aperta after first-trimester valproate exposure. *Prenat Diagn* 1992;12:893–897.

The use of the antiepileptic drug valproic acid during the first trimester is associated with a two- to threefold increase in risk of neural tube defects. Moreover, alpha-fetoprotein screening may be unreliable in women taking valproate. All women of childbearing age taking sodium valproate should be warned about the risk of spina bifida, offered preconceptual counseling, and given an amniocentesis and fetal ultrasound examination when pregnant.

Rietberg CC, Lindhout D: Adult patients with spina bifida cystica: Genetic counselling, pregnancy and delivery. *Eur J Obstet Gynecol Reprod Biol* 1993;52:63–70.

This discussion notes that the risk for parents with spina bifida of having affected offspring is ten times greater (approximately 4%) than that for the general population (approximately 0.1% to 0.3%). In pregnancy, special care is needed in the management of urologic, obstetric, neurologic, and anesthetic problems.

Sabadie P: The Spina Bifida Association of America: Successes and shortcomings. *Birth Defects* 1990;26:108–113.

This article describes the need for a team approach to children with spina bifida and the mission of the Spina Bifida Association of America. It is written by a father of a child with spina bifida and relates his experience with the existing available medical services.

Schweitzer ME, Balsam D, Weiss R: Spina bifida occulta: Incidence in parents of offspring with spina bifida cystica. *Spine* 1993;18:785–786.

This is the first article to disprove the hypothesis that spina bifida occulta is a milder expression of the same genetic abnormality as spina bifida cystica. Spina bifida occulta was noted in 14.5% of parents of children with spina bifida cystica compared to a prevalence of 16.7% in a control group. Because spina bifida occulta appears to be a separate defect with different unrelated genetics, the finding of spina bifida occulta on routine radiographs does not imply an increased risk of having a child with spina bifida cystica.

Tosi LL, Slater JE, Shaer C, et al: Latex allergy in spina bifida patients: Prevalence and surgical implications. *J Pediatr Orthop* 1993;313:709–712.

This is a practical and easy to understand article dealing with the important issue of latex allergy in spina bifida patients. The authors documented in preoperative patients: (1) the prevalence of latex sensitivity, (2) predictors of anaphylactic reaction, and (3) the risk of type I hypersensitivity reaction. Using radioallergosorbent testing, 38% of the spina bifida patients were found to be allergic to latex with 9.7% having had clinically significant allergic reactions. At surgery, rigorous efforts should be made to provide a latex-free environment in all spina bifida patients. Patients with known latex allergy should be premedicated with diphenhydramine, ranitidine, and prednisone at least 1 hour before anesthesia.

Wells TR, Jacobs RA, Senac MO, et al: Incidence of short trachea in patients with myelomeningocele. *Pediatr Neurol* 1990;6:109–111.

Because of the multiple orthopaedic surgeries performed on children with myelomeningocele, the surgeon and anesthesiologist must be aware of this article. Review of chest radiographs revealed that 36% of patients with myelomeningocele have short tracheae. The short tracheae typically are due to a reduced number of tracheal cartilage rings producing a high tracheal bifurcation. Special attention to the short trachea is warranted because of the risk of accidental bronchial intubation and its sequelae.

Fractures

Boytim MJ, Davidson RS, Charney E, et al: Neonatal fractures in myelomeningocele patients. *J Pediatr Orthop* 1991;11:28–30.

This article discusses the risk of neonatal fractures in infants with spina bifida and stresses awareness, pathogenesis, and care in the handling of these children. Infants with high level lesions and significant contractures are at greatest risk to acquire a fracture.

Cuxart A, Iborra J, Melendez M, et al: Physeal injuries in myelomeningocele patients. *Paraplegia* 1992;30:791–794.

This article describes the clinical characteristics, diagnostic difficulties, and treatment of physeal injuries in children with spina bifida. The authors recommend the use of suitable orthoses as a preventive measure and a temporary increase in the length of the orthosis in patients with physeal injuries.

Lock TR, Aronson DD: Fractures in patients who have myelomeningocele. *J Bone Joint Surg* 1989;71A:1153–1157.

Fractures are common in children with myelomeningocele, and the incidence is related to the level of neurologic involvement. Of 76 fractures, 58 were secondary to cast immobilization. Metaphyseal and diaphyseal fractures healed satisfactorily, but physeal fractures often were complicated by delayed union or premature growth arrest.

Ambulation-Rehabilitation

Charney EB, Melchionni JB, Smith DR: Community ambulation by children with myelomeningocele and high-level paralysis. *J Pediatr Orthop* 1991;11:579–582.

The authors concluded that walking can be a realistic goal in many children with myelomeningocele and high-level paralysis. Of the 87 children in this study, 45 (52%) did achieve community ambulation by 5 years of age, while 42 (48%) did not.

Guidera KJ, Smith S, Raney E, et al: Use of the reciprocating orthosis in myelodysplasia. *J Pediatr Orthop* 1993;13:341–348.

The reciprocating gait orthosis (RGO) is useful to maintain upright posture and ambulation in selected patients. Obesity, advanced age, lack of patient or family motivation, scoliosis, and spasticity were significant negative factors in long-term use of the RGO. Good upper extremity strength, trunk balance, previous standing or walking, and active hip flexion were important positive variables.

Liptak GS, Shurtleff DB, Bloss JW, et al: Mobility aids for children with high-level myelomeningocele: Parapodium versus wheelchair. *Dev Med Child Neurol* 1992;34:787–796.

The optimal method for providing mobility for children with myelomeningocele remains controversial. Children in the upright posture using a parapodium were more likely to: (1) develop skin sores of the lower extremities; (2) have dislocated hips; (3) be more obese; and (4) watch more television than children who used a wheelchair. Children using a wheelchair developed skin sores in the gluteal region and knee-flexion contractures. The parapodium was judged by families to be less effective as a mobility aid; however, the upright posture it allows was considered extremely advantageous. A combined approach allowing upright posture and wheeled mobility would appear to be optimal.

McDonald CM, Jaffe KM, Mosca VS, et al: Ambulatory outcome of children with myelomeningocele: Effect of lower-extremity muscle strength. *Dev Med Child Neurol* 1991;33:482–490.

The authors point out the relationship between patterns of muscle strength and mobility. Patients with grade 4 to 5 iliopsoas and quadriceps function were likely to walk, whereas patients with grade 0 to 3 iliopsoas and quadriceps relied on wheelchairs for mobility. Deterioration in mobility was related to decrease in muscle strength and was not age-related.

Phillips DL, Field RE, Broughton NS, et al: Reciprocating orthoses for children with myelomeningocele: A comparison of two types. *J Bone Joint Surg* 1995;77B:110–113.

These authors compared the reciprocating gait orthosis (RGO) and the hip guidance orthosis (HGO) and found both to be cost-effective methods of achieving ambulation for children with high-level myelomeningocele. Younger children preferred the RGO but switched to the HGO as they grew older. Most abandoned both, preferring a wheelchair by early to midteens. The authors recommend walking to their patients, but do not strive unduly for ambulation in every patient.

Steinbok P, Irvine B, Cochrane DD, et al: Long-term outcome and complications of children born with meningomyelocele. *Child Nerv Syst* 1992;8:92–96.

Results of this 20-year, long-term follow-up study reconfirm those of previous studies in which the functional outcome of this population was assessed. Thirty-three percent of the adults were community ambulators, and this correlated well with the presence of intact quadriceps function.

Swank M, Dias LS: Walking ability in spina bifida patients: A model for predicting future ambulatory status based on sitting balance and motor level. *J Pediatr Orthop* 1994;14:715–718.

The authors of this article point out the predictors of community ambulation: sitting balance and motor level. Using these variables, the authors developed a mathematical method to predict which patients are likely to continue to walk into adolescence.

Taylor A, McNamara A: Ambulation status of adults with myelomeningocele. *Z Kinderchir* 1990;45(suppl 1):32–33.

The authors of this article point out the unfortunate realization that children who had been ambulant with orthoses as children often become wheelchair bound as adults. Most of the adults in the study group found knee-ankle-foot orthoses uncomfortable to wear, and almost half of the group developed pressure sores directly related to their orthoses.

Spine

Banta JV: Combined anterior and posterior fusion for spinal deformity in myelomeningocele. *Spine* 1990;15:946–952.

The author recommends anterior and posterior spinal fusion for spinal deformities in patients with myelomeningocele. Anterior fusion of the dysraphic spine allows greater correction of both spinal deformity and pelvic obliquity in addition to contributing significant strength to the fusion mass. Segmental spinal instrumentation with sublaminar and pedicular wiring to custom-contoured Luque rods provides excellent correction and immediate postoperative stability.

Banta JV: The tethered cord in myelomeningocele: Should it be untethered? *Dev Med Child Neurol* 1991;33:173–176.

This article points out that progressive neurologic deterioration may occur after myelomeningocele repair. Magnetic resonance imaging almost invariably demonstrates a conus medullaris in an abnormally low position, whether neurologic symptoms develop or not. Only children presenting with clinical signs and symptoms of tethering are candidates for surgical intervention. Greater use of urodynamic and somatosensory-evoked potential monitoring will help to identify those patients most likely to benefit from surgical de-tethering.

Banta JV, Bonanni C, Prebluda J: Latex anaphylaxis during spinal surgery in children with myelomeningocele. *Dev Med Child Neurol* 1993;35: 543–548.

Intraoperative anaphylaxis to latex involves cutaneous, respiratory, and circulatory changes, which may prove fatal if not promptly recognized and treated. It is estimated that 18% to 40% of children with spina bifida may be affected by latex allergy.

Carstens C, Paul K, Niethard FU, et al: Effect of scoliosis surgery on pulmonary function in patients with myelomeningocele. *J Pediatr Orthop* 1991;11:459–464.

Patients with myelomeningocele and scoliosis frequently have impaired pulmonary function. The authors report ten patients with restricted ventilation disturbance (average 60.9% of the standard value) in whom the vital capacity increased to 66% after surgery.

Fromm B, Carstens C, Niethard FU, et al: Aortography in children with myelomeningocele and lumbar kyphosis. *J Bone Joint Surg* 1992;74B: 691–694.

In children with myelomeningocele who underwent kyphectomy for congenital kyphosis of the lumbar spine, aortography revealed none in whom the aorta followed the spinal curvature. The authors concluded that the aorta is not at risk and that aortography is not usually necessary before kyphectomy, except in patients who have undergone prior abdominal surgery. Noninvasive methods should be used to detect malpositions and malformations of the kidneys.

Hall PV, Lindseth RE, Campbell RL, et al: Scoliosis and hydrocephalus in myelocele patients: The effects of ventricular shunting. *J Neurosurg* 1979;50:174–178.

Progressive scoliosis may be due to shunt malfunction. The importance of neurologic examinations at each visit is stressed.

Karol LA, Richards BS, Prejean E, et al: Hemodynamic instability of myelomeningocele patients during anterior spinal surgery. *Dev Med Child Neurol* 1993;35:261–267.

This article reports six patients in whom sudden intraoperative hemodynamic instability occurred during anterior spinal fusion. Possible etiologies include limited pulmonary reserve, drug reactions, malignant hyperthermia, reaction to blood products, and latex protein allergy.

Lindseth RE: Spine deformity in myelomeningocele, in Tullos HS (ed): *Instructional Course Lectures XL*. Park Ridge, IL, American Academy of Orthopaedic Surgeons, 1991, pp 273–279.

This excellent review summarizes the incidence, etiology, pathophysiology, and treatment of spine deformities in patients with myclomeningocele. These deformities often cause severe disability, thwarting attempts at rehabilitation and negating previous treatment to maintain ambulation.

Lintner SA, Lindseth RE: Kyphotic deformity in patients who have a myelomeningocele: Operative treatment and long-term follow-up. *J Bone Joint Surg* 1994;76A:1301–1307.

After resection of the lordotic segment cephalad to the apical vertebra of a kyphotic deformity, the deformity was reduced by 64%. Although many patients demonstrated recurrence of deformity, only two of 39 patients required a second operation after reaching skeletal maturity.

Martin J, Kumar SJ, Guille JT, et al: Congenital kyphosis in myelomeningocele: Results following operative and nonoperative treatment. *J Pediatr Orthop* 1994;14:323–328.

This article clearly shows that a stable fusion with surgical correction of the kyphosis is preferable to nonsurgical treatment. If surgical treatment is not possible, suitable wheelchair modifications can enable these patients to function with reasonable comfort.

Mazur J, Menelaus MB, Dickens DR, et al: Efficacy of surgical management for scoliosis in myelomeningocele: Correction of deformity and alteration of functional status. *J Pediatr Orthop* 1986;6:568–575.

In 49 patients with myelomeningocele, the authors found that sitting was likely to be improved, but ambulation might be adversely affected after spinal fusion. Patients and their parents should be aware of this potential change.

McLane DG, Herman JM, Gabrieli AP, et al: Tethered cord as a cause of scoliosis in children with a myelomeningocele. *Pediatr Neurosurg* 1990;16:8–13.

In this study, it was recognized that tethered cord causes scoliosis. Spinal stability or improvement can be seen following untethering. Close long-term follow-up is essential to identify those individuals with retethering of their cord.

McMaster MJ: The long-term results of kyphectomy and spinal stabilization in children with myelomeningocele. *Spine* 1988;13:417–424.

A small series (ten patients) treated by kyphectomy and various forms of instrumentation for myelomeningocele kyphosis and followed for a mean of 7 years is presented. A long fusion from the mid thoracic region to the sacrum was necessary to provide long-term stability and to prevent the development of thoracic lordosis. Surgical techniques, risks, and complications are discussed.

Mintz LJ, Sarwark JF, Dias LS, et al: The natural history of congenital kyphosis in myelomeningocele: A review of 51 children. *Spine* 1991;16:S348–S350.

Progression of congenital kyphosis is documented in this article. Progression was related to the severity of the curve: curves $\leq 90°$ progressed 7.7° per year, and those $> 90°$ progressed 12.1° per year. No correlation existed between the rate of curve progression and the frequency of shunt revision or the presence of vertebral anomalies.

Muller EB, Nordwall A: Brace treatment of scoliosis in children with myelomeningocele. *Spine* 1994;19:151–155.

Among 21 children with myelomeningocele and progressive scoliosis who were treated with a Boston brace, the brace slowed or halted progression in 90% of patients with curves of less than 45° but had only a temporary effect on more severe curves. It is recommended that all patients with myelomeningocele be monitored with radiographs so that brace treatment can be instituted early in curves with documented progression.

Muller EB, Nordwall A: Prevalence of scoliosis in children with myelomeningocele in western Sweden. *Spine* 1992;17:1097–1102.

In a cross-sectional study, 69% of 131 patients with myelomeningocele were found to have scoliosis by 6 years of age. The occurrence of scoliosis increased drastically at high levels of dysraphism, from 20% in sacral myelomeningocele to 94% in those with a thoracic myelomeningocele level. The average curve increased from 15° to 33° between the ages of 5 and 10 years, with no significant progression thereafter.

Muller EB, Nordwall A, Oden A: Progression of scoliosis in children with myelomeningocele. *Spine* 1994;19:147–150.

This study of the natural history of scoliosis in children with spina bifida indicates that the chance of developing scoliosis increases with the patient's age and level of paralysis. More progression occurs before 15 years of age. Scoliosis of 40° or more progressed 5° per year. Because of the higher rate of surgical complications, the surgical treatment must start before a severe spinal deformity has developed.

Muller EB, Nordwall A, vonWendt L: Influence of surgical treatment of scoliosis in children with spina bifida on ambulation and motoric skills. *Acta Pediatr* 1992;81:173–176.

The authors of this article confirm that a large percentage (57%) of children lose some of their ambulation capacity after surgical treatment of scoliosis. Intensive attempts to treat these children conservatively to prevent scoliosis progression are suggested, and postoperative physiotherapy is highly advisable.

Samuelsson L, Eklof O: Scoliosis in myelomeningocele. *Acta Orthop Scand* 1988;59:122–127.

This is a review of the prevalence, type, and magnitude of scoliosis in 163 patients with myelomeningocele. Of these patients, 143 developed scoliosis, with 15% being congenital in origin. Scoliosis severity increased with higher neurologic level (particularly above L3) and increasing age. Curve direction correlated with pelvic obliquity, but not with hip dislocation.

Stark A, Saraste H: Anterior fusion insufficient for scoliosis in myelomeningocele: Eight children 2-6 years after the Zielke operation. *Acta Orthop Scand* 1993;64:22–24.

This study showed progressive scoliosis proximal to the level of fusion when anterior fusion with Zielke instrumentation was performed alone. The authors recommend a combined anterior and posterior approach in these patients.

Hip

Broughton NS, Menelaus MB, Cole WG, et al: The natural history of hip deformity in myelomeningocele. *J Bone Joint Surg* 1993;75B:760–763.

In this large series of patients in whom the natural history of hip deformity in myelomeningocele is reviewed, hip dislocation occurred in 28% of children with thoracic neurosegmental level, 38% of those with L1-2 level, 36% of L3, 22% of L4, 7% of L5, and 1% of sacral level. The average hip flexion contracture was significantly greater in those with thoracic (22°) and L1-2 (33°) levels than those with L4 (9°), L5 (5°), or sacral (4°) levels.

Dias LS: Hip deformities in myelomeningocele, in Tullos HS (ed): *Instructional Course Lectures XL.* Park Ridge, IL, American Academy of Orthopaedic Surgeons, 1991, pp 281–286.

This chapter reviews the treatment of hip deformities in myelomeningocele, including soft-tissue procedures for contractures, as well as techniques to manage hip dislocation and subluxation. The author emphasizes the importance of obtaining a concentric, stable reduction and a more balanced musculature with one operation. Stiffness after a single surgical procedure is rare, but it is common after repeated operations.

Fraser RK, Hoffman EB, Sparks LT, et al: The unstable hip and midlumbar myelomeningocele. *J Bone Joint Surg* 1992;74:143–146.

Results of this study confirm previous reports that neurologic level is the most significant determinant of walking ability. All patients with L4 neurologic levels could walk, but only one third of those with L3 lesions could do so. Hip stability did not influence walking ability.

Keggi JM, Banta JV, Walton C: The myelodysplastic hip and scoliosis. *Dev Med Child Neurol* 1992;34:240–246.

Results of this study refute the previous long-standing hypothesis that hip instability contributes to the development of scoliosis or pelvic obliquity. Neurologic instability may be a more important etiologic factor for scoliosis. In neurologically stable patients, unilateral hip instability and scoliosis are comorbid factors, but no causal relationship could be identified.

Phillips DP, Lindseth RE: Ambulation after transfer of adductors, external oblique, and tensor fascia lata in myelomeningocele. *J Pediatr Orthop* 1992;12:712–717.

The authors describe a triple muscle transfer for myelomeningocele patients with hip abductor and extensor weakness. Thirty-seven of 41 patients had an improved gait pattern after the muscle transfers. The need for assistive devices decreased in 21. These muscle transfers are indicated in midlumbar and low lumbar spina bifida patients to improve hip stability, control, balance, and gait pattern.

Sherk HH, Uppal GS, Lane G, et al: Treatment versus non-treatment of hip dislocations in ambulatory patients with myelomeningocele. *Dev Med Child Neurol* 1991;33:491–494.

This article points out the controversy as to whether or not hip dislocations in patients with spina bifida should be treated. Thirty patients with untreated hip dislocations had no pain and excellent hip motion, while six of 11 patients who had undergone open reduction of the hip developed serious perioperative complications, including wound infection, redislocation, and pressure sores from the spica casts.

Tsoi LL, Buck BD, Nason SS, et al: Dislocation of the hip in myelomeningocele. J Bone Joint Surg 1996;78A:664–673.

The McKay procedure was performed in 66 unstable hips in 34 children. The operation helped maintain stability in 37 of 51 hips in children who remained neurologically stable and in eight of 15 hips in children who had progressive loss of neurologic function. The authors recommend the procedure only for documented instability of the hip rather than for all children with myelomeningocele at the third or fourth lumbar level.

Knee and Lower Limb

Fraser RK, Menelaus MB: The management of tibial torsion in patients with spina bifida. *J Bone Joint Surg* 1993;75B:495–497.

Patients with tibial torsion were treated surgically by either closed osteoclasis or tibial osteotomy. Complications occurred in 33% and included delayed unions and infections. Surgery is indicated only in young patients with severe deformities in whom walking is impeded by severe tibial torsion.

Williams JJ, Graham GP, Dunne KB, et al: Late knee problems in myelomeningocele. *J Pediatr Orthop* 1993;13:701–703.

Of 72 adult community ambulators, 17 (24%) had significant knee symptoms. Abnormal stress on the knee commonly leads to medial and anteromedial rotary instability. Eventual degenerative arthritis is likely and may be a factor precluding independent ambulation.

Wright JG, Menelaus MB, Broughton NS, et al: Lower extremity alignment in children with spina bifida. *J Pediatr Orthop* 1992;12:232–234.

A large series of 434 patients was studied to describe the natural history of lower extremity alignment in spina bifida patients. The lower limbs of children with spina bifida had a neutral alignment at birth that gradually increased to 6° of valgus. Valgus of more than 10° was observed in 6% of the population and was unrelated to walking, neurosegmental level, or the use of knee-ankle-foot orthoses.

Wright JG, Menelaus MB, Broughton NS, et al: Natural history of knee contractures in myelomeningocele. *J Pediatr Orthop* 1991;11:725–730.

In this prospective study, knee motion was evaluated from birth to 23 years of age. Fixed flexion contractures of 10° at birth resolved by 9 months of age in all patients, but recurred in patients with upper level lesions. In thoracic/L1–L3 patients, the mean fixed flexion was 10°. Hamstring function had little to do with knee flexion deformities.

Ankle and Foot

Aronson DD, Middleton DL: Extra-articular subtalar arthrodesis with cancellous bone graft and internal fixation for children with myelomeningocele. *Dev Med Child Neurol* 1991;33:232–240.

The authors of this article showed the use of internal fixation and iliac crest bone grafting can improve the success of extra-articular subtalar arthrodesis. Unsatisfactory results were from undercorrection at time of surgery.

Brinker MR, Rosenfeld SR, Feiwell E, et al: Myelomeningocele at the sacral level: Long-term outcomes in adults. *J Bone Joint Surg* 1994; 76A:1293–1300.

Foot deformities present major problems for patients with sacral level spina bifida, and cause a decline in the ability to walk. A decrease in plantarflexion and plantar sensation leads to skin breakdown and infection on the plantar surface of the heels. Fifteen of 36 patients developed osteomyelitis, which led to toe amputations in five, Syme's amputations in two, and below-the-knee amputations in three.

Broughton NS, Graham G, Menelaus MB: The high incidence of foot deformity in patients with high-level spina bifida. *J Bone Joint Surg* 1994;76B:548–550.

The authors describe the high incidence of foot deformity in patients with spina bifida who have no voluntary activity in the motors of the feet. These deformities include equinus, calcaneus, valgus, and varus. Spasticity of muscles controlling the foot was detected in 51% of the calcaneus feet and 17% of the equinus feet.

Drennan JC: Foot deformities in myelomeningocele, in Tullos HS (ed): *Instructional Course Lectures XL*. Park Ridge, IL, American Academy of Orthopaedic Surgeons, 1991, pp 287–291.

This is a comprehensive discussion of the pathogenesis, assessment, and treatment of foot deformities in myelomeningocele.

Gallien R, Morin F, Marquis F: Subtalar arthrodesis in children. *J Pediatr Orthop* 1989;9:59–63.

Subtalar arthrodesis had a large percentage of unsatisfactory results (39%) in children with myelomeningocele. Residual valgus related to deformity in the ankle and forepart of the foot was the most frequent problem.

Georgiadis GM, Aronson DD: Posterior transfer of the anterior tibial tendon in children who have a myelomeningocele. *J Bone Joint Surg* 1990;72A:392–398.

Satisfactory clinical and radiographic results were obtained in 95% of feet treated with posterior transfer of the tendon of the anterior tibial muscle through the interosseous membrane to the calcaneus to prevent or correct a calcaneus deformity. The procedure gave the best results in patients older than 4 years of age and in patients who had fifth lumbar or first sacral motor levels.

Hullin MG, Robb JE, Loudon IR: Ankle-foot orthosis function in low-level myelomeningocele. *J Pediatr Orthop* 1992;12:518–521.

Rigid ankle-foot orthoses (AFOs) were found helpful for low-level myelomeningocele patients with excessive dorsiflexion and knee flexion. Gait analysis showed that the AFO caused a reduction in external knee movement by aligning the knee with the ground reaction force. Knee hypertension could be controlled by a rocker sole. Small changes in the foot-shank angle of the orthosis had a profound effect on knee mechanics.

Maynard MJ, Weiner LS, Burke SW: Neuropathic foot ulceration in patients with myelodysplasia. *J Pediatr Orthop* 1992;12:786–788.

This is an excellent discussion of skin problems in the feet of patients with spina bifida. Clinical indicators that had a strong statistical relationship with eventual development of neuropathic skin changes included foot rigidity, nonplantigrade position, and performance of surgical arthrodesis.

Rodrigues RC, Dias LS: Calcaneus deformity in spina bifida: Results of anterolateral release. *J Pediatr Orthop* 1992;12:461–464.

The authors described an anterior and anterolateral release for the correction of calcaneus deformity. They achieved good results in 81% of their patients with few complications. A 2-week short leg weightbearing cast proved sufficient to promote soft-tissue healing and restore the patients' ability to walk and return to their physical therapy programs.

Section 19

Inflammatory Conditions

John T. Killian, MD

Juvenile Rheumatoid Arthritis

Etiology

Cassidy JT: What's in a name? Nomenclature of juvenile arthritis: A North American view. *J Rheumatol Suppl* 1993;40:4–8.

This is a review of the differences in semantics that still exist between the British and the North American views in juvenile rheumatoid arthritis (JRA).

Miller JJ III: Immunologic abnormalities of juvenile arthritis. *Clin Orthop* 1990;259:23–30.

The various immunologic abnormalities present in juvenile arthritis are discussed. Rheumatoid factor is associated with adult-type rheumatoid arthritis, antinuclear antibodies are associated with an increased incidence of uveitis, and hypogammaglobulinemia may be associated with complicating infections. The limitations of the serologic studies in determining disease prognosis also is outlined.

Nepom B: The immunogenetics of juvenile rheumatoid arthritis. *Rheum Dis Clin North Am* 1991;17:825–842.

This excellent review article presents a state-of-the-art review of the various HLA studies and reviews the evidence for genetic susceptibility to certain forms of JRA.

Pugh MT, Southwood TR, Gaston JS: The role of infection in juvenile chronic arthritis. *Br J Rheumatol* 1993;32:838–844.

These authors discuss the roles of various potential pathogens as infectious agents triggering the onset of juvenile chronic arthritis.

Smith RL: Soluble mediators of articular cartilage degradation in juvenile rheumatoid arthritis. *Clin Orthop* 1990;259:31–37.

The joint degradation that occurs in JRA is related to the alteration of the synovial fluid and articular cartilage components. This article reviews potential mechanisms for the development of arthritis.

Still GF: On a form of chronic joint disease in children. *Clin Orthop* 1990;259:4–10.

This is one of the classic descriptions of the presentation of rheumatoid arthritis in children.

Growth Abnormalities and Nutrition

Henderson CJ, Lovell DJ: Nutritional aspects of juvenile rheumatoid arthritis. *Rheum Dis Clin North Am* 1991;17:403–413.

The authors outline the numerous nutritional abnormalities that are seen in JRA patients and note that over 50% experience some form of malnutrition.

White PH: Growth abnormalities in children with juvenile rheumatoid arthritis. *Clin Orthop* 1990;259:46–50.

The role of growth hormone in treating the growth abnormalities of children with JRA is discussed along with the deformities seen as a result of this problem.

Radiology

Hensinger RN, DeVito PD, Ragsdale CG: Changes in the cervical spine in juvenile rheumatoid arthritis. *J Bone Joint Surg* 1986;68A:189–198.

Patients with pauciarticular disease rarely have symptoms and have only minor changes on radiographs. Stiffness and radiographic findings are common in polyarticular and systemic onset disease. Few patients experience much pain due to their JRA alone.

Reed MH, Wilmot DM: The radiology of juvenile rheumatoid arthritis: A review of the English language literature. *J Rheumatol Suppl* 1991;31:2–22.

This review article outlines the numerous radiologic abnormalities, such as disturbances of growth, joint destruction, alterations in bone density, periostitis, and soft-tissue abnormalities. The role of other imaging modalities in JRA is presented.

Medical Management

Fink CW: Medical treatment of juvenile arthritis. *Clin Orthop* 1990; 259:60–69.

The medical management of JRA, including nonsteroidal anti-inflammatory drugs (NSAIDs) and slow acting antirheumatic drugs, is presented in this review article. The average time for clinical improvement is over 30 days in the 50% of JRA patients who respond to any NSAID within these months.

Furst DE: Toxicity of antirheumatic medications in children with juvenile arthritis. *J Rheumatol Suppl* 1992;33:11–15.

Numerous clinical case presentations are made in this review article on the use of NSAID and disease-modifying antirheumatic drugs (DMARD) in juvenile arthritis. The evolving field of combination medical treatments in JRA also is presented.

Giannini EH, Cassidy JT, Brewer EJ, et al: Comparative efficacy and safety of advanced drug therapy in children with juvenile rheumatoid arthritis. *Semin Arthritis Rheum* 1993;23:34–46.

With nearly two-thirds of patients failing to have resolution of their symptoms with NSAIDs, the clinician should be aware of the next treatment modalities. This randomized, controlled trial presents the results of using D-penicillamine, hydroxychloroquine, and methotrexate. Oral methotrexate is recommended for children with persistent disease.

Rose CD, Doughty RA: Pharmacological management of juvenile rheumatoid arthritis. *Drugs* 1992;43:849–863.

This is a comprehensive review of the various agents currently being prescribed to patients with JRA. Dosages, side effects, and toxicity are reviewed.

Physical Therapy

Rhodes VJ: Physical therapy management of patients with juvenile rheumatoid arthritis. *Phys Ther* 1991;71:910–919.

This review article presents basic material that can be used in developing critical-care pathways in physical therapy in the managment of patients with JRA.

Other Systems

O'Brien JM, Albert DM: Therapeutic approaches for ophthalmic problems in juvenile rheumatoid arthritis. *Rheum Dis Clin North Am* 1989;15:413–437.

This article presents excellent clinical photographs of ophthalmic disasters that may result from ocular inflammation in JRA.

Impairment Evaluation

Duffy CM, Arsenault L, Duffy KN: Level of agreement between parents and children in rating dysfunction in juvenile rheumatoid arthritis and juvenile spondyloarthritides. *J Rheumatol* 1993;20:2134–2139.

This article reviews differences in general assessment of limitations in physical function, psychosocial function, and general symptoms between children with chronic arthritis and their parents. The authors noted a high level of agreement between children with JRA and their parents over a wide range of areas tested.

Howe S, Levinson J, Shear E, et al: Development of a disability measurement tool for juvenile rheumatoid arthritis: The Juvenile Arthritis Functional Assessment Report for Children and Their Parents. *Arthritis Rheum* 1991;34:873–880.

This is one of the questionnaires that currently is being used in the assessment of function in patients with JRA.

Orthopaedic Aspects

Boublik M, Tsahakis PJ, Scott RD: Cementless total knee arthroplasty in juvenile onset rheumatoid arthritis. *Clin Orthop* 1993;286:88–93.

Twenty-three arthroplasties in 14 patients were followed-up an average of 3.9 years. Results were encouraging and comparable to full cemented knee arthroplasties at the 2- to 6-year follow-up.

Cage DJ, Granberry WM, Tullos HS: Long-term results of total arthroplasty in adolescents with debilitating polyarthropathy. *Clin Orthop* 1992; 283:156–162.

Seventeen patients undergoing 29 hip and 13 knee arthroplasties were followed until 11 years after surgery. Thirty-two percent of the hips had gross loosening, and an additional 39% had radiolucent lines more than 2 mm thick. The final modified Harris Hip Rating was 68.

Evans DM, Ansell BM, Hall MA: The wrist in juvenile arthritis. *J Hand Surg* 1991;16B:293–304.

The management and treatment, including injection, synovectomy, arthroplasty, and arthrodesis, of patients with symptomatic synovitis involving the wrist are presented.

Granberry WM: Synovectomy in juvenile rheumatoid arthritis. *Arthritis Rheum* 1977;20:561–564.

Synovectomy is rarely indicated in JRA. The ideal candidate is a child 4 to 5 years of age with only a few joints significantly involved and proliferative, recurrent, unresponsive synovitis with minimal or no destructive changes.

Harris CM, Baum J: Involvement of the hip in juvenile rheumatoid arthritis: A longitudinal study. *J Bone Joint Surg* 1988;70A:821–833.

Patients with polyarticular disease have a 30% incidence of hip involvement. Protusio acetabulae may occur and is associated with a more cephalad vector of migration than is seen in adults.

Jacobsen FS, Crawford AH, Broste S: Hip Involvement in juvenile rheumatoid arthritis. *J Pediatr Orthop* 1992;12:45–53.

Patients with onset of pauciarticular disease after 6 years of age fared worse than those with onset prior to 6 years of age. In the pauciarticular group, age of onset did not affect prognosis. In the systemic group, patients under 6 years of age fared worse.

Moreno-Alvarez MJ, Espada G, Maldonado-Cocco JA, et al: Long-term follow-up of hip and knee soft tissue release in juvenile chronic arthritis. *J Rheumatol* 1992;19:1608–1610.

Soft-tissue releases for appropriate patients can reduce hip and knee flexion contractures and improve function.

Scott RD: Total hip and knee arthroplasty in juvenile rheumatoid arthritis. *Clin Orthop* 1990;259:83–91.

The extensive preoperative planning required for patients requiring total hip or total knee arthroplasty are clearly defined in this article. The role of cementless implants is discussed as well. Component loosening is the most common complication in this study.

Swann M: The surgery of juvenile chronic arthritis. *Clin Orthop* 1990;259:70–75.

This paper outlines the role of a multidisciplinary team in improved surgical outcomes in the management of childhood arthritis.

Witt JD, McCullough CJ: Anterior soft-tissue release of the hip in juvenile chronic arthritis. *J Bone Joint Surg* 1994;76B:267–270.

Seventeen patients with significant fixed flexion deformities involving 31 hips are reviewed. With the use of a more extensive approach, the authors reported satisfactory improvement in symptoms and preservation of range-of-motion in 50% of patients at 5 to 12 years' follow-up.

Witt JD, Swann M, Ansell BM: Total hip replacement for juvenile chronic arthritis. *J Bone Joint Surg* 1991;73B:770–773.

Of 96 primary total hip replacements in 54 patients, a revision procedure was required in 24 hips (25%) at an average of 9.5 years after the primary operation; 17 other hips had radiographic signs of loosening.

Pregnancy

Ostensen M: The effect of pregnancy on ankylosing spondylitis, psoriatic arthritis, and juvenile rheumatoid arthritis. *Am J Reprod Immunol* 1992;28:235–237.

Quiescent JRA was not reactivated by pregnancy. Fetal outcome was not adversely affected by ankylosing spondylitis, psoriatic arthritis, or JRA.

Spondyloarthropathy

Cabral DA, Oen KG, Petty RE: SEA syndrome revisited: A long-term follow-up of children with a syndrome of seronegative enthesopathy and arthropathy. *J Rheumatol* 1992;19:1282–1285.

Seronegative enthesopathy and arthropathy (SEA) syndrome was reviewed in 36 children at an 11-year follow-up. This group of patients lacked rheumatoid factor and antinuclear antibodies but had enthesitis in either arthritis or arthralgia. At 11-year follow-up, 64% had definite or possible seronegative spondyloarthropathy, 10% had JRA, and 13% had noninflammatory diseases. It would appear that children with SEA syndrome are more likely to have juvenile spondyloarthropathy than JRA.

Gran JT, Husby G: Ankylosing spondylitis: Current drug treatment. *Drugs* 1992;44:585–603.

This review article describes the three groups of drugs available in the mainstream treatment of ankylosing spondylitis as represented by sulfasalazine, which is used to suppress disease activity, and steroidal anti-inflammatory drugs (SAIDs), which are used to suppress inflammation; generic analgesics; and muscle relaxants.

Gusis SE, Riopedre AM, Penise O, et al: Protusio acetabuli in seronegative spondyloarthropathy. *Semin Arthritis Rheum* 1993;23:155–160.

These authors found an overall frequency of 32% of protusio acetabuli in children with seronegative spondyloarthropathy but pointed out that its presence does not seem to modify the functional prognoses of these patients.

Levi S, Answell BM, Klenerman L: Tarsometatarsal involvement in juvenile spondyloarthropathy. *Foot Ankle* 1990;11:90–92.

Forty patients with seronegative spondyloarthropathies are reviewed for their osseous involvement in the foot. Spontaneous fusion and obliteration of the tarsometatarsal joints were common.

Juvenile Psoriatic Arthritis

Ansell B, Beeson M, Hall P, et al: HLA and juvenile psoriatic arthritis. *Br J Rheumatol* 1993;32:836–837.

In this study, 70 patients with juvenile psoriatic arthritis (PSA) underwent HLA tissue typing and reclassification of their symptoms based on chronicity and involvement. The authors conclude that there are a number of different subgroups in juvenile PSA.

Hamilton ML, Gladman DD, Shore A, et al: Juvenile psoriatic arthritis and HLA antigens. *Ann Rheum Dis* 1990;49:694–697.

Juvenile PSA is predominantely oligoarticular in presentation but in long-term follow-up, over 82% of the authors' patients demonstrated polyarthritis, and the overall incidence of chronic iridocyclitis was approximately half of that in patients with JRA. This study emphasized an increased incidence of tendonitis and distal interphalangeal joint involvement and an overall greater involvement of weightbearing major joints as opposed to the axial skeleton.

Lyme Disease

Lawrence SJ: Lyme disease: An orthopedic perspective. *Orthopedics* 1992;15:1331–1335.

This is a good overview of Lyme disease.

Rose CD, Fawcett PT, Eppes SC, et al: Pediatric Lyme arthritis: Clinical spectrum and outcome. *J Pediatr Orthop* 1994;14:238–241.

In 44 patients with Lyme arthritis, five different patterns of arthritis were identified. Preceding erythema migrans was seen in 16%, and antinuclear antibodies were positive in 30%. Treatment with amoxicillin, doxycycline, or ceftriaxone obtained complete resolution of articular disease within 2 to 12 weeks. The prognosis for children with clearly defined Lyme arthritis is excellent.

Szer IS, Taylor E, Steere AC: The long-term course of Lyme arthritis in children. *N Engl J Med* 1991;325:159–163.

The authors review the clinical course and long-term outcome of patients who were not initially treated with antibiotics.

Section 20

Disorders of the Hematopoietic System

Walter B. Greene, MD

Sickle Cell Disease

Acurio MT, Friedman RJ: Hip arthroplasty in patients with sickle-cell hemoglobinopathy. *J Bone Joint Surg* 1992;74B:367–371.

Bishop AR, Roberson JR, Eckman JR, et al: Total hip arthroplasty in patients who have sickle-cell hemoglobinopathy. *J Bone Joint Surg* 1988;70A:853–855.

Clarke HJ, Jinnah RH, Brooker AF, et al: Total replacement of the hip for avascular necrosis in sickle cell disease. *J Bone Joint Surg* 1989;71B:465–470.

These three studies document the increased incidence of short-term complications as well as the alarmingly high rate of infection and need for early revision following total hip arthroplasty in patients with sickle cell disease.

Dalton GP, Drummond DS, Davidson RS, et al: Bone infarction versus infection in sickle cell disease in children. *J Pediatr Orthop* 1996;16:540–544.

Review of emergency admissions of 113 children with sickle cell disease and musculoskeletal complaints found four osteoarticular infections in 247 admissions (incidence of 1.6%). If physical examination of a child with sickle cell disease suggests a probable focus of infection, aspiration of the bone or joint should be performed.

Diggs LW: Bone and joint lesions in sickle-cell disease. *Clin Orthop* 1967;52:119–143.

This is a classic reference.

Ebong WW: Pathological fracture complicating long bone osteomyelitis in patients with sickle cell disease. *J Pediatr Orthop* 1986;6:177–181.

The distribution of 266 consecutive skeletal complications seen in 207 Nigerian children with sickle cell disease was as follows: osteomyelitis, 48.5%; aseptic necrosis of the femoral head, 28.2%; septic arthritis, 11.7%; pathologic fracture complicating long bone osteomyelitis, 9.8%; and miscellaneous, 1.8%. Extremities affected by osteomyelitis should be adequately immobilized to prevent pathologic fracture.

Epps CH Jr, Bryant DD III, Coles MJ, et al: Osteomyelitis in patients who have sickle-cell disease: Diagnosis and management. *J Bone Joint Surg* 1991;73A:1281–1294.

This is a detailed outline of difficulties encountered when treating osteomyelitis in patients with sickle cell disease.

Givner LB, Luddy RE, Schwartz AD: Etiology of osteomyelitis in patients with major sickle hemoglobinopathies. *J Pediatr* 1981;99:411–413.

This is a review of reports of culture-proven osteomyelitis in sickle cell anemia. In 84 patients, 68 (74%) were secondary to *Salmonella*, whereas *Staphylococcus* accounted for only 10%.

Greene WB, McMillan CW: Salmonella osteomyelitis and hand-foot syndrome in a child with sickle cell anemia. *J Pediatr Orthop* 1987;7:716–718.

Differentiating osteomyelitis from dactylitis in a child with sickle cell anemia may be difficult. Appropriate screening studies are described.

Hernigou P, Galacteros F, Bachir D, et al: Deformities of the hip in adults who have sickle-cell disease and had avascular necrosis in childhood: A natural history of fifty-two patients. *J Bone Joint Surg* 1991;73A:81–92.

Patients with sickle cell disease who develop osteonecrosis before 10 years of age have a reasonable potential for healing the osteonecrosis. In this group, only five of 14 hips had a Harris hip score of less than 80 points at an average follow-up of 19 years.

Mankad VN, Williams JP, Harpen MD, et al: Magnetic resonance imaging of bone marrow in sickle cell disease: Clinical, hematologic, and pathologic correlations. *Blood* 1990;75:274–283.

Magnetic resonance imaging (MRI) study at the time of sickle cell "crisis" shows that the initiating pathology is a localized marrow of bone area infarction.

Milner PF, Kraus AP, Sebes JI, et al: Osteonecrosis of the humeral head in sickle cell disease. *Clin Orthop* 1993;289:136–143.

In a study of 2,524 patients, the prevalence of osteonecrosis of the humeral head was 5.6%. Similar to osteonecrosis of the femoral head, the prevalence depended on the patient's age and type of sickle cell disease, but disability and pain were less frequent with osteonecrosis of the humeral head, and 79% of the patients were asymptomatic at diagnosis. Concomitant shoulder and hip disease occurred in 76% of SS and 75% of SC patients.

Milner PF, Kraus AP, Sebes JI, et al: Sickle cell disease as a cause of osteonecrosis of the femoral head. *N Engl J Med* 1991;325:1476–1481.

In a radiographic study of 2,890 patients older than 5 years of age, the overall incidence of osteonecrosis was 10%, with the rate dependent on the patient's age and type of sickle cell disease. Patients with SC or Sβ^+ tended to develop osteonecrosis of the femoral head at a later age. Within the SS group, those who were also homozygous for the a-thalassemia gene were 2.4 times more likely to have osteonecrosis. Almost half of the patients were asymptomatic at the time of diagnosis, but in the 5- to 6-year follow-up period, 21% of this group became symptomatic.

Piehl FC, Davis RJ, Prugh SI: Osteomyelitis in sickle cell disease. *J Pediatr Orthop* 1993;13:225–227.

Annual incidence of osteomyelitis in sickle cell disease was 0.36%. Seven of 16 infections were polyostotic. *Salmonella* was the most common organism (13 of 16).

Platt OS, Brambilla DJ, Rosse WF, et al: Mortality in sickle cell disease: Life expectancy and risk factors for early death. *N Engl J Med* 1994;330:1639–1644.

Kaplan-Meier survival curves were calculated based on 7-year follow-up of 3,764 patients of all ages. Median age at death for SS disease was 42 years for males and 48 years for females. For SC disease, the median age at death was 60 years for males and 68 years for females.

Platt OS, Thorington BD, Brambilla DJ, et al: Pain in sickle cell disease: Rates and risk factors. *N Engl J Med* 1991;325:11–16.

Sickle cell "crisis," the most common cause of extremity pain in this disorder, was studied in 3,578 patients followed for an average of 5.1 years. Crisis requiring medical treatment averaged 0.8/year in SS disease, 1.0/year in Sß^0, and 0.4/year in SC and Sß$^+$. Considerable individual variation, however, was observed, and 39% of the patients recorded no episodes.

Sadat-Ali M: Avascular necrosis of the femoral head in sickle cell disease: An integrated classification. *Clin Orthop* 1993;290:200–205.

Based on study of 66 femoral heads with osteonecrosis (ON), four grades of ON were described. Grade I produces minimal symptoms, clinical signs, and radiologic changes; grade IV produces unbearable pain, disability, and marked radiographic changes. Early diagnosis and treatment of patients with grades I and II ON could delay further deterioration of the femoral head.

Stevens MC, Padwick M, Serjeant GR: Observations on the natural history of dactylitis in homozygous sickle cell disease. *Clin Pediatr* 1981;20: 311–317.

In a prospective study, the overall incidence of dactylitis was 45%. Of the affected patients, 41% demonstrated recurrent episodes up to 4 years of age. The problem was not observed after 6 years of age. Cessation of dactylitis coincided with disappearance of hematopoietic marrow in the hands and feet.

Vermylen C, Cornu G: Bone marrow transplantation for sickle cell disease: The European experience. *Am J Pediatr Hematol Oncol* 1994;16:18–21.

Sustained engraftment was observed in 36 of 42 patients who underwent bone marrow transplantation for sickle cell anemia. One patient died of graft versus host disease. The ideal candidate was a young but symptomatic patient with no major chronic organ damage and a healthy HLA identical relative.

Thalassemia

Colavita N, Orazi C, Danza SM, et al: Premature epiphyseal fusion and extramedullary hematopoiesis in thalassemia. *Skeletal Radiol* 1987;16: 533–538.

Premature arrest of the physis occurred in nine of 55 patients who were younger than 10 years old. The proximal humerus was involved in all patients. This complication was associated with delay in beginning transfusion therapy.

Exarchou E, Politou C, Vretou E, et al: Fractures and epiphyseal deformities in beta-thalassemia. *Clin Orthop* 1984;189:229–233.

Of 62 patients with ß-thalassemia, 20 had sustained fractures and 12 had recurrent or multiple fractures. Premature fusion of the physis was observed in 30 patients and most frequently affected the distal tibia and fibula, the proximal humerus, and the distal femur. Deformity was uncommon after fractures, but was frequently caused by asymmetric growth after premature closure of the physis. It should be noted that the transfusion program in this series would be considered substandard by present day criteria.

Giardini C, Angelucci E, Lucarelli G, et al: Bone marrow transplantation for thalassemia: Experience in Pesaro, Italy. *Am J Pediatr Hematol Oncol* 1994;16:6–10.

In a review of 484 thalassemia patients undergoing bone marrow transplantation, the best results were seen in young patients who had not developed hepatomegaly or portal fibrosis, who had received regular chelation therapy before transplantation, and who received an HLA identical donation after undergoing preoperative conditioning. The survival rate, the disease-free survival rate, and rejection rate were 98%, 94%, and 4%, respectively, in 59 patients who met these criteria.

Michelson J, Cohen A: Incidence and treatment of fractures in thalassemia. *J Orthop Trauma* 1988;2:29–32.

In thalassemia patients treated by a transfusion protocol that kept the hemoglobin over 8 g/dl, the incidence of fractures was greater than that reported in the general population; however, the age at injury was older than that reported in earlier series, and fractures occurred with an expected amount of trauma. Fracture healing was uneventful in four patients, but delayed union was observed in one patient who had vitamin C deficiency as a result of chelation therapy.

Piomelli S, Loew T: Management of thalassemia major (Cooley's anemia). *Hematol Oncol Clin North Am* 1991;5:557–569.

Aggressive transfusion programs to normalize hemoglobin levels coupled with chelation therapy to minimize hemosiderosis has markedly altered life expectancy and other problems seen in thalassemia. Growth retardation, endocrine abnormalities, and cardiac dysfunction still occur, but at a markedly reduced rate.

Diamond-Blackfan (Congenital Hypoplastic) Anemia

Alter BP: Thumbs and anemia. *Pediatrics* 1978;62:613–614.

In a review of 200 patients with congenital hypoplastic anemia, 17 had thumb abnormalities that included nine triphalangeal thumbs, three duplicated thumbs, three bifid thumbs, and two subluxed thumbs.

Fanconi Anemia

Minagi H, Steinbach HL: Roentgen appearance of anomalies associated with hypoplastic anemias of childhood: Fanconi's anemia and congenital hypoplastic anemia (erythrogenesis imperfecta). *Am J Roentgenol* 1966;97:100–109.

In a review of 68 patients with Fanconi anemia, the authors recorded nine with radial hemimelia and 25 with deficiencies limited to the hand, either hypoplasia or absence of the thumb. Other skeletal abnormalities were less frequent and included Klippel-Feil syndrome, Sprengel's deformity, hip dislocation, and syndactyly of the toes.

Chronic Granulomatous Disease

Sponseller PD, Malech HL, McCarthy EF Jr, et al: Skeletal involvement in children who have chronic granulomatous disease. *J Bone Joint Surg* 1991;73A:37–51.

Twenty episodes of osteomyelitis in 13 children with chronic granulomatous disease were reviewed. The causative organisms reflected these patients' susceptibility to catalase negative microbes and included *Aspergillus* in seven patients, *Serratia* in five, and *Nocardia* in four. The spine, ribs, hands, and feet were the most common sites. Best results were obtained with preoperative imaging to define the extent of the infection, temporary withholding of antibiotics to obtain reliable intraoperative cultures, and thorough debridement.

The International Chronic Granulomatous Disease Cooperative Study Group: A controlled trial of interferon gamma to prevent infection in chronic granulomatous disease. *N Engl J Med* 1991;324:509–516.

In a multicenter, blinded study, recombinant interferon resulted in a 72% reduction in the rate of serious infection.

Shwachman-Diamond Syndrome

Aggett PJ, Cavanagh NP, Matthew DJ, et al: Shwachman's syndrome: A review of 21 cases. *Arch Dis Child* 1980;55:331–347.

Dhar S, Anderton JM: Orthopaedic features of Shwachman syndrome: A report of two cases. *J Bone Joint Surg* 1994;76A:278–282.

Exocrine pancreatic insufficiency and cyclic neutropenia are the hallmarks of Schwachman-Diamond syndrome. A variable degree of short stature and delayed bone age are also universally present. Radiographic changes of metaphyseal chondrodysplasia are recorded in about half of the patients. Coxa vara and osteonecrosis, misdiagnosed as Legg-Calvé-Perthes disease, has also been observed.

Acquired Immunodeficiency Syndrome (AIDS)

Falloon J, Eddy J, Wiener L, et al: Human immunodeficiency virus infection in children. *J Pediatr* 1989;114:1–30.

Pizzo PA: Pediatric AIDS: Problems within problems. *J Infect Dis* 1990;161:316–325.

The salient features of these two review articles include the following. The vast majority of children with acquired immunodeficiency syndrome (AIDS) are born to human immunodeficiency virus (HIV)-infected mothers. Approximately 25% to 30% of children born to HIV-infected women will become HIV-seropositive. Twenty percent to 50% of children who are congenitally infected develop symptoms in the first year of life. Some aspects of opportunistic infections that occur in children are different from those seen in adults with AIDS.

Greene WB, DeGnore LT, White GC: Orthopaedic procedures and prognosis in hemophilic patients who are seropositive for human immunodeficiency virus. *J Bone Joint Surg* 1990;72A:2–11.

Although HIV infection has been virtually eliminated in children with hemophilia, this study provides background material that can be used when confronting the question of elective surgery in an HIV-positive patient. The rate of nosocomial infection and the results of surgical therapy were not adversely affected in 30 hemophiliacs who were, HIV-positive; however, abnormal postoperative fever without the expected elevation in white blood cell count was seen in five patients. Preoperative assessment of immune competence should be factored into the decision-making process.

Persuad D, Chandwani S, Rigaud M, et al: Delayed recognition of human immunodeficiency virus infection in pre-adolescent children. *Pediatrics* 1992;90:688–691.

The authors evaluated 32 HIV-infected children, whose initial diagnosis was made in midchildhood (median age 6.1 years, range 4 to 9 years). Twenty-four were symptomatic at evaluation, and most of these presented with recurrent bacterial infections or hematologic abnormalities. The mode of infection was perinatal in 22, by blood products in eight, and by sexual abuse in two.

Gaucher Disease

Amstutz HC, Carey EJ: Skeletal manifestations and treatment of Gaucher's disease: Review of twenty cases. *J Bone Joint Surg* 1966;48A:670–701.

Although this article was written at a time when there was limited understanding of Gaucher disease, the detailed account of the skeletal manifestations in 20 patients makes it a worthy review. Pain was most frequent in the hip, knee, shoulder, and spine. The femur was the first bone to show changes and the most frequently involved. Periosteal reaction was associated with systemic signs mimicking infection. Reconstructive surgery carried a significant risk of hemorrhage and infection.

Barton NW, Brady RO, Dambrosia JM, et al: Replacement therapy for inherited enzyme deficiency: Macrophage-targeted glucocerebrosidase for Gaucher's disease. *N Engl J Med* 1991;324:1464–1470.

Figueroa ML, Rosenbloom BE, Kay AC, et al: A less costly regimen of alglucerase to treat Gaucher's disease. *N Engl J Med* 1992;327:1632–1636.

Mankin HJ: Editorial: Gaucher's disease: A novel treatment and an important breakthrough. *J Bone Joint Surg* 1993;75B:2–3.

These three articles outline the exciting development of aglucerase as a substitute for the deficient enzyme glucocerebrosidase. Early investigators have observed consistent decrease in splenic and hepatic volume and increased hemoglobin concentration and platelet counts. Whether changes in the skeleton will be reversed is unclear. Trials using reduced dosages have been stimulated by the astronomic cost of the medicine.

Bell RS, Mankin HJ, Doppelt SH: Osteomyelitis in Gaucher disease. *J Bone Joint Surg* 1986;68A:1380–1388.

Delay in diagnosis leading to an unsatisfactory outcome was observed in three of five patients. Atypical organisms were commonly encountered. It should be noted that although osteomyelitis is surprisingly uncommon in Gaucher disease, it may be difficult to diagnose because the presenting signs and symptoms may be similar to those in a Gaucher crisis.

Horev G, Kornreich L, Hadar H, et al: Hemorrhage associated with "bone crisis" in Gaucher's disease identified by magnetic resonance imaging. *Skeletal Radiol* 1991;20:479–482.

Katz K, Mechlis-Frish S, Cohen IJ, et al: Bone scans in the diagnosis of bone crisis in patients who have Gaucher disease. *J Bone Joint Surg* 1991;73A:513–517.

These two articles outline the clinical course and explain the pathogenesis of a Gaucher crisis, also known as pseudosteomyelitis. Hemorrhage in the intramedullary canal initates the crisis. The resultant pain is acute in onsct and relatively well-localized. Fever often is present, and the white blood cell count and the erythrocyte sedimentation rate are elevated.

Katz K, Horev G, Grunebaum M, et al: The natural history of the femoral head in children and adolescents who have Gaucher disease. *J Bone Joint Surg* 1996;78A:14–19.

Six patients (ten hips) with osteonecrosis of the femoral head were treated with bed rest and nonweightbearing with crutches only in the symptomatic stage of the bone crisis. At an average follow-up of 13 years, the Mose rating was good in one, fair in two, and poor in seven. Despite poor radiographic ratings, all six patients were asymptomatic and did not require assistance with daily activities.

Katz K, Cohen IJ, Ziv N, et al: Fractures in children who have Gaucher disease. *J Bone Joint Surg* 1987;69A:1361–1370.

This study analyzed 23 fractures occurring in nine children at an average age of 12 years (range 6 to 18 years). Two thirds of the fractures occurred at a site that had been affected by a crisis 2 to 12 months previously. Common locations included the distal femur, proximal tibia, and base of the femoral neck. Delayed union and malunion were common.

Katz K, Sabato S, Horev G, et al: Spinal involvement in children and adolescents with Gaucher disease. *Spine* 1993;18:332–335.

Nineteen patients with Gaucher disease presented with back pain at an average age of 13 years (range 6 to 18 years). Nine patients had nonspecific mild pain in the thoracic spine that lasted for 2 to 5 days. Three patients had severe pain typical of Gaucher crisis. Pathologic fractures typically had the insidious onset of pain 1 to 2 months prior to diagnosis. Central vertebral collapse and anterior wedge compression were the two fracture patterns. Compression fractures caused development of progressive kyphosis and spinal cord compression.

Zimran A, Kay A, Gelbart T, et al: Gaucher disease: Clinical, laboratory, radiologic, and genetic features of 53 patients. *Medicine* 1992;71:337–353.

This study provides an excellent analysis of the presenting symptoms, chronic problems, laboratory and radiologic abnormalities, disease progression, and site of genetic mutation in 53 patients with Type I Gaucher disease. The most common symptom at presentation is an abnormality of coagulation. Bone pain or fracture heralding the disease is uncommon, but skeletal involvement is a major cause of the long-term morbidity and disability. Clinical heterogeneity is correlated with specific genotypes.

Langerhans Cell Histiocytosis (Eosinophilic Granuloma of Bone)

In the past, orthopaedic textbooks typically included this condition in the chapter on tumors. Langerhans cell histiocytosis, however, is not a neoplasm, at least not in the classic sense. The characteristic cell is a component of the mononuclear-phagocytic system. The disease probably results from a reactive immunologic process causing bone and/or soft tissue destruction.

Bollini G, Jouve JL, Gentet JC, et al: Bone lesions in histiocytosis x. *J Pediatr Orthop* 1991;11:469–477.

Sixty-two patients with Langerhans cell histiocytosis were grouped into solitary bony involvement (39), multiple osseous lesions (9), and visceral tissue involvement (14). Patients who only had bony lesions demonstrated progressive improvement that was independent of treatment. Surgical treatment of bony lesions is advocated only if there is a pathologic fracture or risk of instability.

Dimentberg RA, Brown KL: Diagnostic evaluation of patients with histiocytosis X. *J Pediatr Orthop* 1990;10:733–741.

This study reviews 52 patients grouped into three categories: bone involvement with no soft-tissue involvement (32); bone and soft-tissue involvement (14), and soft-tissue involvement only (6). Two patients died of a secondary malignancy, possibly related to low-level radiotherapy. Diligent follow-up and less aggressive treatment of patients without organ dysfunction is advocated. The authors outline an excellent approach to the initial evaluation and follow-up examination.

Favara BE: Langerhans' cell histiocytosis pathobiology and pathogenesis. *Semin Oncol* 1991;18:3–7.

This is a good review of current thinking concerning the ontogeny and pathogenesis of Langerhans cell histiocytosis.

Raney RB Jr, D'Angio GJ: Langerhans' cell histiocytosis (histiocytosis X): Experience at the Children's Hospital of Philadelphia, 1970-1984. *Med Pediatr Oncol* 1989;17:20–28.

In 64 patients with Langerhans cell histiocytosis, 33 had localized lesions, 22 had multifocal disease without organ dysfunction, and nine had multifocal disease with organ dysfunction. Recurrence was infrequent (7%) in those with localized disease and all survived. In multifocal disease without organ dysfunction, recurrence was frequent (74%), but 21 of the 22 survived. Of nine patients with organ dysfunction, only three survived. Chemotherapy should be reserved for patients with organ dysfunction or persistent symptoms.

Sessa S, Sommelet D, Lascombes P, et al: Treatment of Langerhans-cell histiocytosis in children: Experience at the Children's Hospital of Nancy. *J Bone Joint Surg* 1994;76A;10:1513–1525.

Forty children with Langerhans cell histiocytosis were evaluated. Localized disease involving one or more bones (30) had better prognosis than multifocal disease that involved both bone and soft tissue (10). The low recurrence rate noted in this study led the authors to recommend avoidance of intensive therapeutic measures, if possible, and long-term follow-up to identify development of additional lesions.

Thrombocytopenia With Absent Radius (TAR) Syndrome

Hall JG: Thrombocytopenia and absent radius (TAR) syndrome. *J Med Genet* 1987;24:79–83.

This study reviewed the clinical spectrum in 100 patients. By definition, the radius was absent (bilateral in 99%). The thumb was always present, but was hypoplastic in 51%. Lower extremity abnormalities were most common about the knee and included genu varum (32%), patellar abnormalities (14%), and stiff knee (9%). Onset of thrombocytopenia was usually by 6 weeks of age, but may be delayed. Thrombocytopenia typically resolved by early childhood without need for steroids or splenectomy.

Schoenecker PL, Cohn AK, Sedgwick WG, et al: Dysplasia of the knee associated with the syndrome of thrombocytopenia and absent radius. *J Bone Joint Surg* 1984;66A:421–427.

The authors provide a detailed description of lower extremity abnormalities in 21 patients with TAR syndrome. Genu varum associated with flexion contracture and internal tibial torsion was the most common abnormality. Recurrent varus was frequently observed after realignment procedures.

Hemophilia

Arnold WD, Hilgartner MW: Hemophilic arthropathy: Current concepts of pathogenesis and management. *J Bone Joint Surg* 1977;59A:287–305.

This is a landmark article.

Aronstam A, Browne RS, Wassef M, et al: Clinical features of early haemarthroses in severely affected adolescent haemophiliacs. *Clin Lab Haematol* 1984;6:9–15.

The authors analyzed 690 bleeds into the knees, ankles, and elbows of severe hemophiliacs who were promptly transfused. Stiffness, pain, and tenderness were common complaints. There was a direct relationship between the restriction of joint motion and time taken for complete restoration of function, the mean of which was 3.6 days for elbows, 2.5 for knees, and 1.1 for ankles.

DeGnore LT, Wilson FC: Surgical management of hemophilic arthropathy, in Barr JS Jr (ed): *Instructional Course Lectures XXXVIII.* Park Ridge, IL, American Academy of Orthopaedic Surgeons, 1989, pp 383–388.

This article reviews the results and hematologic management of patients with hemophilia who are undergoing surgery.

Erken EH: Radiocolloids in the management of hemophilic arthropathy in children and adolescents. *Clin Orthop* 1991;264:129–135.

Siegel HJ, Luck JV, Siegel ME, et al: Hemarthosis and synovitis associated with hemophilia: Clinical use of P-32 chromic phosphate synoviorthesis for treatment. *Radiology* 1994;190:257–261.

Siegel HJ, Luck JV, Siegel ME, et al: P-32 chromic phosphate colloid radiosynovectomy for hemarthrosis and synovitis in hemophilia. Abstract for XXI International Congress of the World Federation of Hemophilia, 1994.

These three articles analyze the results of radioactive synovectomy in patients with hemophilia. In their study, Erken and associates used yttrium Y 90, an agent that has a relatively short half-life (2.7 days), whereas chromic phosphate P 32, an agent with a half-life of 14 days was used in the latter two studies. All studies showed a reduced rate of hemarthoses; however, the results were not quite as good as that following a surgical synovectomy. On the other hand, radioactive synovectomy can be repeated easily, requires significantly less expensive transfusion therapy, and has low morbidity.

Greene WB: Synovectomy of the ankle for hemophilic arthropathy. *J Bone Joint Surg* 1994;76A:812–819.

Open synovectomy of the ankle resulted in marked decrease in the rate of hemarthroses. In contrast to the knee, the postoperative rehabilitation in these patients was relatively easy, even when using conventional modalities.

Green WB, DeGnore LT, White GC: Orthopaedic procedures and prognosis in hemophilic patients who are seropositive for human immunodeficiency virus. *J Bone Joint Surg* 1990;72A:2–11.

Although functional results were similar to those in hemophilic patients treated before 1982, subsequent progression or infection with

HIV occurred in most patients. Acquired immunodeficiency syndrome (AIDS) was diagnosed in six. A more rapid progression to AIDS was seen in patients who had a lower CD4 lymphocyte count preoperatively. Pre-operative evaluation of the CD4 lymphocyte count and the response to intradermal skin-test antigens provides additional information concerning immunologic competence.

Greene WB, McMillan CW: Nonsurgical management of hemophilic arthropathy, in Barr JS Jr (ed): *Instructional Course Lectures XXXVIII*. Park Ridge, IL, American Academy of Orthopaedic Surgeons, 1989, pp 367–381.

This article reviews mechanisms of normal clotting and disorders of coagulation, as well as the pathogenesis, radiographic evaluation, and nonsurgical management of joint and muscle bleeds in patients with hemophilia.

Greene WB, Yankaskas BC, Guilford WB: Roentgenographic classifications of hemophilic arthropathy: Comparison of three systems and correlation with clinical parameters. *J Bone Joint Surg* 1989;71A:237–244.

In 105 knees, three radiographic classifications of hemophilic arthropathy were compared. Statistical analysis showed that a four-sign, seven-point classification was as good as more complex grading systems. Radiographic signs that correlated with clinical signs of arthropathy included subchondral irregularity, joint narrowing, marginal erosions, and joint surface incongruity.

Hoyer LW: Hemophilia A. *N Engl J Med* 1994;330:38–47.

This article is a comprehensive review of the molecular structure of factor VIII, the pathophysiology of inhibitors, and medical management of bleeding episodes.

Montane I, McCollough NC III, Lian EC-Y: Synovectomy of the knee for hemophilic arthropathy. *J Bone Joint Surg* 1986;68A:210–216.

Synovectomy of the knee was performed in 13 patients. The incidence of hemarthrosis was markedly decreased, and progression of the arthropathy was slowed; however, ten patients lost an average of 41° of motion.

Nicol RO, Menelaus MB: Synovectomy of the knee in hemophilia. *J Pediatr Orthop* 1986;6:330–333.

Ten children underwent synovectomy of the knee with marked reduction in the frequency and severity of bleeding. Continuous passive motion was important in postoperative management.

Rivard GE, Girard M, Bélanger R, et al: Synoviorthesis with colloidal ^{32}P chromic phosphate for the treatment of hemophilic arthropathy. *J Bone Joint Surg* 1994;76A:482–488.

Ninety-two synoviortheses (destruction of synovial tissue by intraarticular injection of a radioactive agent) were performed in 48 patients. Frequency and severity of bleeding episodes were decreased; range of motion improved or remained stable in 50% and continued to decrease in 50%. Radiographic scores worsened progressively, but patients' level of satisfaction with the result was high.

Triantafyllou SJ, Hanks GA, Handal JA, et al: Open and arthroscopic synovectomy in hemophilic arthropathy of the knee. *Clin Orthop* 1992; 283:196–204.

Synovectomy of the knee was performed using open technique in eight patients and arthroscopic technique in five. Patients undergoing arthroscopic synovectomy also received continuous passive motion as part of their postoperative management. Both techniques reduced the rate of hemarthroses, but the arthroscopic group had better postoperative motion.

Leukemia

Appell RG, Bühler T, Willich E, et al: Absence of prognostic significance of skeletal involvement in acute lymphocytic leukemia and non-Hodgkin lymphoma in children. *Pediatr Radiol* 1985;15:245–248.

In 72 children with acute lymphocytic leukemia and malignant non-Hodgkin's lymphoma, no correlation in survival rate was noted in children without skeletal involvement at diagnosis, those with involvement of less than three bones, and those with involvement of three or more bones.

Heinrich SD, Gallagher D, Warrior R, et al: The prognostic significance of the skeletal manifestations of acute lymphoblastic leukemia of childhood. *J Pediatr Orthop* 1994;14:105–111.

In 83 children with leukemia, 56% had pain in their extremities at diagnosis. Radiographic skeletal abnormalities at diagnosis included metaphyseal bands in 30%, periosteal reaction in 21%, osteoporosis in 20%, diffuse permeative bone destruction in 18%, sclerotic changes in 6%, and lytic defects in 4%. Patients without radiographic skeletal abnormalities and those with five or more lesions had a significantly lower 5-year survival rate compared to children with one to four radiographic changes at diagnosis.

Ostrov BE, Goldsmith DP, Athreya BH: Differentiation of systemic juvenile rheumatoid arthritis from acute leukemia near the onset of disease. *J Pediatr* 1993;122:595–598.

Ten children, who initially were referred for a rheumatologic evaluation but who later were diagnosed as having leukemia, were compared to a group of children with systemic juvenile rheumatoid arthritis (JRA). Lymphadenopathy, splenomegaly, and hepatomegaly were equivalent in both groups. Musculoskeletal night pain was observed in children with leukemia, but morning stiffness was the pattern in those with JRA. Nonarticular bone pain was found in all of the patients with leukemia, but was not seen in those with JRA. Patients with leukemia frequently had other abnormalities on radiographs besides the joint effusions noted in the patients with arthritis.

Rogalsky RJ, Black GB, Reed MH: Orthopaedic manifestations of leukemia in children. *J Bone Joint Surg* 1986;68A:494–501.

The presenting complaints of 107 patients involved the musculoskeletal system in 20.6% and included pain in the extremities, back pain, osteomyelitis, septic arthritis, or fracture. Radiographic abnormalities at presentation were even more frequent and included osteopenia in 24.3%, lytic lesions in 18.7%, metaphyseal bands in 7.5%, sclerotic lesions in 3.7%, and periosteal reaction alone in 1.9%.

Section 21

Tumors

Robert M. Bernstein, MD
William L. Oppenheim, MD

Evaluation and Diagnosis

General

Black B, Dooley J, Pyper A, et al: Multiple hereditary exostoses: An epidemiologic study of an isolated community in Manitoba. *Clin Orthop* 1993;287:212–217.

Screening of 266 persons for multiple hereditary exostosis (MHE) revealed the condition in 21 children (19.4%) and 14 adults (8.5%). Forty-one percent of children had lesions detectable before 10 years of age, 74% of which were characteristically sessile. Although lesions of the knee were most common, sites previously thought to be uncommon, such as the metatarsals, hands, and spine, were involved in 40%. Severity and multiplicity of lesions in successive generations point to an oncogenic gene origin.

Brown KL: Limb reconstruction with vascularized fibular grafts after bone tumor resection. *Clin Orthop* 1991;262:64–73.

After canine study comparing conventional grafts to vascularized fibular grafts, the author recommends vascularized fibular grafts as ideal for diaphyseal defects of more than 10 cm, especially in very young children; in instances of poor vascularization; or when bone healing is delayed by chemotherapeutic agents. To maximize hypertrophy, external fixation is used to immobilize the graft.

Cara JA, Canadell J: Limb salvage for malignant bone tumors in young children. *J Pediatr Orthop* 1994;14:112–118.

Limb-salvage surgery was performed in 47 children; allografts were used in 26, autografts in seven, and nonbiologic material in seven. The overall survival rate was 76.6%. The most serious complications were infection (four) and osteosynthesis anchorage detachment (eight).

Gebhardt MC, Ready JE, Mankin JH: Tumors about the knee in children. *Clin Orthop* 1990;255:86–110.

In addition to discussing the differential diagnosis, this article includes an excellent discussion of patient evaluation including history, physical examination, radiographic evaluation, and subsequent staging. The most frequent benign lesions were osteochondroma, nonossifying fibroma, and chondroblastoma. Osteosarcoma was the most common malignancy. Although most pediatric patients with knee pain have an infectious, traumatic, or developmental cause, a high index of suspicion must be maintained in any child with complaints about the knee.

Glasser DB, Duane K, Lane JM, et al: The effect of chemotherapy on growth in the skeletally immature individual. *Clin Orthop* 1991;262:93–100.

The authors studied the immediate and long-term effects of chemotherapy on height in 122 patients treated for osteosarcoma and Ewing's sarcoma. During the year of treatment, only 15% of patients grew at the expected rate. Nutritional status scores were also significantly affected. In those patients followed to skeletal maturity, 16% lost more than one standard deviation in height, and 80% changed less than one standard deviation. However, the mean heights were well within the normal range for American adults.

Goldwein JW: Effects of radiation therapy on skeletal growth in childhood. *Clin Orthop* 1991;262:101–107.

The physical effects of radiation on skeletal growth include physeal growth arrest, degenerative joint changes, scoliosis, and abnormal dentition. Psychological effects are also discussed.

Gonzalez-Herranz P, Burgos-Flores J, Ocete-Guzman JG, et al: The management of limb-length discrepancies in children after treatment of osteosarcoma and Ewing's sarcoma. *J Pediatr Orthop* 1995;15:561–565.

Of 15 children with limb-length discrepancies after treatment of sarcoma, ten required limb lengthening (average 8.1 cm), two had shortening of the contralateral femur, and two had femoral-tibial epiphysiodeses.

Biopsy

Simon MA, Biermann JS: Biopsy of bone and soft-tissue lesions. *J Bone Joint Surg* 1993;75A:616–621.

This excellent review of biopsy techniques emphasizes the importance of a carefully planned biopsy, taking into consideration location and diagnostic yield. Open and closed techniques are discussed as well as tissue examination.

Simon MA, Finn HA: Diagnostic strategy for bone and soft-tissue tumors. *J Bone Joint Surg* 1993;75:622–631.

This is a thorough review of current diagnostic strategy, including history, physical examination, radiographs, and staging tests. Ultrasound, scintigraphy, computerized tomography (CT), magnetic resonance imaging (MRI), and angiography are highlighted. Simple algorithms for the workup of bone and soft-tissue tumors are provided.

Imaging

Bohndorf K, Reiser M, Lochner B, et al: Magnetic resonance imaging of primary tumours and tumour-like lesions of bone. *Skeletal Radiol* 1986;15:511–517.

The authors reviewed the radiographic, CT, and MRI findings in 81 patients with primary bone tumors. While plain radiographs and CT were better at determining cortical destruction, MRI was superior in demonstrating extraosseous extension. Plain radiographs were more useful in formulating a differential diagnosis.

Ghelman B: Radiology of bone tumors. *Orthop Clin North Am* 1989;20:287–312.

The radiographic, CT, and MRI appearances of a variety of bone tumors are described. Excellent illustrations of various imaging techniques are provided with accompanying explanations.

Gillespy T III, Manfrini M, Ruggieri P, et al: Staging of intraosseous extent of osteosarcoma: Correlation of preoperative CT and MR imaging and pathologic macroslides. *Radiology* 1988;167:765–767.

MR imaging was significantly more accurate than CT in evaluating the extent of intraosseous tumor.

Staging

Springfield DS: Staging systems for musculoskeletal neoplasia, in Schafer M (ed): *Instructional Course Lectures 43*. Rosemont, IL, American Academy of Orthopaedic Surgeons, 1994, pp 537–542.

The author provides a thorough review of the various staging systems currently in use for both soft-tissue and skeletal neoplasia, including the American Joint Committee for Cancer Staging, the Musculoskeletal Tumor Society System, and the Hajdu System. The advantages and limitations of each are discussed.

Allografts

Alman BA, DeBari A, Krajbich JI: Massive allografts in the treatment of osteosarcoma and Ewing sarcoma in children and adolescents. *J Bone Joint Surg* 1995;77A:54–64.

Allograft reconstructions were performed in 26 patients, with good or excellent results in 18 (69%), fair results in four, and failure in four. Twenty patients (77%) had at least one complication other than limb-length discrepancy and 14 (54%) had at least one fracture of the allograft. Although the rate of complications is higher than in adults, allograft reconstruction is a useful option for the management of skeletally immature individuals.

Berrey BH Jr, Lord CF, Gebhardt MC, et al: Fractures of allografts: Frequency, treatment and end-results. *J Bone Joint Surg* 1990;72A: 825–833.

The authors note a 16% rate of fracture of allografts with a peak incidence between 2 and 3 years postoperatively; 75% of patients ultimately did well despite the interim fractures.

Benign Tumors

Aneurysmal Bone Cyst

Freiberg AA, Loder RT, Heidelberger KP, et al: Aneurysmal bone cysts in young chldren. *J Pediatr Orthop* 1994;14:86–91.

After curettage and bone grafting of seven aneurysmal bone cysts in children from 2.9 to 10.6 years of age, 71% recurred; 100% of "aggressive" or "active" cysts recurred. The time to recurrence was rapid, averaging 8 months. The authors recommend counseling of the parents with respect to the high rate of recurrence and the possible need for multiple procedures.

Marcove RC, Sheth DS, Takemoto S, et al: The treatment of aneurysmal bone cyst. *Clin Orthop* 1995;311:157–163.

Of 55 patients with either primary or secondary aneurysmal bone cysts treated by cryotherapy 82% were cured after one treatment and 96% after a second cryosurgery.

Chondroblastoma

Huvos AG, Marcove RC: Chondroblastoma of bone: A critical review. *Clin Orthop* 1973;95:300–312.

This is an excellent review of the literature, including treatment, recurrence rates, radiographic findings, and symptoms.

Springfield DS, Capanna R, Gherlinzoni F, et al: Chondroblastoma: A review of seventy cases. *J Bone Joint Surg* 1985;67A:748–755.

The authors present 70 patients with chondroblastoma, 63 of whom were younger than 30 years of age. The most common site of involvement was the proximal humerus, followed by proximal femur, distal femur, and proximal tibia. Most patients sought medical attention because of aching pain. There were seven recurrences. Treatment recommendations include curettage with or without phenol washing and/or bone grafting. Recurrences can be treated with repeat curettage and marginal excision of extraosseous component.

Chondromyxoid Fibroma

Gherlinzoni F, Rock M, Picci P: Chondroidmyxoid fibroma: The experience at the Istituto Ortopedico Rizzoli. *J Bone Joint Surg* 1983;65A: 198–204.

The authors review their experience with 27 of these rare tumors. With curettage alone, they noted a recurrence rate of 80%, dropping to just 7% with the addition of corticocancellous bone grafting. Histologically, these tumors may be difficult to distinguish from chondrosarcoma.

Enchondroma

Schwartz HS, Zimmerman NB, Simon MA, et al: The malignant potential of enchondromatosis. *J Bone Joint Surg* 1987;69A:269–274.

This is a large retrospective study with long-term follow-up (mean 27.7 years) of patients with Ollier's disease and Maffucci syndrome to determine the rate of malignant degeneration. In patients with Ollier's disease, the incidence of chondrosarcoma was 11% with a projected rate of 25% by 40 years of age. One astrocytoma and one abdominal tumor also were noted. In the seven patients with Maffucci syndrome, four developed six chondrosarcomas, one osteosarcoma, two abdominal malignancies, and one astrocytoma. Of the three patients without malignancy, all were below the age of 28. The authors recommend routine periodic surveillance of the brain and abdomen for occult malignancies.

Eosinophilic Granuloma

Capanna R, Springfield DS, Ruggieri P, et al: Direct cortisone injection in eosinophilic granuloma of bone: A preliminary report on 11 patients. *J Pediatr Orthop* 1985;5:339–342.

Eleven patients with biopsy proven eosinophilic granuloma were treated by one or more injections with methylprednisolone. All lesions completely healed between 12 and 34 months. The authors recommend this method for treatment of solitary lesions.

Greis PE, Hankin FM: Eosinophilic granuloma: The management of solitary lesions of bone. *Clin Orthop* 1990;257:204–211.

The results of 20 patients with solitary eosinophilic granuloma treated over a 30-year period at one institution were reviewed. The treatment was varied and included radiation, curettage with and without bone grafting, and resection. All lesions healed. The authors conclude that solitary eosinophilic granuloma is a benign lesion that can effectively be treated by several methods.

Fibrous Cortical Defect/Nonossifying Fibroma

Arata MA, Peterson HA, Dahlin DC: Pathological fractures through nonossifying fibromas: Review of the Mayo Clinic experience. *J Bone Joint Surg* 1981;63A:980–988.

In this large series (23 patients) of pathologic fractures through histologically confirmed nonossifying fibroma, all but one occured in the lower extremity, with the distal tibia most commonly involved. Radiographically, the lesion involved more than 50% of the bone in both planes in every patient. Treatment involved cast immobilization followed by biopsy at a later date, curettage with or without bone grafting, or segmental resection of fibular lesions.

Giant Cell Tumor

Kransdorf MJ, Sweet DE, Buetow PC, et al: Giant-cell tumor in skeletally immature patients. *Radiology* 1992;184:233–237.

In this large series of giant cell tumors in skeletally immature patients, the metaphyseal region was involved in 96%, and epiphyseal extension was noted in only three patients.

Picci P, Manfrini M, Zucchi V, et al: Giant-cell tumor of bone in skeletally immature patients. *J Bone Joint Surg* 1983;65A:486–490.

Six skeletally immature patients with histologically confirmed giant cell tumor are presented, representing 1.8% of all giant cell tumors at that institution. Metaphyseal involvement was predominant in all six patients and epiphyseal involvement was confirmed in five of six. Treatment varied widely.

Osteoblastoma

Beauchamp CP, Duncan CP, Dzus AK, et al: Osteoblastoma: Experience with 23 patients. *Can J Surg* 1992;35:199–202.

Demographics, symptoms, radiographic appearence, and treatment were reviewed for 23 patients. Age at diagnosis ranged from 15 months to 52 years, with most patients presenting at age 30 years or younger. Twenty-one patients were successfully treated by intralesional curettage with or without bone grafting. Of note were a recurrence in one patient 17 years after initial treatment and a 30-year persistence in one patient.

Gitelis S, Schajowicz F: Osteoid osteoma and osteoblastoma. *Orthop Clin North Am* 1989;20:313–325.

This is a concise review of these two lesions including their diagnosis and treatment. Osteoblastoma can be unpredictable and thus should be treated with en bloc resection.

Kroon HM, Schurmans J: Osteoblastoma: Clinical and radiologic findings in 98 new cases. *Radiology* 1990;175:783–790.

The radiographic, CT, and MR features of osteoblastoma are described.

Myles ST, MacRae ME: Benign osteoblastoma of the spine in childhood. *J Neurosurg* 1988;68:884–888.

The authors present ten patients with osteoblastoma of the spine. Nine occured in the posterior elements. Complete relief of pain was achieved in all but two patients with complete excision or incomplete excision with bone grafting. There were no recurrences.

Tonai M, Campbell CJ, Ahn GH, et al: Osteoblastoma: Classification and report of 16 patients. *Clin Orthop* 1982;167:222–235.

The authors classified these lesions as vertebral, central "benign," "aggressive," and periosteal based on radiographic and histologic evidence. Curettage and marginal excision were curative for most lesions. Aggressive lesions required wide local resection.

Osteochondroma

Masada K, Tsuyuguchi Y, Kawai H, et al: Operations for forearm deformity caused by multiple osteochondromas. *J Bone Joint Surg* 1989;71B:24–29.

The authors provide a classification of forearm deformities in multiple osteochondromas as a guide for specific surgical recommendations. Depending on the classification, they used a variety of procedures, including excision of the lesion, radial osteotomy, ulnar lengthening, and radial head excision. They noted better functional results in younger patients.

Peterson HA: Deformities and problems of the forearm in children with multiple hereditary osteochondromata. *J Pediatr Orthop* 1994;14:92–100.

This is a comprehensive review of the various surgical techniques available to treat forearm deformities. The author notes that surgical intervention improves cosmetic appearance more than function. Aggressive treatment to prevent further progression of deformity, functional impairment, and radial head dislocation is strongly advocated.

Schmale GA, Conrad EU III, Raskind WH: The natural history of hereditary multiple exostoses. *J Bone Joint Surg* 1994;76A:986–992.

This is the largest series of patients with hereditary multiple exostoses to date. The material is the result of a database in the state of Washington, including 113 patients from 46 kindreds. It reviews the median age at diagnosis (3 years), overall prevalence (1:50,000), penetrance (96%), functional status, and anatomic distribution. One patient developed a chondrosarcoma (0.9%), but 76 patients were below the age of 40 at latest follow-up.

Taniguchi K: A practical classification system for multiple cartilaginous exostosis in children. *J Pediatr Orthop* 1995;15:585–591.

Forty-one patients were classified into three groups: group I, no involvement of the distal forearm, group II, involvement of the distal forearm without shortening of the radius or ulna, and group III, involvement of the distal forearm with shortening of the radius or ulna. The classification proved useful in estimating severity and identifying patients at high risk for malignant transformation.

Osteoid Osteoma

Kneisl JS, Simon MA: Medical management compared with operative treatment for osteoid-osteoma. *J Bone Joint Surg* 1992;74A:179–185.

This is the first reported series on the efficacy of medical management using nonsteroidal anti-inflammatory medications (NSAIDs). Twelve patients were treated with NSAIDs. Three ultimately required surgical resection of the nidus. Six were cured with no relapse after stopping the medication and three were pain free but still under medical treatment. The authors conclude that medical treatment is often as effective as surgical treatment.

Thompson GS, Wong KM, Konsens RM, ct al: Magnetic resonance imaging of an osteoid osteoma of the proximal femur: A potentially confusing appearance. *J Pediatr Orthop* 1990;10:800–804.

This case report emphasizes that care must be taken in interpretation of MRI in disorders in which secondary bone marrow changes occur to avoid erroneous diagnoses and possibly incorrect operative procedures.

Voto SJ, Cook AJ, Weiner DS, et al: Treatment of osteoid osteoma by computed tomography guided excision in the pediatric patient. *J Pediatr Orthop* 1990;10:510–513.

The nidus of an osteoid osteoma was disrupted and removed by the use of CORB biopsy system guided by computed tomography scan in nine patients. At an average 42.5-month follow-up, seven had complete resolution of pain and two required en bloc excisions with bone grafting.

Ward WG, Eckardt JJ, Shayestehfar S, et al: Osteoid osteoma diagnosis and management with low morbidity. *Clin Orthop* 1993;291:229–235.

A "burr-down" technique is described in which successive burring through reactive bone is used to identify the nidus, which is removed with curettes and burrs. The technique requires precise preoperative anatomic localization by thin-section computed tomography scans. This technique was used successfully in 15 patients, with no local recurrences.

Unicameral Bone Cyst

Moreau G, Letts M: Unicameral bone cyst of the calcaneus in children. *J Pediatr Orthop* 1994;14:101–104.

Six children with pathologically confirmed unicameral bone cysts of the calcaneus were treated successfully with bone grafting (either autogenous or allograft). Steroid injection failed in one patient, but whether calcaneal cysts are unresponsive to steroid therapy remains inconclusive.

Oppenheim WL, Galleno H: Operative treatment versus steroid injection in the management of unicameral bone cysts. *J Pediatr Orthop* 1984;4:1–7.

The authors compare patients treated by steroid injection to those treated surgically (primarily curettage and bone grafting). Recurrence or persistance were common in both groups although major complications were higher in the surgical group. The authors recommend steroid injection as the treatment of choice because of its simplicity and low morbidity.

Scaglietti O, Marchetti PG, Bartolozzi P: Final results obtained in the treatment of bone cysts and methylprednisolone acetate (Depo-Medrol) and a discussion of results achieved in other bone lesions. *Clin Orthop* 1982;165:33–42.

The authors present the results of 163 patients with unicameral cysts treated by injection with steroids with excellent results. Similar results occured in patients treated for eosinophilic granuloma. Poor results occured in patients with aneurysmal bone cysts.

Smith RW, Smith CF: Solitary unicameral bone cyst of the calcaneus: A review of twenty cases. *J Bone Joint Surg* 1974;56A:49–56.

In this large series of unicameral cysts of the calcaneus, nonoperative treatment is recommended initially. If this fails, curettage and bone grafting is the treatment of choice.

Malignant Tumors

Adamantinoma

Keeney GL, Unni KK, Beabout JW, et al: Adamantinoma of long bones: A clinicopathologic study of 85 cases. *Cancer* 1989;64:730–737.

The authors describe the clinical and histologic findings in 85 patients. Age at diagnosis was most commonly in the second decade. Factors associated with recurrent or metastatic disease were a lack of squamous differentiation on histologic examination, male sex, pain, and short duration of symptoms. Wide en bloc resection was their treatment of choice.

Ewing's Sarcoma

Bacci G, Toni A, Avella M, et al: Long-term results in 144 localized Ewing's sarcoma patients treated with combined therapy. *Cancer* 1989;63:1477–1486.

In 144 consecutive patients with a minimum of 5 years' follow-up, better results were noted in patients treated by a combined approach of surgery, chemotherapy, and radiation than in those patients treated only by chemotherapy and radiation.

Maygarden SJ, Askin FB, Siegal GP, et al: Ewing's sarcoma of bone in infants and toddlers: A clinicopathologic report from the Intergoup Ewing's Study. *Cancer* 1993;71:2109–2118.

The authors review 19 patients younger than 3 years of age with Ewing's sarcoma. This lesion is rare in this age group (2.6% of all Ewing's sar-comas) and shows a marked predominance for female gender (79%). However, survival rates were almost identical to those of older patients.

O'Connor MI, Pritchard DJ: Ewing's sarcoma: Prognostic factors, disease control, and the reemerging role of surgical treatment. *Clin Orthop* 1991;262:78–87.

This is an excellent review of the current treatment of Ewing's sarcoma, including the importance of multi-agent systemic chemotherapy, radiation therapy, and surgical resection. Poor prognostic factors include large tumor size, pelvic lesions, and poor response to chemotherapy.

Chondrosarcoma

Young CL, Sim FH, Unni KK, et al: Chondrosarcoma of bone in children. *Cancer* 1990;66:1641–1648.

The authors reviewed 47 patients with chondrosarcoma that developed before the age of 17 years. The most common site was the proximal humerus (35%). In general, the tumors were low grade and resembled their counterparts in the adult population both histologically and radiographically. En bloc resection was the only procedure that prevented local recurrence, and there were no metastases in those with long-term follow-up.

Osteosarcoma

Bechler JR, Robertson WW Jr, Meadows AT, et al: Osteosarcoma as a second malignant neoplasm in children. *J Bone Joint Surg* 1992;74A: 1079–1083.

Nine patients had osteosarcomas that developed in a previously irradiated site at an average of 10 years after initial treatment. Six patients died within 3 years of diagnosis of the osteosarcoma. Plans for tumor therapy should take into account the risk of this usually fatal complication.

Eckardt JJ, Eilber FR, Rosen G, et al: Endoprosthetic replacement for stage IIB osteosarcoma. *Clin Orthop* 1991;270:202–213.

Of 100 patients with grade IIB osteosarcoma, 78 were treated with limb salvage and endoprosthetic replacement. There were only three amputations after endoprosthetic replacement; one each for mechanical failure, infection, and recurrence. The best results involved distal femoral replacement. Those patients treated after 1984 (and thus receiving adjuvant chemotherapy) had a significantly improved probability of survival compared to those not receiving adjuvant chemotherapy, confirming earlier reports. The authors calculate that the probability of endoprosthetic survival was 2.5 times greater than the probability of patient survival, and believed that complications could be satisfactorily managed.

Glasser DB, Lane JM, Huvos AG, et al: Survival, prognosis, and therapeutic response in osteogenic sarcoma: The Memorial Hospital experience. *Cancer* 1992;69:698–708.

The authors reviewed 279 consecutive patients with stage II osteosarcoma of the appendicular skeleton to determine predictors of long-term survival. Histologic response to chemotherapy was the only independent predictor of outcome. The effect of location of the primary tumor appeared to be related to the ability to provide local control.

Harris NL, Eilert RE, Davino N, et al: Osteogenic sarcoma arising from bony segments following Ilizarov femoral lengthening through fibrous dysplasia. *J Pediatr Orthop* 1994;14:123–129.

This report of osteosarcoma formation in a 15-year-old boy with fibrous dysplasia raises two questions: (1) whether the biologic stimulus of distraction oteogenesis through abnormal metaplastic bone increases the risk of malignant neoplasia; and (2) whether distraction osteogenesis through dysplastic bone is contraindicated because the regenerate tissue does not form normal bone.

Kozakewich H, Perez-Atayde AR, Goorin AM, et al: Osteosarcoma in young children. *Cancer* 1991;67:638–642.

In this large series of osteosarcomas occurring in children under the age of 6 years, no significant differences were noted when compared to osteosarcoma in older patients. Survival rate dramatically increased to 67% from 20% after 1972 with the introduction of high dose methotrexate with leukovorin rescue.

Link MP, Goorin AM, Miser AW, et al: The effect of adjuvant chemotherapy on relapse-free survival in patients with osteosarcoma of the extremity. *N Engl J Med* 1986;314:1600–1606.

Definitive study in which patients were randomized postoperatively to multi-agent chemotherapy or no chemotherapy. There was a significant improvement in relapse-free survival in the chemotherapy group (66%) versus the nonchemotherapy group (17%).

Marina NM, Pratt CB, Rao BN, et al: Improved prognosis of children with osteosarcoma metastatic to the lung(s) at the time of diagnosis. *Cancer* 1992;70:2722–2727.

Patients were retrospectively reviewed and separated into one of three categories based on treatment (single and two-agent chemotherapy versus standard multiagent therapy with occasional thoracotomy for pulmonary metastases versus intensive multiagent therapy with thoracotomy for all patients with pulmonary metastases). There were no survivors in the former two groups at 3 years, whereas there was a 50% estimated probability of survival at 3 years in the latter group (seven of 18 patients alive 19 months to 7 years after diagnosis). The authors conclude that aggressive multimodal chemotherapy coupled with aggressive surgical resection of pulmonary metastases improves the prognosis.

Meyer WH, Malawer MM: Osteosarcoma: Clinical features and evolving surgical and chemotherapeutic strategies. *Pediatr Clin North Am* 1991;38:317–348.

This is a comprehensive review of the characteristics of osteosarcoma and its evaluation and treatment. There is an extensive bibliography.

Simon MA, Aschliman MA, Thomas N, et al: Limb-salvage treatment versus amputation for osteosarcoma of the distal end of the femur. *J Bone Joint Surg* 1986;68A:1331–1337.

The authors retrospectively compare the results of limb-salvage treatment versus above knee amputation or hip disarticulation in patients with osteosarcoma of the distal end of the femur. There were similar rates of metastases and death in all groups. Local recurrence was slightly higher in the limb-salvage patients than the above knee ampuation patients. No recurrences occurred in the hip disarticulation patients.

Soft-Tissue Sarcomas

Donaldson SS: Rhabdomyosarcoma: Contemporary status and future directions. *Arch Surg* 1989;124:1015–1020.

Using data from the Intergroup Rhabdomyosarcoma Study (IRS) I, the author presents an overall view of the current staging and treatment of this lesion.

Lange TA: The evaluation of a soft-tissue mass in the extremities, in Barr JS Jr (ed): *Instructional Course Lectures XXXVIII.* Park Ridge, IL, American Academy of Orthopaedic Surgeons, 1989, pp 391–398.

The author presents a logical sequence for the workup of a soft-tissue mass in the extremities. A simple algorithm is described using various imaging modalities including radiographs, MRI, ultrasound, and bone scan.

Makley JT: Preoperative staging techniques for soft-tissue neoplasms, in Barr JS Jr (ed): *Instructional Course Lectures XXXVIII.* Park Ridge, IL, American Academy of Orthopaedic Surgeons, 1989, pp 399–405.

The usefulness of various modalities in the staging of soft-tissue neoplasms is discussed.

Malignant Fibrous Histiocytoma

Raney RB Jr, Allen A, O'Neill J, ct al: Malignant fibrous histiocytoma of soft tissue in childhood. *Cancer* 1986;57:2198–2201.

This series of seven patients is the largest in the literature. Surgical removal is the key to successful therapy. In those patients with incomplete excision, chemotherapy and radiation therapy provided some response but their roles remain to be defined.

Spanier SS, Floyd J: A clinicopathologic comparison of malignant fibrous histiocytoma and liposarcoma, in Barr JS Jr (ed): *Instructional Course Lectures XXXVIII.* Park Ridge, IL, American Academy of Orthopaedic Surgeons, 1989, pp 407–417.

This is an excellent description of these lesions and their subtypes.

Rehabilitation

Cammisa FP Jr, Glasser DB, Otis JC, et al: The Van Nes tibial rotationplasty: A functionally viable reconstructive procedure in children who have a tumor of the distal end of the femur. *J Bone Joint Surg* 1990;72A:1541–1547.

Twelve patients with Van Ness rotationplasties had survival rates comparable with those for above-knee amputees and those with endoprosthetic replacement. Functional testing showed that these patients peformed as well as those with endoprosthetic replacement and better than those with amputation.

Catani F, Capanna R, Benedetti MG, et al: Gait analysis in patients after Van Nes rotationplasty. *Clin Orthop* 1993;296:270–277.

Ten patients treated for distal femoral malignancies by Van Ness rotationplasty underwent gait analysis. Although gait was not normal, the rotationplasty provided a smooth and coordinated gait pattern.

Eckardt JJ, Safran MR, Eilber FR, et al: Expandable endoprosthetic reconstruction of the skeletally immature after malignant bone tumor resection. *Clin Orthop* 1993;297:188–202.

Twelve patients treated with expandable endoprostheses were observed until death or revision. Seven patients underwent a total of 11 expansions, one required a revision-expandable prosthesis, and four did not require expansion. Ten complications occurred in eight patients; seven were associated with failure of the expansion mechanism.